Orthopedics: Principles of Diagnosis and Treatment

Orthopedics: Principles of Diagnosis and Treatment

Edited by Johan Saunders

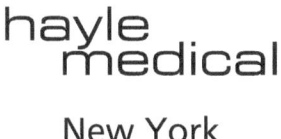

New York

Hayle Medical,
750 Third Avenue, 9th Floor,
New York, NY 10017, USA

Visit us on the World Wide Web at:
www.haylemedical.com

ISBN: 978-1-63241-537-0

Cataloging-in-Publication Data

Orthopedics : principles of diagnosis and treatment / edited by Johan Saunders.
    p. cm.
Includes bibliographical references and index.
ISBN 978-1-63241-537-0
1. Orthopedics. 2. Orthopedics--Diagnosis. 3. Orthopedics--Treatment. I. Saunders, Johan.
RD731 .O78 2019
616.7--dc23

Table of Contents

Preface

Orthopedic surgery is a branch of surgery that involves both surgical and nonsurgical procedures to deal with musculoskeletal trauma, degenerative diseases, sports injuries, spine diseases, tumors, etc. Sub-specialties of orthopedic surgery include shoulder and elbow surgery, total joint reconstruction, musculoskeletal oncology, orthopedic trauma, spine surgery, etc. Common procedures involved in these include knee replacement, arthroscopy of shoulder and knee, hip replacement and repair of fractures, besides many others. Research in orthopedic surgery seeks to develop less invasive surgical procedures and construct durable and more efficient implanted components. Some of the diverse topics covered in this book address the varied procedures and sub-specialties that fall under orthopedic surgery. The aim of this book is to present researches that have transformed this field and aided its advancement. It is a vital tool for all researching and studying this field.

After months of intensive research and writing, this book is the end result of all who devoted their time and efforts in the initiation and progress of this book. It will surely be a source of reference in enhancing the required knowledge of the new developments in the area. During the course of developing this book, certain measures such as accuracy, authenticity and research focused analytical studies were given preference in order to produce a comprehensive book in the area of study.

This book would not have been possible without the efforts of the authors and the publisher. I extend my sincere thanks to them. Secondly, I express my gratitude to my family and well-wishers. And most importantly, I thank my students for constantly expressing their willingness and curiosity in enhancing their knowledge in the field, which encourages me to take up further research projects for the advancement of the area.

Editor

Radiological and functional outcome in unstable, osteoporotic trochanteric fractures stabilized with dynamic helical hip system

**Ram Chander Siwach · Rajesh Rohilla ·
Roop Singh · Rohit Singla · Sukhbir Singh Sangwan ·
Paritosh Gogna**

Abstract A dynamic hip screw (DHS) remains the implant of choice for stabilization of trochanteric fractures because of its favourable results and low rate of non-union or hardware failure, but complication rates of the DHS are higher in unstable and osteoporotic trochanteric fractures. The proponents of the dynamic helical hip system (DHHS) report that it has the potential to decrease the cut-out rates in such fractures as helical blade allows compaction in osteoporotic femoral head which in itself improves anchorage. The purpose of the present study was to evaluate the radiological and functional outcome of DHHS in unstable and osteoporotic trochanteric fractures. This was a prospective observational study. The mean age of the 51 patients (24 men and 27 women) was 72.8 years. Fractures were type AO31A2.2 in 28 patients and AO31A2.3 in 23 patients. According to DEXA scans, 41 patients had osteoporosis and 10 patients had osteopenia. Osteoporosis was grade 3 in 36 patients and grade 2 in 15 patients according to Singh's index. The mean follow-up was 1.84 years. The average sliding of the lag screw was 3.6 mm (range 2–10 mm). The mean operative time was 54.74 (range 48–65) min. The average tip–apex distance was 20.24 mm (range 12–28 mm). All but one fractures united. The average time to union was 13.14 (range 11–24) weeks. There were four mechanical complications namely late helical blade migration ($n = 1$), late medialization of shaft ($n = 2$) and varus collapse with cut through ($n = 1$). No patient was noted to have a plate pull-out. The average Harris hip score was 92.87 (range 76–97). The use of a DHHS for stabilization of unstable(AO31A2), osteoporotic trochanteric fractures in the elderly patients was associated with reliable rates of union and functional outcome and a decreased incidence of screw cut-out and side plate pull-out.

Keywords Dynamic helical hip system · Osteoporosis · Unstable fracture · Pertrochanteric fracture · DHS

Introduction

Pertrochanteric fractures are common problems in elderly patients. Operative stabilization permits early mobilization and minimizes complications of prolonged recumbency [1]. Stable pertrochanteric fractures are preferably fixed by sliding hip screws [2–4]. In general, for the treatment of unstable pertrochanteric fractures, two options exist: extramedullary or intramedullary stabilization [5]. Each device has its advantages and disadvantages. The advantage of extramedullary fixation, such as dynamic hip screw (DHS), is the relatively simple, safe and forgiving surgical technique [5]. The DHS remains the implant of choice because of its favourable results and low rates of non-union or hardware failure [2–4], but the complication rates of the DHS are higher in *unstable* pertrochanteric fractures; despite the widespread use of the DHS, cut-out rates of 5–17 % have been reported in the literature [3, 6–8]. The most common mode of failure of a DHS is *cut-out* of the lag screw from the femoral head [9, 10] followed by *lift-off* of the plate from the femur [3, 4, 11]. Wolfgang et al. [12] reported a 19 % mechanical and technical complication rate with unstable pertrochanteric fractures treated with

R. C. Siwach · R. Rohilla (✉) · R. Singh · R. Singla ·
S. S. Sangwan · P. Gogna
Department of Orthopaedic Surgery, Paraplegia and
Rehabilitation, Pt. B.D. Sharma PGIMS, 9-J/28, Medical
Enclave, Rohtak 124001, Haryana, India
e-mail: drrajeshrohilla@rediffmail.com

sliding hip screw device. Moreover, osteoporosis, associated with pertrochanteric fractures in elderly patients, also presents a problem for stable osteosynthesis of the fracture [13].

A number of variations of basic sliding hip screws have been proposed because of such complications in elderly patients with AO31A2, 31A3 type fractures; in these excessive collapse can lead to shortening and hardware failure [5, 13]. One proposal was to improve implant anchorage in the femoral head by the use of a helical blade. The shape of the blade leads to improved rotational stability of the femoral head and neck fragment, which is vital for reducing the risk of cut-out, and may contribute to fewer delayed unions or varus angulation in unstable pertrochanteric fractures [14, 15]. The tip of the blade allows for *compaction* of the bone when it is inserted, which is thought responsible for improving anchorage in femoral head [16, 17]. Another study reported that the DHS with fixed angle locking screws (locking side plate) would reduce the risk of DHS failure and would be particularly useful in patients with osteoporotic bone or for patients with less stable fracture configurations [9]. The dynamic hip helical system (DHHS), designed by AO/ASIF, merges the concept of locking side plate, helical blade and dynamic hip screw. Several biomechanical studies have shown that helical blade has the potential to decrease the cut-out rate [14, 15], but few clinical studies have been reported. The purpose of the present study was to evaluate the radiological and functional outcome in elderly patients with unstable pertrochanteric fractures treated with the DHHS. The main outcome measures of the study were union rate, cut-out, the average sliding of the blade and functional outcome.

Materials and methods

All patients presenting with unstable pertrochanteric fractures to the authors' institute, a tertiary level centre, between January 2009 and June 2010 were included in the present prospective study. The study was approved by the Institutional Review Board. The *inclusion criteria* were: (1) age over 50 years, (2) unstable pertrochanteric fracture according to AO classification (Fracture AO31A2), (3) all patients with bone mineral density (T-score <-1) and Singh's index grade ≤ 3 [18] and (4) a minimum follow-up of 1 year. Patients with reverse oblique fractures (AO31A3), stable fractures (AO31A1), fractures extending into subtrochanteric region and pathological fractures were excluded from the study. Fractures were categorized as stable or unstable on the basis of AO/ASIF classification. Fractures from AO31A1.1 to AO31A2.1 are classified as stable pertrochanteric fractures, and fractures from

AO31A2.2 to AO31A3.3 are classified as unstable fractures [14]. Out of 172 pertrochanteric fractures, fifty-one patients with unstable pertrochanteric fractures stabilized with the DHHS met the inclusion criteria. The study included only type AO31A2.2 and type AO31A2.3 fractures. There were 24 men and 27 women with an average age of 72.8 years (range 60–85 years; standard deviation ± 6.82 years). The right hip was involved in 18 patients and the left in 33 patients. Forty-six patients had fallen, and 5 patients were injured after road traffic accidents. Anteroposterior and lateral radiographs including the full extent of femur from hip joint to knee joint were obtained. Preoperative radiographs were assessed by three blinded observers not associated with treatment for fracture classification. Fractures were classified using AO/ASIF classification and were type A2.2 in 28 patients and A2.3 in 23 patients. To estimate the bone mineral density (BMD), a DEXA scan of contralateral hip was obtained and the value of T-score was noted. The T-score was <-2.5 in 41 patients, and 10 patients had a T-score between -1 to -2.5. The Singh's index was assessed from anteroposterior radiographs of the contralateral hip. The Singh's index was grade 3 in 36 patients and grade 2 in 15 patients. The average time interval from injury to operation was 6 (range 3–10) days.

The helical blade is available in lengths of 65–145 mm with the outer diameter of 12.5 mm. The barrel angle varies from 130° to 150° and measures 25 and 38 mm in length. The 135° DHHS barrel used in this study had a 9-mm long key that engages the blade shaft to prevent rotation and a locking side plate. This is different from the standard DHS, where the screw shaft engages the barrel over its entire length. The procedures were performed by the three senior authors of the study. The implant was fixed as per the recommended technique. The locking side plate in DHHS is a combi-hole design allowing non-locking or locking screws to be used. Initially, one cortical screw was inserted to allow directional compression at fracture site, followed by the insertion of locking screws. In the majority of patients, this practice was followed. For most patients, an indirect reduction was attempted, but no attempt was made to reduce the posteromedial fragment if it required extensive soft tissue dissection for fixation. In all cases, efforts were made to achieve optimum positioning of the tip of the screw in the subchondral bone of the femoral head with a combined tip–apex distance measuring <25 mm on anteroposterior and lateral radiographs. Antibiotic prophylaxis was given as per institutional protocol. Patients were taught and encouraged to do pain-free intermittent quadriceps, hip and knee flexion exercises starting on the second postoperative day. Partial weight bearing was allowed with a walker aid and advanced to as tolerated by the patient with full weight bearing encouraged after 12 weeks.

Patients were followed at 6, 12, 24, 52 and 100 weeks and then once a year until last follow-up. Functional outcomes were assessed using the *Harris hip score* [19]. Union was defined as bridging of three of the four cortices and disappearance of fracture line on the plain radiographs for a patient who was able to bear full weight. Non-union was defined as a fracture that did not heal within six months. Radiological parameters (sliding, screw/blade cutout, varus/valgus angulation, side plate pull-out) were recorded. The *sliding of helical blade* was determined by measuring the length of the root (R) of the blade and that of thread (T) on radiograph as reported by Hardy et al. [3].

Results

The mean operative time was 54.74 (range 48–65) min. The mean follow-up was 20.4 (range 12–28) months. The average sliding of lag screw was 3.6 mm (range 2–10 mm). The average tip–apex distance was 20.24 mm (range 12–28 mm). In two cases, it was more than 25 mm (26 and 28 mm). The average time to union was 13.14 (range 11–24) weeks (Figs. 1, 2). Two fractures had delayed union at 20 and 24 weeks, respectively. One patient had a varus collapse of the fracture. This patient had type AO31A2.3 fracture with grade 3 Singh's index, but this patient was lost to follow-up. All other fractures healed uneventfully. There were four mechanical complications: late helical blade migration ($n = 1$), late medialization of shaft ($n = 2$) and varus collapse with cut through ($n = 1$) (Table 1). All mechanical complications occurred in different patients. Medialization of shaft was seen at the second month follow-up, weight bearing was delayed in these two cases for 3 months. No patient had side plate pull-out. There were no deep infections or deep venous thromboses. The average Harris hip score was 92.87 (range 76–97). In the final grading as per Harris hip score, 42 patients had excellent results (score 90–100), 6 had good results (score 80–100) and 3 had fair outcome (score 70–80).

Discussion

The best treatment for unstable pertrochanteric fractures remains controversial. The diversity of fixation devices available for treatment of unstable pertrochanteric fractures illustrates the difficulties encountered in the actual treatment. Intramedullary devices have mechanical and biological advantages in such fractures [20]. The dynamic hip screw (DHS) remains the implant of choice because of its favourable results and low rate of non-union or hardware failure [2], but complication rates of the DHS are higher in unstable pertrochanteric fractures; despite the widespread use of the DHS, cut-out rates of 5–17 % have been reported in the literature [3, 6–8]. The DHS is often linked to a high incidence of therapeutic failure in patients with pertrochanteric fractures and a severe degree of osteoporosis [1, 11, 13]. Complications have been associated with cut-out of lag screw from femoral head predominantly, particularly in unstable pertrochanteric fractures [3, 21]. Most mechanical failures involve progressive varus deformity at the fracture site. This may increase tension on the side plate screws, leading to failure of screw–bone interface. The side plate pull-out has been reported in patients with severe osteoporosis [4, 11]. The majority of patients ($n = 41$) in the present study had osteoporosis, and only 4 % patients had fixation failure. No patient had a side plate pull-out in the present study, which may be attributed to the concept of a *locking side plate*. Strauss et al. [15] reported that the biomechanical advantages seen with helical blade fixation of the femoral head compared to sliding hip screw designs

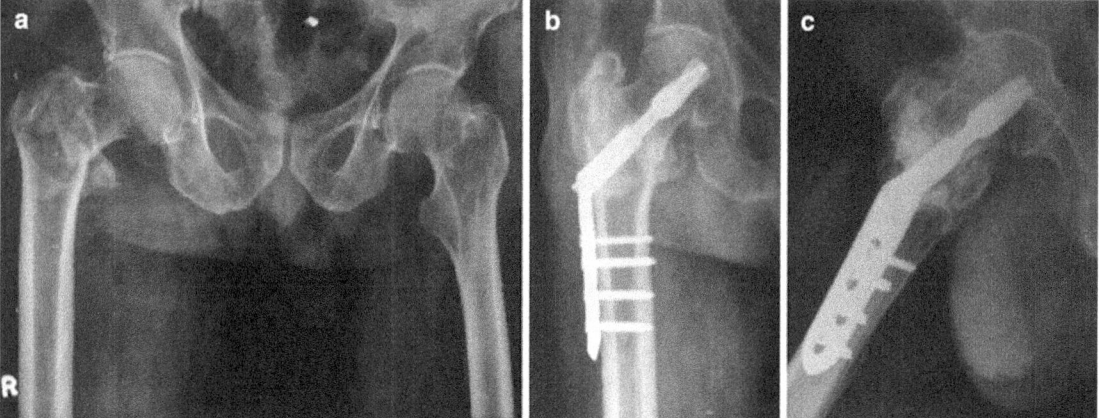

Fig. 1 **a** Preoperative anteroposterior radiograph in a 82-year-old male showing 31A2.2 pertrochanteric fracture. **b** Follow-up anteroposterior radiograph of the same patient showing union. **c** Follow-up lateral radiograph of the same patient showing union

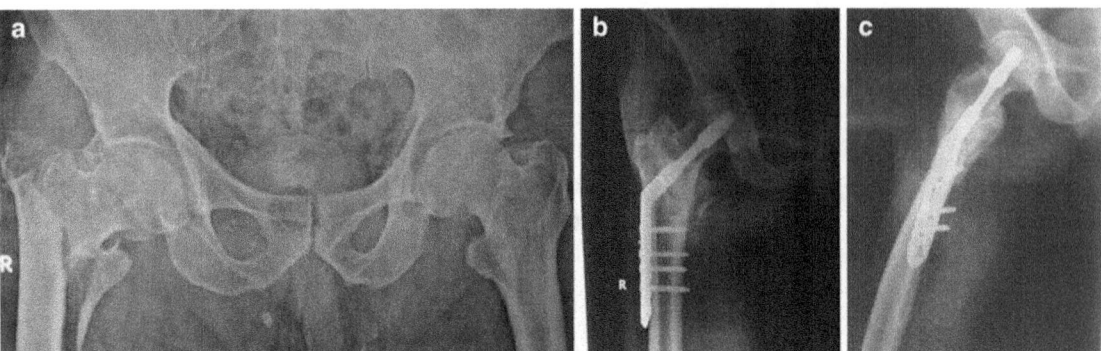

Fig. 2 a Preoperative anteroposterior radiograph in a 75-year-old male showing 31A2.3 pertrochanteric fracture. **b** Follow-up anteroposterior radiograph of the same patient showing union. **c** Follow-up lateral radiograph of the same patient showing union

Table 1 Complications in the present study

Complication	Number of patients (%)
Non-union	1 (2)
Delayed union	2 (4)
Late helical blade migration	1 (2)
Varus collapse	1 (2)
Late medialization of shaft	2 (4)

may be useful in managing fractures in patients with poor bone quality. We, as a consequence of this review, are also of the opinion that the dynamic helical hip system (DHHS) is a reliable alternative in stabilization of *osteoporotic* pertrochanteric fractures.

In general, for treatment of unstable pertrochanteric fractures, two options exist: extramedullary or intramedullary stabilization [5]. The minimally invasive intramedullary technique is reported to be associated with less blood loss and a lower infection rate; the implant allows early full weight bearing because of its favourable biomechanical properties [5, 19], but screw cut through in 8 % and re-operation in 7.1 % patients have been reported in unstable pertrochanteric fractures treated with proximal femoral nail (Table 2) [20, 22]. Screw cut through was observed in 2 % patients in the present study. Union was achieved in all patients except in one case which was lost to follow-up. Eighty-six per cent in the present study had good to excellent functional outcome with mean Haris hip score of 92.87, which is comparable to average scores (83–90) reported in the literature [23–25]. Barton et al. [21] reported a randomized study comparing long gamma nail and sliding hip screw in treatment of type AO31A2 fractures and concluded sliding hip screw should remain a gold standard for the treatment of such fractures. We report that the DHHS is a reliable alternative for stabilization of *unstable pertrochanteric* fractures. Only two patients in the present study had a tip–apex distance more than 25 mm. The importance of the tip–apex distance is likely to be

greater in patients with unstable pertrochanteric fracture [21]. Although the apex–tip distance is originally described for the standard DHS, we have used this method in the present study also to assess the implant position. Reduction in cut-out numbers will not be accomplished by newer implants since implant design cannot make up for suboptimal fracture reduction or poor implant position [5].

Several biomechanical studies have shown an advantage of the helical blade over a screw type implant for unstable and osteoporotic pertrochanteric fractures. Strauss et al. [15] concluded that fixation of the femoral head with a helical blade was biomechanically superior to fixation with a standard sliding hip screw in a cadaveric, unstable pertrochanteric hip fracture model. In a cellular polyurethane foam surrogate model of the femoral head, Sommers et al. [26] demonstrated that the helical blade of the pertrochanteric fixation nail provided the greatest resistance to cut-out compared to the lag screw design of the extramedullary dynamic hip screw and the intramedullary gamma nail. Jewell et al. [9] compared the standard DHS design with a DHS fixed to shaft of femur with locking plate and concluded that a locking screw DHS would be particularly useful in patients with osteoporotic bone and in patients with less stable fracture configurations. Windolf et al. [27] compared the mechanical performance of the DHS and helical blade in paired cadaveric specimens under dynamic loading. They noted 100 % cut-out in the DHS group, but only 50 % cut-out in the helical blade group. They also noted increased fracture collapse in the helical blade group. The compressed bone around the helical blade theoretically provides improved resistance to cut-out relative to the osteoporotic, non-compressed bone surrounding the DHS [17]. Additionally, these spiral blade implants may provide better rotational control of the fracture construct, especially when the lag screw is placed in an eccentric position [26].

Late *helical blade migration* was seen in an otherwise asymptomatic patient at the sixth month of follow-up that

Table 2 Comparison of studies reporting treatment of unstable trochanteric fractures

	Implant	Average age (years)	Unstable fractures (%)	Operation time (min)	Cut-out (varus) (%)
Hardy et al. [3]	DHS	80	74	57	15
Bucicuto et al. [8]	CHS	81	100	63	15
Adams et al. [4]	SHS	81	53	61	3
Al-yassari et al. [20]	PFN	84	77	–	8
Banan et al. [22]	PFN	79	83	–	8.7
Fitzpatrick et al. [29]	DHHS	80.41	5	34.52	None
Present study	DHHS	72.8	100	54.74	2

had little impact on fracture healing. The tip–apex distance in this case was 16 mm. A similar late migration of tip of the helical blade was reported by Gardner et al. [14] after pertrochanteric fixation nail in elderly patients with pertrochanteric fractures. All position changes occurred within first 6 weeks postoperatively, with no subsequent detectable migration or telescoping with no significant differences between stable and unstable fractures [14]. Gardner et al. also reported reverse migration of blade in 8 % cases and intra-articular penetration in one patient. We did not observe reverse migration of blade in the present study. The average sliding of lag screw was 3.6 mm (range 2–10 mm) in the present study, which was lower than a previous study using the DHS alone [28]. This supports the concept of a fixed angle implant and bone construct with a locking side plate, both of which provides stable fixation in unstable pertrochanteric fracture. Fitzpatrick et al. [29] in their randomized controlled trial have reported the average sliding of 7.4 mm with dynamic helical blade group. Short shaft engagement of helical blade could have led to the binding of the blade in the barrel. This could explain the lesser degree of sliding obtained in the present study.

The literature has few clinical studies evaluating the role of a DHHS in extra-capsular fractures of femur. Fitzpatrick et al. [29] conducted a randomized prospective study on 51 patients comparing the locking helical blade with a dynamic hip screw. They found out no significant difference in the radiographic outcomes of pertrochanteric hip fractures treated with either of these implants. The helical blade group had two failures with central cut through which they relate to a defect in rotational control mechanism. The limitation in their study was that eighty per cent of their fractures were stable in nature (40 out of 51), but the present study included unstable osteoporotic pertrochanteric fractures only.

The present study also has its own limitations; the number of patients is too small to resolve the current controversies. The present study does not have a control group. The surgeries were conducted by surgeons of varied lengths of experience but may have the advantage of the results of the present study applicable to a majority of orthopaedic surgeons performing hip surgery.

Conclusion

In the present clinical study, the use of a DHHS for stabilization of unstable (AO31A2), osteoporotic pertrochanteric fractures in the elderly patients was associated with reliable rates of union and functional outcome and decreased incidence of screw cut-out and side plate pull-out as compared to standard DHS.

References

1. Cleveland H, Bosworth DM, Thompson FR (1947) Interpertrochanteric fractures of the femur; a survey of treatment in traction and by internal fixation. J Bone Joint Surg 29:1049–1067
2. Rao JP, Banzon MT, Weiss AB, Rayhack J (1983) Treatment of unstable interpertrochanteric fractures with anatomic reduction and compression hip screw fixation. Clin Orthop Relat Res 175:65–71
3. Hardy DC, Descamps PY, Krallis P, Fabeck L, Smets P, Bertens CL et al (1998) Use of an intramedullary hip-screw compared with a compression hip-screw with a plate for interpertrochanteric femoral fractures: a prospective, randomized study of one hundred patients. J Bone Joint Surg Am 80:618–630
4. Adams CL, Robinson CM, Court-Brown CM, McQueen MM (2001) Prospective randomized controlled trial of an intramedullary nail versus dynamic screw and plate for interpertrochanteric fractures of the femur. J Orthop Trauma 15:394–400
5. Schipper IB, Marti RK, van der Werken C (2004) Unstable pertrochanteric femoral fractures: extramedullary or intramedullary fixation. Review of literature. Injury 35:142–151
6. Nordin S, Zulkifli O, Faisham WI (2001) Mechanical failure of Dynamic Hip Screw (DHS) fixation in interpertrochanteric fracture of the femur. Med J Malaysia 56(D):12–17
7. Simpson AH, Varty K, Dodd CA (1989) Sliding hip screws: modes of failure. Injury 20(4):227–231
8. Buciuto R, Uhlin B, Hammerby S, Hammer R (1998) RAB-plate versus Richards CHS plate for unstable pertrochanteric hip fractures. A randomized study of 233 patients with 1-year follow-up. Acta Orthop Scand 69:25–28
9. Jewell DPA, Gheduzzi S, Mitchell MS, Miles AW (2008) Locking plates increase the strength of the dynamic hip screws. Injury 39:209–212

10. Stern R (2007) Are there advances in the treatment of extracapsular hip fractures in the elderly? Injury 38(3):S77–S87

11. Laohapoonrungsee A, Arpornchayanon O, Phornputkal C (2005) Two hole side plate DHS in the treatment of inter-pertrochanteric fracture: results and complications. Injury 36:1355–1360

12. Wolfgang GL, Bryant MH, O'Neil JP (1982) Treatment of intertrochanteric fracture of the femur using sliding screw plate fixation. Clin Orthop Relat Res 163:148–158

13. Stromsoe K (2004) Fracture fixation problems in osteoporosis. Injury 35:107–113

14. Gardner MJ, Briggs SM, Kopjar B, Helfet DL, Lorich DG (2007) Radiographic outcomes of interpertrochanteric hip fractures treated with the pertrochanteric fixation nail. Injury 38:1189–1196

15. Strauss E, Frank J, Lee J, Kummer FJ, Tejwani N (2006) Helical blade versus sliding hip screw for treatment of unstable interpertrochanteric hip fractures: a biomechanical evaluation. Injury 37:984–989

16. Wahnert D, Gudushauri P, Schiuma D, Richards G, Windolf M (2010) Does cancellous bone compaction due to insertion of a blade implant influence the cut-out resistance? A biomechanical study. Clin Biomech (Bristol, Avon) 25:1053–1057

17. Windolf M, Muths R, Braunstein V, Gueorguiev B, Hänni M, Schwieger K (2009) Quantification of cancellous bone-compaction due to DHS Blade insertion and influence upon cut-out resistance. Clin Biomech (Bristol, Avon) 24(1):53–58

18. Singh M, Nagrath AR, Maini PS (1970) Changes in trabecular pattern of the upper end of the femur as an index of osteoporosis. J Bone Joint Surg Am 52:457–467

19. Ahmad AM, Xypnitos NF, Giannoudis PV (2011) Measuring hip outcomes: common scales and checklists. Injury 42:259–264

20. Al-yassari G, Langstaff RJ, Jones JW, Al-Lami M (2002) The AO/ASIF proximal femoral nail (PFN) for the treatment of unstable pertrochanteric femoral fracture. Injury 33:395–399

21. Barton TM, Gleeson R, Topliss C, Greenwood R, Harries WJ, Chesser TJ (2010) A comparison of the long gamma nail with the sliding hip screw for treatment of AO/OTA 31-A2 fractures of the proximal part of the femur: a prospective randomized trial. J Bone Joint Surg Am 92:792–798

22. Banan H, Al-Sabti A, Jimulia T, Hart AJ (2002) The treatment of unstable, extracapsular hip fractures with the AO/ASIF proximal femoral nail (PFN)-our first 60 cases. Injury 33:401–405

23. Luo XP, He SQ, Li ZA (2011) Case control studies on locking plates and dynamic hip screw in the treatment of interpertrochanteric hip fractures. Zhongguo Gu Shang 24:242–244

24. Lavini F, Renzi-Brivio L, Aulisa R, Cherubino F, Di Seglio PL, Galante N et al (2008) The treatment of stable and unstable proximal femoral fractures with a new pertrochanteric nail: results of a multicentre study with the Veronail. Strategies Trauma Limb Reconstr 3(1):15–22

25. Karn NK, Singh GK, Kumar P, Shrestha B, Singh MP, Gowda MJ (2006) Comparison between external fixation and the sliding hip screw in the management of pertrochanteric fracture of femur in Nepal. J Bone Joint Surg 88:1347–1350

26. Sommers MB, Roth C, Hall H, Kam BC, Ehmke LW, Krieg JC et al (2004) A laboratory model to evaluate cutout resistance of implants for perpertrochanteric fracture fixation. J Orthop Trauma 18(6):361–368

27. Windolf M, Braunstein V, Dutoit C, Schwieger K (2009) Is a helical shaped implant a superior alternative to the Dynamic Hip Screw for unstable femoral neck fractures? A biomechanical investigation. Clin Biomech (Bristol, Avon) 24(1):59–64

28. Jacobs RR, McClain O, Armstrong HJ (1980) Internal fixation of interpertrochanteric hip fractures: a clinical and biomechanical study. Clin Orthop Relat Res 146:62–70

29. Fitzpatrick DC, Sheerin DV, Wolf BR, Wuest TK (2011) A randomized, prospective study comparing interpertrochanteric hip fracture fixation with dynamic hip screw and dynamic helical hip system in a community practice. Iowa Orthop J 31:166–172

2

Open reduction internal fixation of lateral humeral condyle fractures in children. A series of 105 fractures from a single institution

Andreas Leonidou · Krissen Chettiar ·
Simon Graham · Pouya Akhbari · Konstantinos Antonis · Eleftherios Tsiridis · Omiros Leonidou

Abstract Lateral humeral condyle fractures account for 17 % of the distal humeral condyle fractures. Displaced and/or rotated fractures require appropriate reduction and stabilisation. There are, however, a number of controversies in the surgical management of these patients. The aim of the present study was to review the results of patients with a displaced lateral humeral condyle fracture treated with open reduction and internal fixation (ORIF). We retrospectively reviewed children treated with ORIF of lateral humeral condyle fractures at a single institution over a period of 13 years. All cases were identified through the trauma register. Case notes and radiographs were retrieved. Fracture classification, mode of fixation, time to union, and final outcomes at the latest follow-up were reviewed. One hundred and five lateral condyle fractures were identified in 76 male and 29 female patients. Average age was 6.2 years. Ninety-two were Milch type II and 13 Milch type I. According to the Jacob's classification, 38 were type II and 67 type III. All fractures were treated with open reduction and fixation with K-wires. Average time to radiological union was 33 days. Follow-up ranged between 2 and 8 years (average 3.2 years). Radiological hypertrophy of the lateral condyle was present in 45 cases (42 %). Three patients developed a pseudo-cubitus varus deformity. Further four patients developed a true cubitus varus.

There was one case of superficial infection of the K-wires and one case of delayed union. At the latest follow-up, 96 % of the patients achieved an excellent final result and 4 % a good final result. Our results demonstrate that fracture union and excellent final outcomes can be expected in all patients using our protocol, whereby all patients with a displaced fracture are managed by ORIF with K-wire fixation, with the wires only being removed after there is evidence of radiological union. Compared to recent reports of closed reduction internal fixation, this series demonstrates good results with no complications directly relating to the open reduction technique. *Level of evidence* Case series, Level IV.

Keywords Lateral condyle fractures · ORIF · Radiological union · Lateral spurring

A. Leonidou (✉) · K. Antonis · O. Leonidou
First Department of Trauma and Orthopaedics, Athens Paediatric Hospital "Agia Sophia", Thivon and Papadiamantopoulou, Goudi, 11527 Athens, Greece
e-mail: leonidou@doctors.org.uk

A. Leonidou · K. Chettiar · S. Graham · P. Akhbari · E. Tsiridis
Division of Surgery, Academic Department of Orthopaedics and Trauma, Aristotle University Medical School, Thessaloníki, Greece

Introduction

Lateral condyle fractures of the distal humerus are the second most common fractures at the elbow in the paediatric population usually between the ages of 6–10 years old making up 5–20 % of fractures in children [1, 2].

The diagnosis can be difficult both radiologically and clinically, with loss of function occurring, due to extension into the articular surface. The result of an incorrectly treated lateral condylar physeal injury may not be evident until months or years after the initial index injury [3].

The Milch classification is widely used, and they are; type I and type II according to whether the fracture exited through the capitellar–trochlear groove or through the trochlear, respectively [4]. Cotton noted that the fragment was commonly displaced outward and backwards [5]. The Jacob classification dictates whether surgical intervention is required. A Jacob I is non-displaced, II is displaced by 2 mm, but not malrotated. Type III is displacement with malrotation [6]. The aim of lateral humeral condyle fracture treatment is to ensure healing of the fracture and to prevent pseudoarthrosis, malunion, deformities and functional disorders [3]. Traditionally, undisplaced stable fractures were treated in cast immobilisation with observation. Articular fractures that have a hinge may be treated with closed reduction and percutaneous pinning. In certain situations, an arthrogram or an MRI scan may help define articular congruity and adequacy of the reduction [3, 7].

Fractures that are unstable, malrotated and displaced by over 2 mm usually undergo open reduction internal fixation usually with wires, smooth pins or screws [8, 9]. Debate persists as to how much displacement and fracture instability is required before open reduction and internal fixation (ORIF) is indicated [2, 10]. Recently published studies further challenge the necessity of open reduction of a displaced fracture, advocating good results following close reduction and internal fixation (CRIF) of completely displaced and rotated fragments [9].

The aim of the present study was to review the results of patients with a displaced lateral humeral condyle fracture treated with ORIF over a 13-year period at a paediatric tertiary referral centre.

Methods

A retrospective study of all patients presenting with a displaced paediatric lateral humeral condyle fracture to our tertiary Paediatric Orthopaedic Unit between 1993 and 2011 was conducted. Approval to perform our study was obtained by the Institutional Ethics Committee for Human Research.

Initial assessment of the patients was performed in the Accident and Emergency Department of our Institution. The injured limb was examined for deformity, wounds and neurovascular integrity. Antero–posterior, oblique and lateral radiographs of the elbow were routinely performed. Fractures were classified using the Milch as well as the Jacob classification. The acceptable displacement for conservative management in an above elbow plaster of Paris (POP) cast was up to 2 mm. Patients who were treated conservatively were closely followed up with radiographs every week to ensure that the fracture has not displaced. The POP cast was removed upon radiological union— typically between 4 and 6 weeks—and physiotherapy commenced.

Following anaesthetic assessment, all patients with a displaced lateral humeral condyle fracture were consented and listed for ORIF with Kirschner wires (K-wires) in the operating theatre. All fractures were treated by a Consultant Paediatric Orthopaedic Surgeon as earlier as starvation status and emergency theatres facility allowed access. A single dose of intravenous prophylactic antibiotics was administered at the anaesthetic induction, as per hospital policy, and tourniquet was used. The fracture was identified and reduced via a dorsolateral approach to the distal humerus, through the interval between brachioradialis and triceps. The joint surface was accurately reduced with minimal dissection of soft tissues from the distal fragment in order to reduce the risk of avascular necrosis of the capitellum. The reduction was stabilised with two divergent K-wires that were left outside the skin. Subsequently, an above elbow POP in neutral position was applied.

Patients were followed up weekly until radiological union of the fracture was evident (Fig. 1), and thereafter, the wires and the POP were removed in the outpatient department without the use of general or local anaesthetic. Following the removal of plaster, all patients were mobilised with intensive physiotherapy focusing on elbow full range of movement (ROM), mainly with active movement exercises.

According to the institutional protocols, our patients were followed up until skeletal maturity to assess residual or late deformities. At the final follow-up appointment before discharge, the patient's outcome was assessed clinically for ROM and deformity and radiologically. Also, the patients were asked about any residual pain and whether or not they were happy performing daily life activities and sports. The results were graded according to the criteria suggested by Hardacre et al. (Table 1) [11].

Results

One hundred and five patients with a displaced paediatric lateral humeral condyle fracture were identified and included in the study, 76 males and 29 females. The age of the patients ranged between 3 and 13 years, with a mean of 6.2 years. All included cases were the result of low-energy closed injuries. In relation to the Milch's classification, 13 fractures were classified as Milch I and 92 as Milch II. According to the Jacobs classification for displacement, 38 fractures were classified as type II and 67 as type III.

The mean time to radiological union of the fracture and therefore removal of the wires was 33 days (4.7 weeks). Radiological union ranged between 21 and 56 days. (3–8 weeks). All the K-wires were removed in the outpatient department.

One patient had a superficial infection around the K-wires, which responded well and eventually resolved with the administration of oral antibiotics. The majority of the fractures demonstrated radiological union between 4

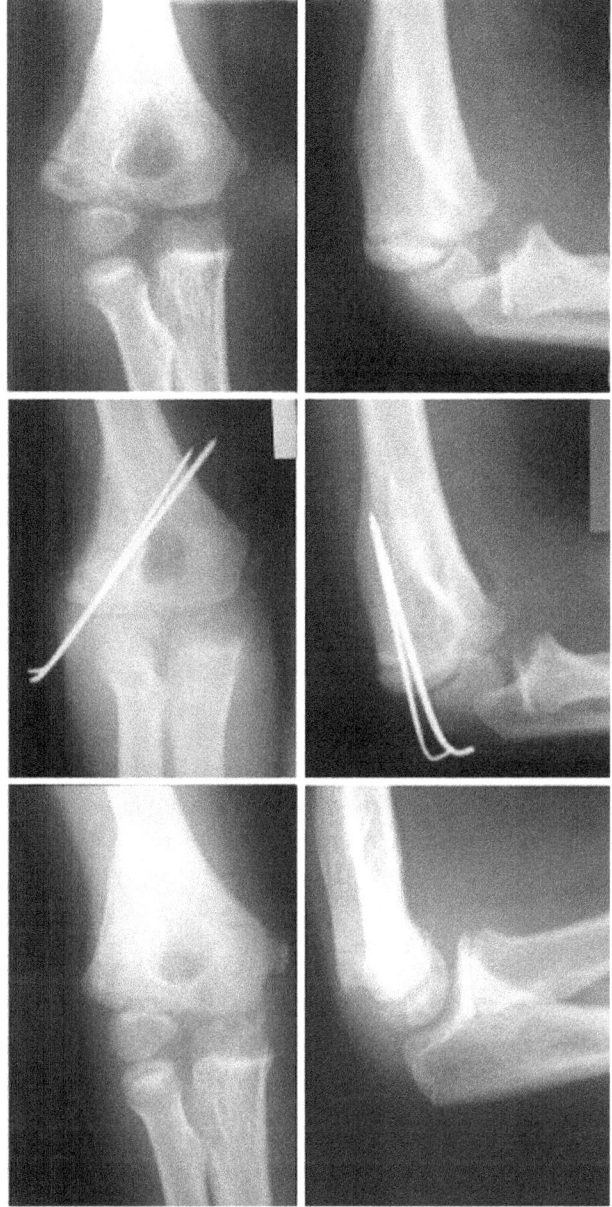

Fig. 1 9-year-old male, fracture healed at 5 weeks, X-ray at 1 year demonstrates healing with lateral hypertrophy

Table 1 Assessing the results of treatment in patients with lateral humeral condyle fractures as described by Hardacre et al. [10]

Excellent Result	No symptoms + Full ROM + No alteration in the carrying angle
Good Result	ROM deficit < 15o of complete extension + minimal alteration in the carrying angle + pain apart from arthritic/neurological pain
Poor Result	Disabling loss of motion, conspicuous alteration of carrying angle, arthritic symptoms, ulnar neuritis, non-union and avascular necrosis.

and 6 weeks with the exception of one patient with a Jacob III fracture who reached 8 weeks.

Follow-up ranged between 2 and 8 years with an average of 3.2 years. At the final appointment, all patients had achieved full range of movement of the elbow joint. Furthermore, there were no cases of residual pain, and all patients were happy performing daily life activities and participating in sports. None of the patients in this series developed a non-union or a malunion.

Following our management lateral spurring (hypertrophy of the lateral condyle) occurred in 45 cases (42 %). As a result of lateral spurring, 3 patients developed a pseudo-cubitus varus deformity. Further, 4 patients developed a true cubitus varus of less than 5°. In all cases of lateral spurring and cubitus varus, there was no pain or interference with daily activities, and sports and no corrective intervention was required. None of the patients developed a fishtail deformity. Figures 2 and 1 demonstrate, respectively, a case where the fracture healed without radial hypertrophy and a case that lateral spurring occurred. According to the criteria by Hardacre et al, 101 patients (96 %) achieved an excellent final result, 4 patients (4 %) achieved good final results, and no patient achieved a poor result.

Discussion

The results of our study demonstrate that open reduction and K-wire fixation of displaced (>2 mm) lateral humeral condyle fractures leads to excellent clinical and radiological results without any significant complications. The necessity of reduction and stabilisation of displaced and/or rotated lateral condyle fractures has been well established in the literature [3, 10, 12]. There are, however, a number of controversies in the surgical management of these patients.

The first controversy is as to whether displaced and rotated lateral condyle fractures should be managed with ORIF or with CRIF [10]. Advocates of close reduction hypothesise that ORIF might be unnecessary in many cases and that it might even lead to avascular necrosis as a result of extensive soft tissue dissection [10]. Song et al. [9] prospectively looked at 63 patients with lateral condyle fractures of the humerus. They attempted closed reduction internal fixation using K-wires in all of them, but in 13 cases ORIF was required. Their success rate for fixation was 73 % with no cases of non-union or malunion. They suggested that CRIF often results in effective treatment for displaced lateral condyle fractures. However, in their study, only 3 of the 6 patients with a Jacob III fracture were managed with closed reduction [9]. In a subsequent study, Song et al. [13] prospectively looked at 24 Jacob III lateral condyle fractures. Of these, 18 were managed with CRIF

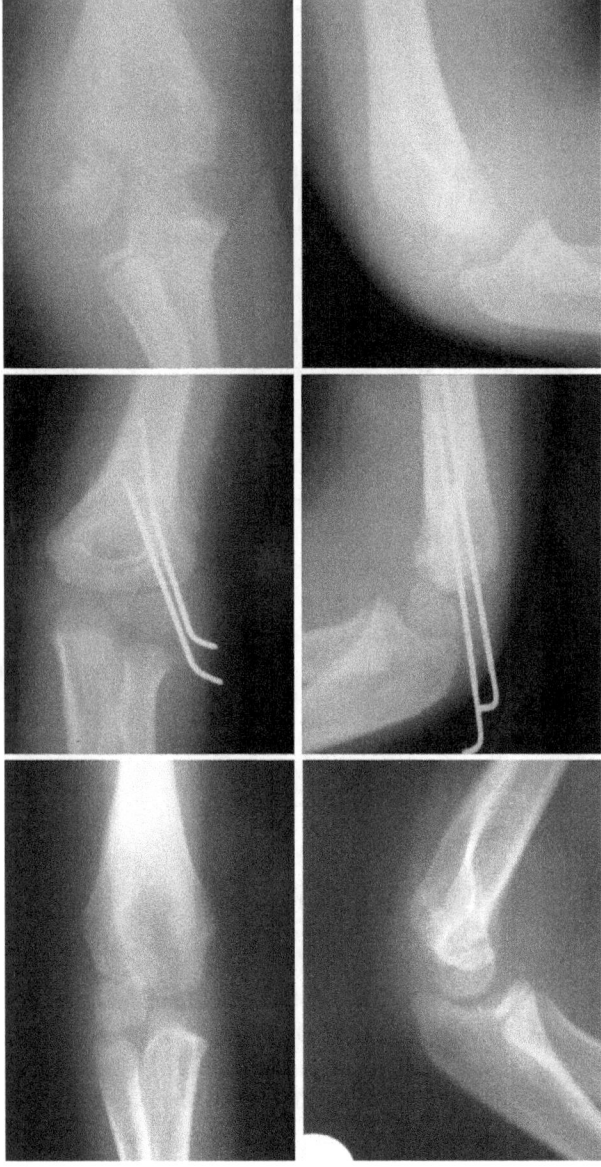

Fig. 2 6-year-old male, fracture healed at 5 weeks, X-ray at 1 year demonstrates healing without lateral hypertrophy

and 6 with ORIF using K-wires. It is of note that out of the 6 cases of ORIF, 3 were the results of the surgeon's lack of confidence and experience, according to the authors [13]. The vast majority of the cases in both studies by Song et al. [9, 13] were managed by one experienced paediatric orthopaedic surgeon, suggesting that close reduction could work better in the hands of more experienced surgeons. In our study, we presented 67 cases of Jacob III fractures treated successfully with ORIF with only one case of delayed union and no cases of avascular necrosis. We therefore advocate for ORIF in all displaced lateral condyle fracture as our results demonstrated union and good functional outcome in all patients with no significant complications.

A second controversy exists as to when the K-wires should be removed. Thomas et al. [12] managed 104 cases of displaced lateral condyle fractures of the humerus with ORIF and K-wire fixation. They advocated that 3 weeks of K-wire stabilisation is sufficient for the fracture to heal and therefore removed all the wires and began elbow mobilisation after the elapse of this period [12]. The authors reported only one case of delayed union in a patient whose K-wires were removed at 19 days [12]. In the present study, we removed the K-wire only after radiological union was evident. Even though we had cases with union and subsequent removal of wires at 3 weeks, the mean time to radiological union of the fracture was 33 days (4.7 weeks). Consequently, we advise for the K-wires to be removed once radiological union is evident. In agreement to our suggestion is the recent paper by Song and Waters [10]. The authors mentioned that displaced fractures should be stabilised until they are healed radiographically [10].

In our study, all the K-wires were left exposed. It has been stipulated that leaving the wires exposed could increase the risk of infection with reported incidences varying from 1 to 28 % [8]. The authors of the present study believe that leaving the wires exposed carries the advantage of wire removal in the outpatient department instead of administrating a further general anaesthetic to the patient. Furthermore, from our series, only 1 case out of 105 (0.9 %) developed a superficial infection around the K-wires, which was successfully treated with oral antibiotics. There were no cases of deep infection. In agreement to our practice is the study by Das De et al. [8], which advocates for leaving the wires exposed following ORIF of a lateral condyle fracture. In our study, all patients received a single dose of prophylactic antibiotics at induction. It has been debated whether prophylactic antibiotics should be used for percutaneous wiring of fractures and some authors advise against it [14, 15]. Nevertheless, in our cohort, all patients underwent open reduction and subsequent wire fixation, and therefore, the authors felt that prophylactic antibiotics should be used, which is in accordance with our institutional policy. Several authors are in agreement that prophylactic antibiotics should be used for open orthopaedic procedures where a foreign material is inserted [16, 17].

Bony overgrowth (lateral spurring) over the lateral condyle is a distinct radiological finding commonly seen in children following a fracture of the lateral condyle of the humerus [12, 18]. A recent study by Pribaz et al. [19] consisting of 212 lateral condyle fractures treated by various methods, demonstrated that 73 % of the patients developed some degree of lateral spur. The development and size of the spur was positively correlated with the degree of initial fracture displacement [19]. Furthermore, they noted that lateral spurring was more common in patients treated surgically (incidence 91 %) compared with those managed conservatively (incidence 59 %). However, they did not find a significant difference between those managed with CRIF compared with ORIF [19]. The authors concluded that the increased incidence of spurring in the surgically treated group is related to the increased fracture displacement at the time of the injury [19]. In our series, 44 cases (42 %) of the patients developed lateral spurring. Similar incidence of lateral spurring (40 %) was reported in the study by Thomas et al. [12]. As a sequela of lateral spurring, 3 of our patients developed a pseudo-cubitus varus deformity at the elbow. Although the patients were able to feel the spur, it was pain free and did not affect their range of movements nor interfered with their daily activities and sports, which is in accordance to the published literature [12, 19].

Cubitus varus angulation has been a documented complication of lateral condyle fractures [20–22]. The incidence of cubitus varus is not positively related to either surgical or conservative management [20]. The deformity is most of the times benign and very rarely causes symptoms and requires surgical correction [20–22]. In our study, four patients (4 %) developed a true cubitus varus of less than 5°. This was mainly a cosmetic deformity not affecting patients' quality of life, and therefore, no corrective osteotomies were required.

Growth disturbance can occur after a lateral humeral condyle fracture in the form of a partial lateral growth plate closure or partial closure of the centre of the physis. In the latter case, a persistent gap between the lateral condylar physis and the trochlea could lead to a sharp angle wedge deformity also known as "fishtail deformity" [3]. Fishtail deformity can lead to cubitus varus and usually does not cause any functional problems or requires surgical intervention [3]. Several authors have correlated fishtail deformity with inadequately reduced fractures [23, 24]. In our cohort, all the patients were treated with open reduction, and none of them subsequently developed a fishtail deformity. This further emphasises the importance of achieving accurate anatomic reduction in these patients.

Treatment of lateral humeral condyle fractures should ensure that patients are not exposed to unnecessary radiation. During the operation, screening must be kept to a minimum and the patient should be covered with a lead radioprotective apron. During follow-up, only one radiograph per week until bone healing is established and then 6 months—yearly radiographs until skeletal maturity when indicated. Different authors report low effective doses of radiation following an elbow radiograph between 0.01 and 0.05 mSV, which is the equivalent period of natural background radiation of a few days and carries no

increased risk for severe complications and cancer development [25, 26].

In 1971, Hardacre et al. [11] presented their criteria for grading the outcomes following treatment of lateral humeral condyle fractures, taking into consideration symptoms, range of motion and deformity. These criteria have been used in several other studies for assessing outcomes in lateral condyle fractures [2, 9, 13]. In the author's opinion, this grading system as used in the present study was easy to utilise and corresponded well with the patient's clinical outcome.

To the best of our knowledge, this study presents the third larger single-centre series of surgical management of paediatric lateral condyle fractures recorded in the English language over the last 20 years. The good follow-up of our patients provides useful information on the outcome of the surgical management of displaced lateral condyle fractures. The main limitation of the study was its retrospective nature.

Our results demonstrate that fracture union and excellent final outcomes can be expected in all patients using our protocol, whereby all patients with a displaced fracture are managed by ORIF with K-wire fixation, with the wires only being removed after there is evidence of radiological union. Physiotherapy as soon as possible after the immobilisation period is important as it has been shown to be related with fewer complications, fewer residual symptoms and faster gains in range of motion and strength [27]. The authors believe that the Jacob classification system is sufficient to guide treatment with focus on the necessity to reduce fractures displaced more than 2 mm. On the basis of the good outcomes and no significant complications in cases of Jacob III fractures, we advocate for open reduction of these injuries as opposed to the proposed closed reduction by some studies. Furthermore, our results confirm that lateral spurring—even though frequent—does not cause any symptoms. Our study adds evidence on the outcomes of surgically treated lateral humeral condyle fractures and contributes to the clarification of the associated controversies.

Acknowledgments No financial support was received for this study.

5. References

1. Bauer AS, Bae DS, Brustowicz KA, Waters PM (2013) Intra-articular corrective osteotomy of humeral lateral condyle malunions in children: early clinical and radiographic results. J Pediatr Orthop 33(1):20–25
2. Marcheix PS, Vacquerie V, Longis B, Peyrou P, Fourcade L, Moulies D (2011) Distal humerus lateral condyle fracture in

children: when is the conservative treatment a valid option? Orthop Traumatol Surg Res 97(3):304–307

3. Rockwood CA, Wilkins KE, Beaty JH, Kasser JR (2006) Rockwood and Wilkins' fractures in children, 6th edn. Lippincott Williams & Wilkins, Philadelphia, xv, p. 1200

4. Milch H (1964) Fractures and fracture dislocations of the humeral condyles. J Trauma 4:592–607

5. Cotton FJ (1902) IX Elbow fractures in children. Fractures of the lower end of the humerus; lesions and end results, and their bearing upon treatment. Ann Surg 35(3):365–399

6. Jakob R, Fowles JV, Rang M, Kassab MT (1975) Observations concerning fractures of the lateral humeral condyle in children. J Bone Joint Surg Br 57(4):430–436

7. Beltran J, Rosenberg ZS (1997) MR imaging of pediatric elbow fractures. Magn Reson Imaging Clin N Am 5(3):567–578

8. Das De S, Bae DS, Waters PM (2012) Displaced humeral lateral condyle fractures in children: should we bury the pins? J Pediatr Orthop 32(6):573–578

9. Song KS, Kang CH, Min BW, Bae KC, Cho CH, Lee JH (2008) Closed reduction and internal fixation of displaced unstable lateral condylar fractures of the humerus in children. J Bone Joint Surg Am 90(12):2673–2681

10. Song KS, Waters PM (2012) Lateral condylar humerus fractures: which ones should we fix? J Pediatr Orthop 32(Suppl 1):S5–S9

11. Hardacre JA, Nahigian SH, Froimson AI, Brown JE (1971) Fractures of the lateral condyle of the humerus in children. J Bone Joint Surg Am 53(6):1083–1095

12. Thomas DP, Howard AW, Cole WG, Hedden DM (2001) Three weeks of Kirschner wire fixation for displaced lateral condylar fractures of the humerus in children. J Pediatr Orthop 21(5):565–569

13. Song KS, Shin YW, Oh CW, Bae KC, Cho CH (2010) Closed reduction and internal fixation of completely displaced and rotated lateral condyle fractures of the humerus in children. J Orthop Trauma 24(7):434–438

14. Subramanian P, Kantharuban S, Shilston S, Pearce OJ (2012) Complications of Kirschner-wire fixation in distal radius fractures. Tech Hand Upper Extrem Surg 16(3):120–123

15. Formaini N, Jacob P, Willis L, Kean JR (2012) Evaluating the use of preoperative antibiotics in pediatric orthopaedic surgery. J Pediatr Orthop 32(7):737–740

16. Bratzler DW, Dellinger EP, Olsen KM, Perl TM, Auwaerter PG, Bolon MK et al (2013) Clinical practice guidelines for antimicrobial prophylaxis in surgery. Am J Health Syst Pharm Off J Am Soc Health Syst Pharm 70(3):195–283

17. Boxma H, Broekhuizen T, Patka P, Oosting H (1996) Randomised controlled trial of single-dose antibiotic prophylaxis in surgical treatment of closed fractures: the Dutch Trauma Trial. Lancet 347(9009):1133–1137

18. Koh KH, Seo SW, Kim KM, Shim JS (2010) Clinical and radiographic results of lateral condylar fracture of distal humerus in children. J Pediatr Orthop 30(5):425–429

19. Pribaz JR, Bernthal NM, Wong TC, Silva M (2012) Lateral spurring (overgrowth) after pediatric lateral condyle fractures. J Pediatr Orthop 32(5):456–460

20. So YC, Fang D, Leong JC, Bong SC (1985) Varus deformity following lateral humeral condylar fractures in children. J Pediatr Orthop 5(5):569–572

21. Skak SV, Olsen SD, Smaabrekke A (2001) Deformity after fracture of the lateral humeral condyle in children. J Pediatr Orthop B 10(2):142–152

22. Weiss JM, Graves S, Yang S, Mendelsohn E, Kay RM, Skaggs DL (2009) A new classification system predictive of complications in surgically treated pediatric humeral lateral condyle fractures. J Pediatr Orthop 29(6):602–605

23. Rutherford A (1985) Fractures of the lateral humeral condyle in children. J Bone Joint Surg Am 67(6):851–856

24. Launay F, Leet AI, Jacopin S, Jouve JL, Bollini G, Sponseller PD (2004) Lateral humeral condyle fractures in children: a comparison of two approaches to treatment. J Pediatr Orthop 24(4):385–391

25. International Commission on Radiological Protection (ICRP) (2001) Radiation and your patient: a guide for medical practitioners. Ann ICRP 31(4):5–31

26. Crawley MT, Rogers AT (2000) Dose-area product measurements in a range of common orthopaedic procedures and their possible use in establishing local diagnostic reference levels. Br J Radiol 73(871):740–744

27. Cincinatti Children's Hospital Medical Centre (2007) Evidence-based guideline for loss of elbow motion following surgery or trauma in children aged 4–18. Cincinnati Child Hosp Med Cent 21(9):1–9

3

The effect of HIV infection on the incidence and severity of circular external fixator pin track sepsis: a retrospective comparative study of 229 patients

Nando Ferreira · Leonard Charles Marais

Abstract Pin track sepsis is a common complication of circular external fixation. HIV status has been implicated as an independent risk factor for the development of pin track infection and has been cited as a reason not to attempt complex limb reconstruction in HIV-positive patients. This retrospective review of patients treated with circular external fixators looked at the incidence of pin track sepsis in HIV-positive, HIV-negative and patients whose HIV status was unknown. The records of 229 patients, 40 of whom were HIV-positive, were reviewed. The overall incidence of pin track sepsis was 22.7 %. HIV infection did not affect the incidence of pin track sepsis ($p = 0.9$). The severity of pin track sepsis was not influenced by HIV status ($p = 0.9$) or CD_4 count ($p = 0.2$). With the employment of meticulous pin insertion techniques and an effective postoperative pin track care protocol, circular external fixation can be used safely in HIV-positive individuals.

Keywords HIV · Pin track sepsis · Complication · Ilizarov · Circular external fixator

Introduction

External fixation, and circular external fixation in particular, has evolved as an indispensible component of contemporary trauma and limb reconstruction surgery. Owing to its minimally invasive nature, circular fixators are being used increasingly in the management of skeletal trauma. In injuries associated with soft tissue compromise, such as periarticular fractures of the tibia, circular fixation has been shown to decrease the incidence of deep infection [1–6]. Its use is well established in the reconstruction of post-traumatic, post-infective bone defects and congenital deformities. This treatment modality is, however, associated with its own set of complications of which the most frequent is pin track sepsis with the reported incidences ranging from 11.3 to 100 % [4, 7–15].

Pin track sepsis is often the first clinical manifestation of a vicious cycle of pin loosening and sustained pin site infection. It is a misconception that pin track sepsis result in pin loosening; pin loosening is more often the inciting event that leads to pin site infection [14, 16–19]. Failure of the pin–bone interface can have catastrophic consequences and may lead to failure of the reconstruction and, ultimately, limb ablation in some. A meticulous approach to pin and wire insertion combined with a structured protocol of pin site care has been shown to decrease the incidence of pin track sepsis [4, 20, 21]. Certain patient factors may, however, influence the incidence and severity of pin track sepsis. Poor diabetic control and HIV infection have both been implicated as independent risk factors for the development of pin track infection [7, 15, 22–24].

HIV infection was previously considered to be a relative contraindication for the use of external fixators. A recent study from Malawi investigating the use of monolateral external fixators in tibial trauma found an increased incidence and severity of pin track sepsis in HIV-positive patients [22–24]. This study is cited frequently against limb reconstruction with external fixation in HIV-positive patients. The use of circular fixators, in particular, has been avoided in HIV-positive patients due to the prolonged periods of treatment required.

N. Ferreira (✉) · L. C. Marais
Tumour Sepsis and Reconstruction Unit, Department of Orthopaedic Surgery, Greys Hospital, Nelson R. Mandela School of Medicine, University of KwaZulu-Natal, Pietermaritzburg 3201, South Africa
e-mail: Nando.Ferreira@kznhealth.gov.za

South Africa has the highest incidence of HIV infection in the world. The 2011 National Antenatal Sentinel Survey reported a national prevalence of 17.3 %, with areas like KwaZulu-Natal approaching 25 % [25]. The majority of these patients are between 20 and 50 years old. South Africa also has one of the highest incidences of road traffic accidents in the world, affecting mostly young adults [26, 27]. The HIV pandemic in South Africa, combined with the high incidence of trauma, has resulted in many HIV-positive patients requiring treatment for complex trauma or a need for post-traumatic limb reconstruction. Of note is that the overall fracture prevalence is increased in HIV-positive compared to HIV-negative patients [28–30].

This retrospective review aims to compare the rate and severity of pin track sepsis in HIV-positive and HIV-negative patients treated with circular external fixators. The research proposal was reviewed and approved by the local ethics committee. An extensive literature review revealed this current study to be the largest yet to compare the incidence of pin track sepsis in HIV-positive and HIV-negative patients. It is currently also the only study investigating the effect of HIV infection on the incidence and severity of pin track sepsis with the use of circular external fixators.

Materials and methods

The study population consisted of all patients who were treated with circular external fixators at our institution between July 2008 and December 2012. Patients were included if they had completed treatment and had the external fixator removed. Patients were excluded if the external fixator was not applied at our institution or if the records were insufficient for the required data.

All patients were offered voluntary HIV counseling and testing. The CD_4 count of all HIV-positive patients was measured. Patients with CD_4 counts below 350 cells/mm^3 were started on highly active antiretroviral therapy (HAART) in accordance with South African national antiretroviral treatment guidelines.

The fixator design and application followed the general principles as outlined by Catagni with the emphasis on construction of a stable frame configuration [31–36]. Particular attention was paid to atraumatic pin and wire insertion. Recognized anatomical safe zones were used and insertion was carried out with as little heat and energy transfer as possible [31, 36, 37]. Postoperative pin track care followed the protocol previously set out by Ferreira and Marais [21]. Outpatient follow-up was scheduled at two to four weekly intervals until frame removal. At every clinic visit, the progress was assessed and any complications, including pin track sepsis, were documented. Pin site

Table 1 Checketts–Otterburn classification

Grade	Characteristics	Treatment
Minor infection		
1	Slight redness, little discharge	Improved pin site care
2	Redness of the skin, discharge, pain and tenderness in the soft tissue	Improved pin site care, oral antibiotics
3	Grade 2 but no improvement with oral antibiotics	Affected pin or pins resited and external fixation can be continued
Major infection		
4	Severe soft tissue infection involving several pins, sometimes with associated loosening of the pin	External fixation must be abandoned
5	Grade 4 but radiographic changes	External fixation must be abandoned
6	Infection after fixator removal. Pin track heals initially, but will subsequently break down and discharge in intervals. Radiographs show new bone formation and sometimes sequestra	Curettage of the pin tract

infections were graded according the Checketts and Otterburn classification (Table 1) [38].

A retrospective review was undertaken and the variables recorded included patient demographics, HIV status, CD_4 count and use of antiretroviral medication, indications for circular fixation, type of external fixator used, pin track complications and treatment of these complications. Results were analyzed using the independent t test, one-way ANOVA test and the Kruskal–Wallis H test to ascertain whether HIV infection had any effect on the incidence or severity on pin track sepsis.

Results

The records of 274 patients were reviewed. Forty-five patients were excluded because the external fixators had not yet been removed. Therefore, 229 patients (163 males and 66 females) were included: The mean age was 34.5 years (standard deviation ± 15.4, range 6–71 years); mean time in external fixation was 22.9 weeks (SD ± 14.7, range 6–104 weeks).

The external fixators applied consisted of 71 Ilizarov fixators (Smith and Nephew, Memphis, TN), 91 Truelok fixators (Orthofix, Verona, Italy), 65 Taylor Spatial Frames (Smith and Nephew, Memphis, TN) and two TL-Hex fixators (Orthofix, Verona, Italy) (Table 2). The indications for the use of the external fixators are listed in Table 3.

Table 2 External fixators applied

	HIV+	HIV−	Unknown	Total
Ilizarov	14	44	13	71
Truelok	21	65	5	91
Taylor Spatial Frame	5	57	3	65
TL-Hex	0	2	0	2
Total	40	168	21	229

Table 3 Circular external fixator indications

Indications	HIV+	HIV−	Unknown
Complex trauma	7	21	3
Periarticular fracture	17	50	12
Non-union	5	25	2
Bone transport	1	7	1
Bone defect	2	3	
Limb lengthening		1	
Chronic osteomyelitis	3	5	
Deformity correction	5	56	3
Total	40	168	21

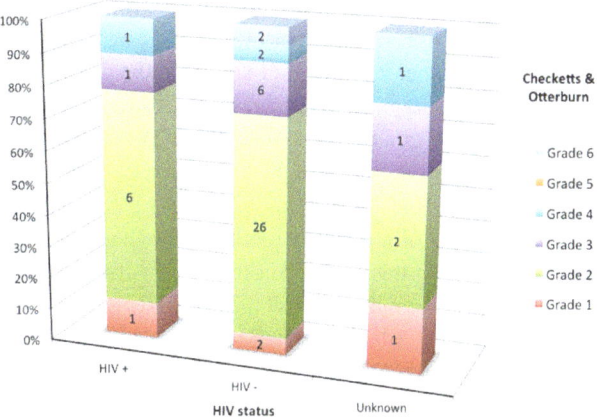

Fig. 1 Pin track infection grades in HIV+, HIV− and Unknown groups

mm^3 (D $\pm$ 162.4, range 82–682 cells/mm^3) and 25 (62.5 %) patients were receiving HAART. Our data showed that CD_4 count had no influence on either the incidence ($p = 0.57$) or severity ($p = 0.21$) of pin track sepsis in the HIV-positive group.

The patients were divided into groups according to their HIV status. A third group was made up of patients who refused HIV testing and designated as the unknown group. The HIV-positive group consisted of 40 (17.5 %) patients. The mean age was 37.2 years (SD $\pm$ 10.2, range 8–56 years). Time in the external fixator averaged 26 weeks (SD $\pm$ 16.6, range 6–77 weeks). The HIV-negative group consisted of 168 (73.4 %) patients. The mean age was 33.2 (SD $\pm$ 16.5, range 6–71 years) and time in the external fixator averaged 33.2 weeks (SD $\pm$ 16.5, range 6–71 weeks). The group whose HIV status was unknown consisted of 21 (9.2 %) patients. Their mean age was 39.7 years (SD $\pm$ 13.1, range 17–59 years) and time in external fixation averaged 18.9 weeks (SD $\pm$ 10.2, range 7–50 weeks). There was no statistically significant difference between the three groups in terms of age ($p = 0.09$) or time in the external fixator ($p = 0.18$).

Pin track infection occurred in 52 (22.7 %) out of 229 patients. In the subgroups, nine (22.5 %) patients in the HIV-positive group ($n = 40$), 38 (22.6 %) patients in the HIV-negative group ($n = 168$) and five (23.8 %) patients in the unknown group ($n = 21$) developed pin track sepsis. Checketts and Otterburn grades for the three groups are shown in Fig. 1. There was no statistically significant difference in the incidence of pin track sepsis between the three groups ($p = 0.94$). Furthermore, the three groups had no statistically significant differences in terms of severity of pin track sepsis ($p = 0.9$).

A subgroup analysis of the HIV-positive patients ($n = 40$) was undertaken. Mean CD_4 count was 347.4 cells/

Discussion

Pin track sepsis remains a common complication with the use of external fixators [7, 15]. Quoted incidences range from 11.3 to 100 % [9–13]. Mostafavi reported a 71 % incidence of pin site infection in reconstructive surgery [11].

The use of meticulous pin insertion techniques and the implementation of an evidence-based pin track care protocol can reduce the incidence of pin track sepsis with circular external fixation in reconstructive surgery to approximately 25 % [4]. Our results compare favorably to previously published figures with an overall pin track sepsis incidence of 22.7 % (52 out of 229) observed in this series.

Several factors have been implicated in the development of pin track sepsis [4, 21]. They include frame design and biomechanics, pin and wire insertion techniques, point of commencement of pin track care and the specific care protocol employed [7, 8, 12, 13, 40]. Strategies to reduce pin track sepsis should include measures aimed at optimization of these factors. Some non-modifiable risk factors have also been associated with pin site infection. These include diabetes mellitus and HIV infection [7, 15, 22–24].

HIV infection has prompted many orthopedic and trauma surgeons to avoid the use of circular external fixators for the purpose of limb reconstruction in HIV-positive patients. Norrish and Harrison published the first data comparing pin track infection with the use of monolateral external fixators in HIV-positive and HIV-negative patients [22, 24, 39]. They reported on 13 HIV-positive and 34 HIV-negative patients and found significantly more infections requiring pharmaceutical or surgical intervention in the HIV-positive group. Our results differ in that we could show no correlation between the incidence or severity of pin track sepsis and HIV status. Our results do correlate with the findings of no correlation between CD_4 count and the severity of pin track infection in HIV-positive patients. The low patient numbers and wide CD_4 range could explain the apparent lack of relationship and more research is required.

In conclusion, while pin track sepsis is a common complication with the use of circular external fixators, we did not find that the incidence or severity of pin track sepsis was influenced by HIV infection or degree of immune compromise. This finding should not preclude the use of circular external fixators for complex trauma and limb reconstruction in HIV-positive individuals.

References

1. Bone L, Stegemann P, McNamara K, Seibel R (1993) External fixation of severely comminuted and open tibial pilon fractures. Clin Orthop 292:101–107
2. Chin TYP, Bardana D, Bailey M, Williamson OD, Miller R, Edwards ER, Esser MP (2005) Functional outcome of tibial plateau fractures treated with the fine-wire fixator. Injury 36:1467–1475
3. Dendrinos GK, Kontos S, Katsenis D, Dalas A (1996) Treatment of high-energy tibial plateau fractures by the Ilizarov circular fixator. J Bone Joint Surg Br 78-B:710–717
4. Ferreira N, Marais LC (2012) Pin tract sepsis: incidence with the use of circular fixators in a limb reconstruction unit. SA Orthop J 11(1):10–18
5. Kapoor SK, Kataria H, Patra SR, Boruah T (2010) Capsuloligamentotaxis and definitive fixation by an ankle-spanning Ilizarov fixator in high-energy pilon fractures. J Bone Joint Surg Br 92-B:1100–1106
6. Kataria H, Sharma N, Kanojia RK (2007) Small wire external fixation for high-energy tibial plateau fractures. J Orthop Surg 15(2):137–143
7. Bibbo C, Brueggeman J (2010) Prevention and management of complications arising from external fixation pin sites. J Foot Ankle Surg 49:87–92
8. Davies R, Holt N, Nayagam S (2005) The care of pin sites with external fixation. J Bone Joint Surg Br 87-B:716–719
9. DeJong ES, DeBerardino TM, Brooks DE, Nelson BJ, Campbell AA, Bottoni CR, Pusateri AE, Walton RS, Guymon CH, McManus AT (2001) Antimicrobial efficacy of external fixator pins coated with a lipid stabilized hydroxyapatite/chlorhexidine complex to prevent pin tract infection in a goat model. J Trauma 50:1008–1014
10. Cavusoglu AT, Er MS, Inal S, Ozsoy MH, Dincel MS, Sakaogullari A (2009) Pin site care during circular external fixation using two different protocols. J Orthop Trauma 23:724–730
11. Mostafavi HR, Tornetta P III (1997) Open fractures of the humerus treated with external fixation. Clin Orthop Relat Res 337:187–197

12. Parameswaran AD, Roberts CS, Seligson D, Voor M (2003) Pin tract infection with contemporary external fixation: how much of a problem? J Orthop Trauma 17:503–507
13. Patterson MM (2005) Multicentre pin care study. Orthop Nurs 24(5):349–360
14. Piza G, Caja VL, Gonzalez-Veijo MZ, Navarro A (2004) Hydroxyapatite-coated external-fixation pins. The effect on pin loosening and pin-tract infection in leg lengthening for short stature. J Bone Joint Surg Br 86-B:892–897
15. Rogers LC, Bevilacqua NJ, Frykberg RG, Armstrong DG (2007) Predictors of postoperative complications of Ilizarov external ring fixators in the foot and ankle. J Foot Ankle Surg 46(5):372–375
16. Harding AK, Toksvig-Larsen S, Tagil M, W-Dahl A (2010) A single dose zolendronic acid enhances pin fixation in high tibial osteotomy using the hemicallotasis technique. A double-blind controlled randomized study in 46 patients. Bone 46:649–654
17. Moroni A, Heikkila J, Magyar G, Toksvig-Larsen S, Giannini S (2001) Fixation strength and pin tract infection of hydroxyapatite-coated tapered pins. Clin Orthop Relat Res 388:209–217
18. Moroni A, Aspenberg P, Toksvig-Larsen S, Falzarano G, Giannini S (1998) Enhanced fixation with hydroxyapatite coated pins. Clin Orthop Relat Res 346:171–177
19. Moroni A, Cadossi M, Romagnoli M, Faldini C, Giannini S (2008) A biomechanical and histological analysis of standard versus hydroxyapatite-coated pins for external fixation. J Biomed Mater Res 86B:417–421
20. Antoci V, Ono CM, Antoci V Jr, Raney EM (2008) Pin-tract infection during limb lengthening using external fixation. Am J Orthop 37(9):E150–E154
21. Ferreira N, Marais LC (2012) Prevention and management of external fixator pin tract sepsis. Strat Traum Limb Recon 7:67–72. doi:10.1007/s11751-012-0139-2
22. Harrison WJ (2009) Open tibia fractures in HIV positive patients. Malawi Med J 21(4):174–175
23. Lubega N, Harrison WJ (2010) Orthopaedic and trauma surgery in HIV positive patients. Orthop Trauma 24(4):298–302
24. Norrish AR, Lewis CP, Harrison WJ (2007) Pin-track infection in HIV-positive and HIV-negative patients with open fractures treated by external fixation. J Bone Joint Surg 89B:790–793
25. The 2011 national antenatal sentinel HIV and Syphilis prevalence survey in South Africa. http://www.doh.gov.za/docs/presenta tions/2013/Antenatal_Sentinel_survey_Report2012_final.pdf
26. http://www.who.int/gho/road_safety/en/index.html
27. Global status report on road safety 2013.pdf http://www.who.int/ violence_injury_prevention/road_safety_status/2013/en/index. html
28. Hansen AB, Gerstoft J, Kronborg G, Larsen CS, Pedersen C, Pedersen G, Obel N (2012) Incidence of low and high-energy fractures in persons with and without HIV infection: a Danish population-based cohort study. AIDS 26(3):285–293. doi:10. 1097/QAD.0b013e32834ed8a7
29. Shiau S, Broun EC, Arpadi SM, Yin MT (2013) Incident fractures in HIV-infected individuals: a systematic review and meta-analysis. AIDS 27(12):1949–1957. doi:10.1097/QAD.0b013e 328361d241
30. Triant VA, Brown TT, Lee H, Grinspoon SK (2008) Fracture prevalence among human immunodeficiency virus (HIV)-infected versus non-HIV-infected patients in a large U.S. healthcare system. J Clin Endocrinol Metab 93:3499–3504. doi:10.1210/jc. 2008-0828
31. Catagni MA (2009) Treatment of fractures, nonunions, and bone loss of the tibia with the Ilizarov method, 5th edn. Il quadratino, Italy
32. Bronson DG, Samchukov ML, Birch JG, Browne RH, Ashman RB (1998) Stability of external circular fixation: a multi-variable

biomechanical analysis. Clin Biomech 13:441–448
33. Fragomen AT, Rozbruch SR (2007) The mechanics of external fixation. HSSJ 3:13–29. doi:10.1007/s11420-006-9025-0
34. Ilizarov GA (1990) Clinical application of the tension-stress effect for limb lengthening. Clin Orthop 250:8–26
35. Mullins MM, Davidson AW, Goodier D, Barry M (2003) The biomechanics of wire fixation in the Ilizarov system. Inj Int J Care Inj 34:155–157
36. Watson MA, Mathias KJ, Maffulli N (2000) External ring fixators: an overview. Proc Inst Mech Eng 214:459–470
37. Nayagam S (2007) Safe corridors in external fixation: the lower

leg (tibia, fibula, hindfoot and forefoot). Strat Traum Limb Recon 2:105–110
38. Checketts RG, MacEachern AG, Otterburn M (2000) Pin track infection and the principles of pin site care. In: Goldberg A, De Bastiani A, Apley AG (eds) Orthofix external fixation in trauma and orthopaedics. Springer, Berlin, pp 97–103
39. Harrison WJ, Lewis CP, Lavy CBD (2004) Open fractures of the tibia in HIV positive patients: a prospective controlled single-blind study. Inj Int J Care Inj 35:852–856
40. Holmes SH, Brown SJ (2005) Skeletal pin site care. Orthop Nurs 24(2):99–107

4

Nailing treatment in bone transport complications

C. Biz · C. Iacobellis

Abstract A series of cases of reamed intramedullary nailings carried out after complications in regenerated bone and docking site had occurred in bone transport is presented here. Nine patients (femur = 5; tibia = 4) had treatment with resection after open fractures or infection and underwent bone transport. The mean length of regenerated bone was 9.5 cm (range 6–18 cm). After bone transport, the fixator remained in place for a mean period of 12.8 months (range 8–24 months). In six cases (femur 4; tibia 2), the thickness of the cortical wall of the regenerate column was insufficient, and in two of these, there was, in addition, nonunion of the docking site. In the two tibial cases, nailing was carried out shortly after the fixator had been removed and after refracture of the regenerated bone had occurred due to insufficient cortical thickness. In one femur, nailing was carried out for nonunion of the docking site. Follow-up involved clinical and X-ray checks. The mean follow-up was 3.9 years (range 2–6 years). In all cases, union and with complete corticalization of the regenerate column was observed at an average 6 months after nailing (range 4–11 months). Infection occurred in one tibia 4 months after nailing. The infection was treated with antibiotics, and the nail was subsequently removed. We conclude that nailing is a potential solution for regenerated bone and docking site problems but, if used after prolonged periods of external fixation, may necessitate antibiotic therapy for at least 10 days after the fixator has been removed.

C. Biz · C. Iacobellis (✉)
Orthopaedic Clinic, Department of Surgery, Oncology and Gastroenterology DiSCOG, University of Padua,
Via Giustiniani 2, 35128 Padua, Italy
e-mail: claudio.iacobellis@unipd.it

Keywords Bone transport · Distraction osteogenesis · External fixator · Intramedullary nailing

Introduction

Bone transport for segmental resections in the treatment for infected nonunion, osteomyelitis, or after bone loss in open fractures remains a major undertaking for orthopedic surgeons [1–4]. For long-bone diaphyseal defects larger than 5 cm, with or without a soft-tissue defect, specialized management is needed [5]. The use of vascularized bone grafts [6, 7], allograft bone transplantation, or bone transport by an external fixator alone or over an intramedullary nail has been reported in [8–10]. Bone transport with a circular or monolateral external fixator represents a standard method for managing lower limb bone defects and for limb lengthening [11–14]. These methods induce two biological processes: distraction osteogenesis, the new production of bone from a corticotomy, and transformational osteogenesis, where the mechanical stimulation of an abnormal bony interface regenerates normal bony continuity and achieves consolidation [15, 16]. Further, the regenerated bone formed by bone transport is mechanically stronger to that formed by bone grafting but there is a risk of refracture after frame removal [17]. Distraction osteogenesis by the Ilizarov technique [18–20], subsequently modified by Cattaneo et al. [21], has been used successfully in all long bones since its introduction [17, 22–26]. In contrast, bone transport using a monolateral external fixator achieves a similar result through distraction of callus (callotasis) that is obtained from a subperiosteal osteotomy [27]. Compared with a circular frame, this device has the advantage of being lighter and a simpler application. There is also less soft-tissue transfixation by pins, thereby allowing early physical exercise and partial weight-bearing [28]. Use of hydroxyapatite-coated pins decreases pin site-related problems [9, 29].

Bone transport carries advantages of minimal soft-tissue trauma, almost limitless reconstruction of bone defects and elimination of donor site morbidity [30, 31]. The process of bone transport using an external fixator alone is still a lengthy and uncomfortable process. It is a labor-intensive surgical procedure and subjects to many complications with considerable treatment times [32–36]. Despite the versatility of distraction osteogenesis, both patients and orthopedic surgeon are prompted to remove the external fixator early to decrease discomfort and complications [37] of which the most frequent are nonunion at the docking site [38], fracture of regenerated bone due to the lack of internal stabilization, failure of distraction osteogenesis, and recurring infection [39, 40]. Simpson and Kenwright [41] report a fracture rate of 9.4 % in a series of 180 lengthening segments; O'Carrigan [42] reports an 8 % fracture rate in 650 patients with 986 lengthening segments, and Danziger [43] had refracture of the femur in 6 of 18 patients. Lavini [38] had axial deviation in 17.6 % in a series of 17 cases. In our previous study of 100 consecutive cases of bone transport using the Ilizarov method, we found 1 % refracture of the newly formed bone segment of the tibia, 17 % nonunion at the docking site in 10 femurs and 7 tibias, 10 % bone transport arrest due to the failure of distraction osteogenesis in 2 femurs and 8 tibias, and 4 % of cases had recurring infection [22]. Furthermore, paresthesiae (9 %) [32, 44], angulation, and deformity of the newly formed bone column (2–17 %) [22, 38, 44], and neighboring joint contractures due to increased soft-tissue tension and joint stiffness (10–28 %) [22, 44], are encountered frequently during lengthening and bone transport.

One solution to some of these complications is the insertion of an intramedullary nail in order to support the regenerated bone during the consolidation phase and facilitate the removal of the external fixator after the distraction phase of lengthening. However, intramedullary nailing after bone transport with a circular or monolateral external fixator is still controversial as there is a risk of infection. Specifically, when combining external and internal fixation, the risk of deep infection has been reported between 3 and 15 % [45, 46]. Other methods employed to shorten the external fixation treatment period have been described: docking site stimulation with autogenous bone graft, bone marrow injection, electric or magnetic field stimulation, ultrasound stimulation, and the use of bone growth stimulating factors [47].

This retrospective study was carried out on a sample of patients treated with reamed intramedullary nailing after bone transport with the aim of assessing the evolution of union and the incidence of infection and major complications after surgery.

Materials and methods

This is a retrospective review of a case series. All subjects participating in this study were counselled over the risks and benefits of the procedure; informed consent for inclusion in this retrospective case series was obtained. Between 2006 and 2010, nine patients (eight males, one female; average age 35.5 years; range 25–57) underwent bone transport for bone loss after open fractures and infection. All patients had bone defects of >5 cm after resection and debridement. There were no specific exclusion criteria. Five femurs and four tibias were involved. In all cases, samples were taken for culture. These included no fewer than four swabs both before and during surgery. The cause of infection was identified as *Staphylococcus aureus* in six cases and *Pseudomonas aeruginosa* in 3. Subsequent antibiotic therapy was carried out, according to the culture and sensitivity results, for a minimum 6-week period or until the erythrocyte sedimentation rate and C-reactive protein level had returned to normal [48].

Six patients were treated using the Ilizarov circular fixator (Amplimedical s.p.a, Milan, Italy) and 3 with a monolateral rail fixator (Limb Reconstruction System Orthofix SRL, Verona, Italy). The types of transport through healthy tissue were descending (proximal–distal) in two cases (femurs), ascending in four cases (one femur, three tibias), double transport in two femurs (with mid-diaphyseal contact of transported bone ends at the docking site from proximal and distal metaphyseal osteotomies), and in one tibia (twin transport from a double proximal osteotomy). The mean length of regenerated bone was 9.5 cm (range 6–18). At the end of transport, the fixator was kept in place for a mean period of 12.8 months (range 8–24). In all cases, the docking site was exposed, the interposed tissue was removed, and if small residual gaps were seen between the two bone ends, cancellous bone was taken from the ipsilateral iliac crest and grafted. We observed spontaneous healing of the skin defects at the docking site; plastic surgical cover was not required. Reaming and nailing (Synthes nail) were carried out in six cases (four femurs, two tibias; cases 1–4, 6, 9) for which the thickness of the cortical wall of the regenerated bone was deemed insufficient (Fig. 1) and removal of the fixator would have created a high risk of fracture. In two of these six patients (cases 4 and 9), nonunion of the docking site was diagnosed additionally. In another patient (case 3; Fig. 2), a bony bridge had formed between the intended docking site and transport segment causing an arrest of transport and varus and procurvatum deformity of the regenerated bone.

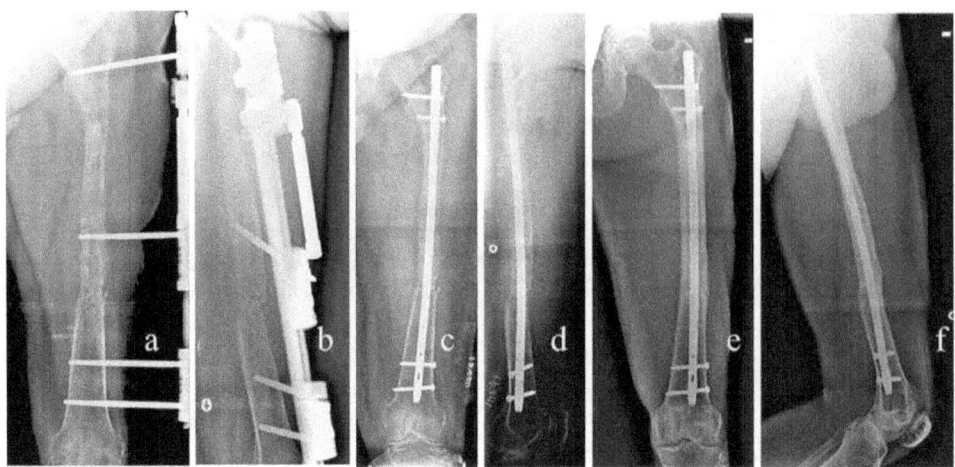

Fig. 1 Case 2: **a**, **b** preoperative X-ray, **c**, **d** postoperative checkup, **e**, **f** follow-up 5 years later

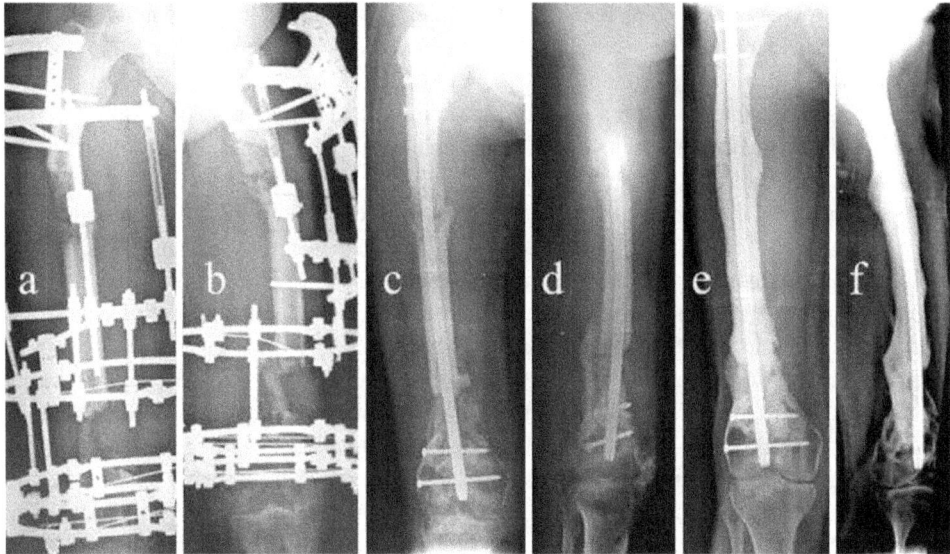

Fig. 2 Case 3: **a**, **b** preoperative X-ray; bony bridge in the docking site, arrest of transport, varus, and procurvatus of the regenerated bone, **c**, **d** follow-up 40 days later, **e**, **f** follow-up 4 years later

For this case, as well as intramedullary nailing, the docking site was filled with autogenous bone grafts. In two patients (cases 5 and 7, both tibial defects), nailing was carried out for refracture of regenerated bone, which occurred soon after fixator removal. In one patient (case 8, femoral defect), intramedullary nailing was carried out for nonunion of the docking site. In all cases, the fixator was removed prior to nailing and a plaster cast was applied for 10 days. Details of the cases are summarized in Table 1.

Patients were followed up at 2-month intervals until X-rays showed corticalization with bone thickness equal to that of the bone adjacent to the regenerated bone and/or consolidation of the docking site. The functional outcome measures were recorded, they are as follows: an observable limp, stiffness of the principal joints (defined as >70° loss of knee flexion or >15° loss of knee extension, >50° loss of

ankle motion, all as compared with the normal contralateral side), and the ability to fully weight-bearing pain-free. The limb and bone segment was assessed radiologically for axial deformity, union, and for signs of infection after nailing. Fractures after nail removal were noted. The outcome was considered excellent if the patients were fully weight-bearing, pain-free, without knee and ankle stiffness, and had a normal aligned limb without need for further surgery after the intramedullary nailing had been performed; good if the patients required more surgery to achieve union; and poor if major complications occurred according to Paley's classification [33]. The patients were asked whether they were satisfied with the procedure or would have preferred primary amputation instead of the multiple procedures undertaken to salvage the limb. No statistical analysis was performed as the number of the cases is small.

Table 1 Cases

Case	Gender [age (years)]	Bone, side (L, left; R, right)	Open fracture Gustilo I, II, III	Findings on culture	Bone loss (cm)	Fixator	Transport: A, ascending technique. D, descending T. DL, double-level bone T	External fixator time (months)	Regenerated bone* IC, R	Docking site* C, N
1	M, 32	Femur, R	II	*Staphylococcus aureus*	10	Orthofix	DL	11	IC	C
2	M, 28	Femur, L	I	*Pseudomonas aeruginosa*	6	Orthofix	D	12	IC	C
3	M, 47	Femur, R	II	*Staphylococcus aureus*	9	Ilizarov	D	8	IC	N
4	M, 28	Femur, L	II	*Staphylococcus aureus*	14	Orthofix	DL	11	IC	N
5	M, 57	Tibia, L	I	*Staphylococcus aureus*	6	Ilizarov	A	9	R	C
6	F, 25	Tibia, L	II	*Staphylococcus aureus*	18	Ilizarov	A	24	IC	C
7	M, 44	Tibia, L	II	*Pseudomonas aeruginosa*	7	Ilizarov	DL	10	R	C
8	M, 28	Femur, L	I	*Pseudomonas aeruginosa*	6	Ilizarov	A	13	C	N
9	M, 31	Tibia, L	II	*Staphylococcus aureus*	10	Ilizarov	A	18	IC	N

*C Consolidation, N nonunion, IC insufficient corticalization, R refracture

Results

The mean follow-up was 3.9 years (range 2–6). All cases had undergone resection and bone transport for open fractures after road traffic accidents. Complete corticalization of the regenerate column of bone was achieved on average after 6.5 months (range 4–11) after nailing. The length of regenerated bone was checked before and after nailing, and in no case was shortening of regenerated bone observed. None had major complications, neurovascular injuries, joint subluxations or fracture of the regenerated bone. Using the criteria described earlier, eight patients obtained excellent results and only one patient a good result as further surgery was needed; in this case, infection of the tibia occurred 4 months after nailing despite corticalization (case 5, Fig. 3). The nail was removed and the infection treated. The patient was re-examined 3 years after nail removal and was found to be without signs of recurrence. In three other cases, the nail was removed at the patient's request. One patient was found to have knee stiffness that did not require further surgery. All of the patients were satisfied with the procedure, and none expressed a preference for amputation despite the multiple procedures or length of treatment. The patient outcome data are summarized in Table 2.

Discussion

Several reports in the literature show good results from nailing after or during external fixation. Femoral and tibial nailing with reaming is used commonly after damage control stabilization with external fixation for cases of multiple trauma [16] or open fractures of Gustilo type III [49, 50]. After the removal of the fixator, intramedullary nailing is carried out in the same operating session or delayed to occur after a period of traction [16, 49] or time in plaster [49, 50], (with or without an interim period of antibiotic therapy) for fear that the pins and wire sites could lead to potential deep intramedullary infections. As early as 1956, Bost et al. [51] described a lengthening technique with an inserted nail, involving external devices and Steinmann pins applied to the same bone segment. Forty years later, Paley et al. [52] presented a series of 32 cases of femoral lengthening using external fixators (Ilizarov or Orthofix) over intramedullary nails ensuring the pins or wires did not contact the nail. At the end of the lengthening period, the fixator was removed and the nail locked. Other cases of lengthening where external fixators were combined with intramedullary nails have also been reported [53–55]. In 39 cases of lengthening, Rozbruch et al. [53] reported one deep infection that was treated by nail removal. The authors attributed the low number of infections partly to the fact that the regenerated bone was well vascularized. In 13 lengthenings with fixators and nailing, Bilen et al. [54] had no cases of infection. In 56 lengthenings with fixators and nails which were either unreamed or only very slightly reamed, Park et al. [55] reported no deep infections and only 13 pin track infections, all which resolved with antibiotics. The literature also contains several reports describing intramedullary nails in bony segments already partially resected due to previous infections. Papineau [56] inserted a nail 2 weeks after surgical debridement and later filled the gap with cancellous bone grafts. Several other authors [57–60] have presented cases of bone transport with fixators and nailing. Raschke et al. [57] have adopted a more cautious approach; in four cases of open tibial fractures of Gustilo types II and III, they first proceeded with debridement and application of external

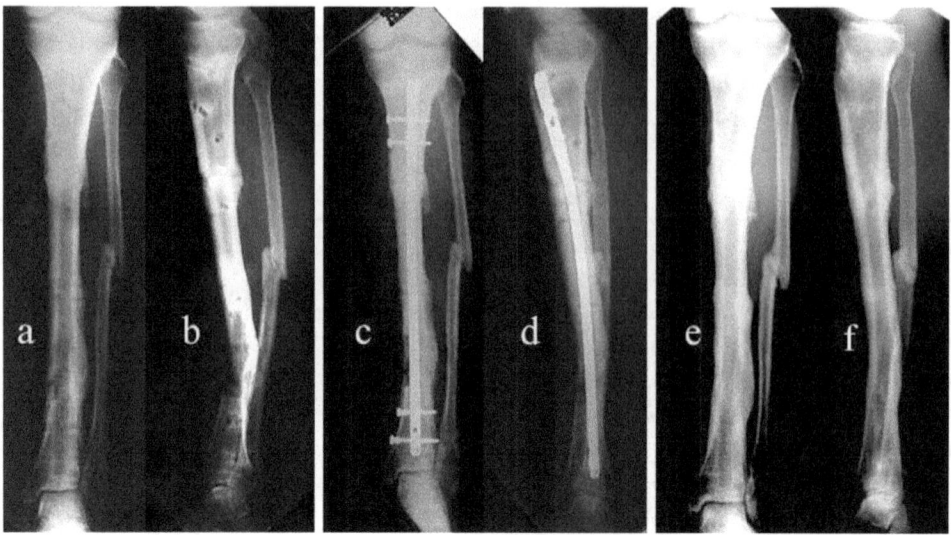

Fig. 3 Case 5: **a, b** preoperative X-ray, 1 month after the removal of the fixator, **c, d** postoperative checkup, **e, f** follow-up 3 years later

Table 2 Results

Case	Follow-up (years) after nailing	Limp	Knee (K) or ankle (A) stiffness	Fully W–B and pain-free	Axial deviation	Infection after nailing	Consolidation after nailing (months)	Removal of the nail	Fractures after nail removal
1	4	No	No K–A	Yes	No	No	10	No	–
2	5	No	No K–A	Yes	No	No	11	No	–
3	4	Yes	Yes K; No A	No	No	No	6	No	–
4	3	No	No K–A	Yes	No	No	8	No	–
5	3	No	No K–A	Yes	No	Yes	4	Yes, after 4 months	No
6	5	No	No K–A	Yes	No	No	6	Yes, after 6 months	No
7	6	No	No K-A	Yes	No	No	4	Yes, after 5 years	No
8	3.5	No	No K–A	Yes	No	No	4	Yes, after 3.5 years	No
9	2	No	No K–A	Yes	no	No	6	No	–

fixators, and after 4–6 weeks inserted locked undreamed intramedullary nails in combination with new monolateral fixators. There were no infections of the medullary canal. In 2002, Lai et al. [15] presented 27 cases of bony transport in femurs and tibias with regenerated bone or docking site problems or refractures. In these cases, with an average of 3–4 weeks after the removal of the fixator, reamed locked nails were inserted. Two cases of infection at the site of the distal docking screws were resolved after nail removal. Eralp et al. [58] presented a series of 17 resections due to chronic osteomyelitis, with antibiotic therapy for 6 weeks and then bone transport with reamed nails and fixators concurrently. They reported three deep infections. In another series of 17 patients, Li et al. [59] used external fixators with reamed nails for bone transport to resolve large defects of the femur which were created after resection for osteomyelitis; the patients were subjected to a 6-week course of antibiotic therapy before bone transport

surgery was performed. They reported 10 superficial pin track infections and one deep intramedullary infection that was treated by the removal of the nail and external fixator and reaming of the medullary canal.

These reports suggest that a nail may be inserted (despite previously infected tissue) if there is interim antibiotic therapy. In our series where bone transport was performed after resection for infection, we inserted the intramedullary nails after an interval of antibiotic therapy. We had one case (case 5) of re-infection after nailing, which we resolved by nail removal after union and antibiotic treatment (Fig. 3). Although some authors [60] believe that the risk of expanding an infection into the medullary cavity increases with the insertion of an intramedullary nail, it is our belief this risk is reduced if the previous site of infection is thoroughly debrided and some time allowed to pass before nailing. This is in order to clear up pin infections that often occur, particularly along screws. Kirschner wires, having a smaller diameter, create less serious infections than those produced by pins. Once the infection is treated and resolved, the nail can be inserted after reaming, which serves as a biological stimulator for the corticalization of the regenerate area. Intramedullary reaming for chronic osteomyelitis results may assist in removing the laminar endosteal sequestra of the tibial canal as well as diminishing the intraosseous pressure; the bone is revascularized through an improved periosteal circulation [61–63]. Several authors have also reported their experience with reaming [64–68] showing that reamed bone has considerable osteoblastic potential, equal to that of the iliac crest [66]. Frölke et al. [66] and Wenisch et al. [67] report that human reaming debris is a source of multipotent stem cells that can grow and proliferate in vitro. In a recent review, Brinker et al. [68] stated that in the cases of nonunion, insertion of a second nail after the first promotes healing as long as the canal is reamed again and a larger nail inserted. These considerations may explain the corticalization effect that we found in our cases.

Bone transport is a reliable method for the reconstruction of bone defects in femur and tibia, and remains a safe treatment dealing with defects after resection for bone infection. Similarly, nailing is a good solution for regenerated bone and docking site problems as long as antibiotic therapy is prescribed, and nailing is carried out at least 10 days after the fixator has been removed. Complications due to deep infections are not common and may be resolved.

There are weaknesses in this case series. We acknowledge the small number of the patients and a potential bias due to its retrospective design being major limitations. The literature is limited on the subject of nailing treatment in bone transport complications. This report adds some support to a successful alternative strategy for the treatment for complications of bone transport with a moderate-term follow-up.

References

1. Mahaluxmivala J, Nadarajah R, Allen PW, Hill RA (2005) Ilizarov external fixator: acute shortening and lengthening versus bone transport in the management of tibial non-unions. Injury Int J Care Injured 36:662–668
2. Reichert JC et al (2009) The challenge of establishing preclinical models for segmental bone defects research. Biomaterials 30:2149–2163
3. Keating JF, Simpsons AH, Robinson CM (2005) The management of fractures with bone loss. J Bone Joint Surg Br 87:142–150
4. Lasanianos NG, Kanakaris NK, Giannoudis PV (2010) Current management of long bone large segmental defects. Orthop Trauma 24:149–163
5. Lin CH et al (1999) Outcome comparison in traumatic lower-extremity reconstruction by using various composite vascularized bone transplantation. Plast Reconstr Surg 104:984–992
6. Capanna J, Campanacci R, Belot DA et al (2007) A new reconstructive technique for intercalary defects of long bones: the association of massive allograft with vascularized fibular autograft. Long-term results and comparison with alternative techniques. Orthop Clin N Am 38:5–60
7. Lawal YZ, Garba ES, Ogirima MO et al (2011) Use of non-vascularized autologous fibula strut graft in the treatment of segmental bone loss. Ann Afr Med 10(1):25–28
8. Ilizarov GA (1989) The tension–stress effect on the genesis and growth of tissues: part 1. The influences of stability of fixation and soft-tissue preservation. Clin Orthop Relat Res 238:249–281
9. Saleh M, Rees A (1995) Bifocal surgery for deformity and bone loss after lower-limb fractures. Comparison of bone–transport and compression–distraction methods. J Bone Joint Surg Br 77:429–434
10. Gordon L, Chiu EJ (1988) Treatment of infected non-unions and segmental defects of the tibia with staged microvascular muscle transplantation of bone-grafting. J Bone Joint Surg Am 70:377–386
11. Aquerreta JD, Forriol F, Canadell J (1994) Complications of bone lengthening. Int Orthop 18:299–303
12. De Backer AI, Mortele KJ, De Keulenaer BL (2004) Picture archiving and communication system: part one: filmless radiology and distance radiology. JBR-BTR 87:234–241
13. De Bastiani G, Aldegheri R, Renzi-Brivio L, Trivella G (1987) Limb lengthening by callus distraction (callotasis). J Pediatr Orthop 7:129–134
14. Paley D (1988) Current techniques of limb lengthening. J Pediatr Orthop 8:73–92
15. Lai KA, Lin CJ, Chen JH (2002) Application of locked intramedullary nails in the treatment of complications after distraction osteogenesis. J Bone Joint Surg Br 84:1145–1149
16. Nowotarski PJ, Turen CH, Brumback RJ, Scaboro JM (2000) Conversion of external fixation to intramedullary nailing for fractures of the shaft of the femur in multiply injured patients. J Bone Joint Surg Am 82:781–788
17. Song HR, Kale A, Park HB, Koo KH, Chae DJ, Oh CW, Chung DW (2003) Comparison of internal bone transport and vascularized fibular grafting for femoral bone defects. J Orthop Trauma 17:203–211
18. Ilizarov GA (1990) Clinical application of the tension–stress effect for limb lengthening. Clin Orthop Relat Res 250:8–26
19. Spinelli R (1989) Segmental bone loss. In: Coombs RG, Sarmiento A (eds) External fixation and functional bracing. Orthotest, London, pp 311–313
20. Tselentakis G, Owen PJ, Naqui SZ et al (2006) Stiffness measurements to assess healing in bone transport: a preliminary report. J Orthop Traumatol 7:84–87
21. Cattaneo R, Villa A, Catagni M, Tentori L (1985) Traitement des pseudarthroses septiques ou non septiques selon la méthode d'Ilizarov en compression monofocale. Rev Chir Orthop 71:223–239
22. Iacobellis C, Berizzi A, Aldegheri R (2010) Bone transport using Ilizarov method: a review of complications in 100 consecutive cases. Strat Traum Limb Recon 5:17–22
23. Maini L et al (2000) The Ilizarov method in infected nonunion of fractures. Injury 31:509–517
24. Rozbruch RS et al (2006) Simultaneous treatment of tibial bone and soft-tissue defects with the Ilizarov method. J Orthop Trauma 20:197–205
25. Rose RE (2002) The Ilizarov technique in the treatment of tibial bone defects. Case reports and review of the literature. West Indian Med J 51:263–267
26. Lerner A, Ullmann Y, Stein H, Peled IJ (2000) Using the Ilizarov

external fixation device for skin expansion. Ann Plast Surg 45:535–537

27. Aldegheri R (1997) Femoral callotasis. J Pediatr Orthop B 6:42–47

28. Caja V, Kim W, Larsson S, Chao EYS (1995) Comparison of the mechanical performance of three types of external fixators: linear, circular and hybrid. Clin Biomech (Bristol, Avon) 10(8):401–406

29. Charalambous CP, Akimau P, Wilkes RA (2009) Hybrid mono-lateral-ring fixator for bone transport in post-traumatic femoral segmental defect: a technical note. Arch Orthop Trauma Surg 129:225–226

30. Cierny G III, Zorn KE (1994) Segmental tibial defects. Comparing conventional and Ilizarov methodologies. Clin Orthop Relat Res 301:118–123

31. Green SA (1994) Skeletal defects. A comparison of bone grafting and bone transport for segmental skeletal defects. Clin Orthop Relat Res 301:111–117

32. Aronson J, Johnson E, Harp JH (1989) Local bone transportation for treatment of intercalary defects by the Ilizarov technique. Biomechanical and clinical considerations. Clin Orthop Relat Res 243:71–79

33. Paley D (1990) Problems, obstacles and complications of limb lengthening by the Ilizarov technique. Clin Orthop 250:81–104

34. Fischgrund J, Paley D, Suber C (1994) Variations affecting time to bone healing during bone lengthening. CORR 301:31–37

35. Linh HB, Feibel RJ (2009) Tibial lengthening over an intra-medullary nail. Tech Orthop 24:279–288

36. Song HR, Cho SH, Koo KH, Jeong ST, Park YJ, Ko JH (1998) Tibial bone defects treated by internal bone transport using the Ilizarov method. Int Orthop 22(5):293–297

37. Wan J, Ling L, Xiang-sheng Z, Zhi-hong L (2013) Femoral bone transport by a monolateral external fixator with or without the use of intramedullary nail: a single-department retrospective study. Eur J Orthop Surg Traumatol 23:457–464

38. Lavini F, Dall'Oca C, Bartolozzi P (2010) Bone transport and compression–distraction in the treatment of bone loss of the lower limbs. Injury, Int J Care Injures 41:1191–1195

39. Wani N, Baba A, Kangoo K, Mir M (2011) Role of early Ilizarov ring fixator in the definitive management of type II, IIIA and IIIB open tibial shaft fractures. Int Orthop 35:915–923

40. Lovisetti G, Sala F, Thabet AM, Catagni MA, Singh S (2011) Osteocutaneous thermal necrosis of the leg salvaged by TSF/Il-izarov reconstruction. Report of 7 patients. Int Orthop 35:121–126

41. Simpson AH, Kenwright J (2000) Fracture after distraction osteogenesis. J Bone Joint Surg Br 82:659–665

42. O'Carrigan T, Paley D, Herzenberg JE (2007) Obstacles in limb lengthening: fractures. In: Rozbruch SR, Ilizarov S (eds) Limb lengthening and reconstruction surgery. Informa Healthcare, New York, pp 675–679

43. Danziger MB, Kumar A, DeWeese J (1995) Fractures after femoral lengthening using the Ilizarov method. J Pediatr Orthop 15:220–223

44. Emara KM, Al Ghafar KA, Al Kersh MA (2011) Methods to shorten the duration of an external fixator in the management of tibial infections. World J Orthop 2(9):85–92

45. Brewster MBS, Mauffrey C, Lewis AC, Hull P (2010) Lower limb lengthening: is there a difference in the lengthening index and infection rates of lengthening with external fixators, external fixators with intramedullary nails or intramedullary nailing alone? A systematic review of the literature. Eur J Orthop Surg Traumatol 20:103–108

46. Sun XT, Easwar TR, Manesh S, Ryu JH, Song SH, Kim SJ, Song HR (2011) Complications and outcomes of tibial lengthening using the Ilizarov method with or without a supplementary nail. JBJS Br 93-B:782–787

47. Mora R, Maccabruni A, Bertani B, Tuvo G, Lucanto S, Pedrotti L (2014) Revision of 120 tibial infected non-unions with bone and soft tissue loss treated with epidermato-fascial osteoplasty according to Umiarov. Injury 45:383–387

48. Cierny G III, Mader JT, Penninck JJ (2003) A clinical staging system for adult osteomyelitis. Clin Orthop Relat Res 414:7–24

49. Blachut PA, Meek RN, O'brien PJ (1990) External fixation and delayed intramedullary nailing of open fractures of the tibial shaft. J Bone Joint Surg Am 75:729–735

50. Cosco F, Risi M, Pompili M, Boriani S (2001) External fixation and sequential nailing in the treatment of open diaphyseal fractures of the tibia. Chir Organi Mov 86:191–197

51. Bost FC, Larsen LJ (1956) Experiences with lengthening of the femur over an intramedullary rod. J Bone Joint Surg Am 38:567–584

52. Paley D, Herzenberg JE, Paremain G, Bhave A (1997) Femoral lengthening over an intramedullary nail. A matched-case comparison with Ilizarov femoral lengthening. J Bone Joint Surg Am 79:1464–1480

53. Rozbruch SR, Kleinman D, Fragomen AT, Ilizarov S (2008) Limb lengthening and then insertion of an intramedullary nail. A case-matched comparison. Clin Orthop Relat Res 466:2923–2932

54. Bilen FE, Kocaoglu M, Eralp L, Balci HI (2010) Fixator-assisted nailing and consecutive lengthening over an intramedullary nail for the correction of tibial deformity. J Bone Joint Surg Br 92:146–1152

55. Park HW, Yang KH, Lee KS, Joo SY, Kwak YH, Kim HW (2008) Tibial lengthening over an intramedullary nail with use of the Ilizarov external fixator for idiopathic short stature. J Bone Joint Surg Am 90:1970–1978

56. Papineau LJ (1973) L'excision-greffe avec fermeture retardé délibérée dans l'osteéomyélite chronique. Nouv Presse Med 41:2573–2755

57. Raschke MJ, Mann JW, Oedekoven G, Claudi BF (1991) Segmental transport after unreamed intramedullary nailing. Clin Orthop Relat Res 282:233–240

58. Eralp L, Kocaoğlu M, Polat G, Bas A, Dirican A, Azam ME (2012) A comparison of external fixation alone or combined with intramedullary nailing in the treatment of segmental tibial defects. Acta Orthop Belg 78:652–659

59. Li Z, Zhang X, Duan L, Chen X (2009) Distraction osteogenesis technique using an intramedullary nail and a monolateral external fixator in the reconstruction of massive postosteomyelitis skeletal defects of the femur. Can J Surg 52:103–111

60. Liodakis E, Kenawey M et al (2011) Comparison of 39 post-traumatic tibia bone transports performed with and without the use of an intramedullary rod: the long-term outcomes. Intern Ortho SICOT 35:1397–1402

61. Klemm K, Henry SL, Seligson D (1988) The treatment of infection after interlocking nailing. Technol Orthop 3:54–61

62. Kouzelis AT, Kourea H, Megas P, Panagiotopoulos E, Marangos M, Lambiris E (2004) Does graded reaming affect the composition of reaming products in intramedullary nailing of long bones? Orthopedics 27(8):852–856

63. Lidgren L, Törholm C (1980) Intramedullary reaming in chronic diaphyseal osteomyelitis: a preliminary report. Clin Orthop Relat Res 151:215–221

64. Chapman MW (1998) The effect of reamed and nonreamed intramedullary nailing on fracture healing. Clin Orthop Relat Res 355(Suppl):S230–S238

65. Hoegel F, Mueller CA, Peter R, Pfister U, Suedkamp NP (2004) Bone debris: dead matter or vital osteoblasts. J Trauma 56:363–367

66. Frölke JP, Nulend JK, Semeins CM, Bakker FC, Patka P, Haarman HJ (2004) Viable osteoblastic potential of cortical reamings from intramedullary nailing. J Orthop Res 22:1271–1275

67. Wenisch S, Trinkaus K, Hild A, Hose D, Herde K, Heiss C, Kilian O, Alt V, Schnettler R (2005) Human reaming debris: a source of multipotent stem cells. Bone 36:74–83

5

Open reduction and pinning for the treatment of Gartland extension type III supracondylar humeral fractures in children

Ahmet Aslan · Mehmet Nuri Konya ·
Aykut Özdemir · Hüseyin Yorgancigil ·
Gökhan Maralcan · Emin Uysal

Abstract In this study, we aim to evaluate the clinical and radiological results of children who were treated with four different surgical approaches. In our clinics between February 2004 and November 2012, the children who underwent surgical treatment for supracondylar humeral fractures and whose data were available with regular follow-up of at least 1 year were included in the study. Clinical outcomes were evaluated for 54 patients with Gartland type 3 extension supracondylar fractures. Functional and cosmetic results of the patients were determined according to the Flynn criteria. Mean age of the patients was 4.9 (between 2 and 14) among which 26 of them were girls and 28 were boys. Mean operation time was 45 (35–85) min. Average length of hospital stay (LHS) was 2.9 (1–7) days. Average duration of splints was 3.5 (2–6) weeks, while the average removal period of the wires was 4.6 (3–8) weeks. Mean consolidation time was 4.6 weeks (3–8). Mean follow-up was 14.36 months.

In our study, we performed 54 patients functional and cosmetic results. While 48 of the patients had satisfying results (excellent, good, or fair), six of them had unsatisfactory (poor) results. The results of this study suggest that clinical results with surgical treatment of Gartland type 3 extension fractures were satisfactory. However, the delay in the surgical treatment may cause a number of complications.

Keywords Children · Humerus · Supracondylar fractures · Surgical approaches · Treatment results

Introduction

Supracondylar humerus fractures are the second common type of pediatric fractures. Supracondylar fractures are 50–60 % of all pediatric elbow fractures. In total, 85 % of these fractures are seen in children between ages of 4–11. Generally, conservative treatment options are preferred in pediatric fractures [1]. Surgical procedures are the treatment of choice in displaced supracondylar humerus fractures [2]. Humerus fractures are a significant part of pediatric fractures due to high incidence, high morbidity, and serious complications [3, 4].

Four different surgical approaches have been described in displaced supracondylar humerus fractures requiring surgical treatment [5, 6]. In the literature, every approach has its own positive aspects and there are some publications reporting good results [6–8]. Although there are comparative studies for some of these surgical approaches, we did not find any study comparing four different approaches. In this study, we aim to evaluate the clinical and radiological results of children who were treated with four different surgical approaches.

A. Aslan (✉) · M. N. Konya · A. Özdemir
Department of Orthopedics and Traumatology, Afyonkarahisar
State Hospital, Orhangazi Mh. Nedim Helvacıoğlu Cd.
Uydukent, 03100 Afyonkarahisar, Turkey
e-mail: draaslan@hotmail.com

H. Yorgancigil
Department of Orthopedics and Traumatology, Faculty of
Medicine, Süleyman Demirel University, Isparta, Turkey

G. Maralcan
Department of Orthopedics and Traumatology, Faculty of
Medicine, Afyon Kocatepe University, Afyonkarahisar, Turkey

E. Uysal
Department of Emergency, Bağcılar Education and Research
Hospital, Istanbul, Turkey

Patients and methods

In our clinics between February 2004 and November 2012, the children who underwent surgical treatment for supra-condylar humeral fracture with available data and regular follow-up of at least 1 year were included in the study. Fractures treated with closed reduction and percutaneous fixation excluded. Initial medical story and neurovascular physical examination were recorded in the emergency room for all patients. Anterior–posterior and lateral radiographs of the elbow were obtained. All the results were recorded. In some patients due to excessive displacement and poor position, we tried to ensure a closed reduction with gentle manipulation until the surgery. All of the patients were hospitalized, and long arm splints were applied. Radiographic control again was followed by the implementation of a long arm splint elbow in 90° flexion. Then, the patients were operated as soon as possible. Open reduction–internal fixation (ORIF) indications were, fractures with high risk of neurovascular injury and engagement of the distal aspect of the proximal fragment in brachial muscles and unsatisfactory closed reductions. In this study, our groups comprise only the patients who need open reduction after failed closed reduction attempts and we only analyzed open reduction and internal fixation patients who underwent closed reduction were excluded from the study. The patients underwent surgical intervention under general anesthesia, often using pneumatic tourniquet, with four different surgical approaches. Our incision choice can be changed about fracture pattern. Nerve injury, vascular injury, fracture pattern displacement, and open fractures are the major patterns of incision choice. The fractures were fixed with at least two lateral or cross Kirschner wires (K-wires) under fluoroscopy control due to fracture pattern and stability and surgeon's preference.

Surgical technique [5, 9–11]

Anterior approach

Transverse or longitudinal incision was made over the antecubital fossa. Subcutaneous tissues were dissected bluntly. With transverse incision distal, fragment's displacement direction can be seen easily. Brachial artery was explored. If any suspicion of neurovascular injury, this is the best approach. In displaced fractures, usually the brachialis muscle is torn and the fracture can be explored easily. Soft tissue interposition was removed. The distal fragment was pulled along the proximal fragment, and the reduction was achieved by applying pressure.

Lateral approach

Incision was made beginning from 5 to 6 cm proximal to 2–3 cm distal to the elbow joint. Dissection was made through biceps and brachialis muscles. If there is any interposition of soft tissues, a manipulation may be required to achieve reduction.

Medial approach

Incision begins 5 cm above the elbow joint, medial to intermuscular septum, and just below the medial epicondyle. Nervus ulnaris was dissected and protected. Fracture line can be found by beneath the triceps and brachialis muscles. Continuity of fracture line was palpated, and reduction was achieved.

Posterior approach

Skin incision was made midline to olecranon starting about 5 cm proximal to the olecranon, giving a slight curve to the distal for 1–2 cm. Ulnar nerve was located to prevent an injury.

Fixation was made by at least two cross or lateral K-wires in all approach. All patients were treated according to the same postoperative protocol. A long-arm cast was applied in the elbow 90° flexion and neutral forearm rotation. Antibiotic prophylaxis with Cefazolin sodium was given 50 mg/kg, four times a day for 24 h. The sutures were removed after 10 days. Postoperative radiological controls were performed on the first, seventh, and thirtieth days. Although it is preferred to remove the K-wires until the end of 4th week, we generally removed the wires between 4th and 5th weeks. Our patients were generally coming from rural and distant areas to authors' hospitals. Usually, patient and family compliance and cooperation were moderate or poor. To prevent some postoperative complications such as losing reduction or refracture, authors have followed some more conservative approach. Active exercises were started according to the fracture healing in radiographs. Modified criteria developed by Flynn [3] were used for evaluation (Table 1).

Statistical analysis

Statistical analysis was performed using SPSS statistical package program (SPSS 19.0 version, SPSS Inc., Chicago, Illinois, USA). Kolmogorov–Smirnov test was used for normal distribution of the data. Pearson's chi-square tests were used in significance analysis. Also we have done power analysis for Pearson's Chi-square test.

Table 1 Modified Flynn Criteria

Outcome	Rating	Cosmetic factor (carrying angle loss in degrees)	Functional factor (movements loss in degree)
Satisfactory	Excellent	0–5	0–5
	Good	6–10	6–10
	Fair	11–15	11–15
Unsatisfactory	Poor	>15	>15

Results

In total, 28 patients (52 %) were male and 26 (48 %) were female. The mean age was 4.9 years. The patients were distributed between the ages of two and 14. The peak range was between 4 and 8 years of age (58.7 %). The fractures were at the right elbow in 54 % of the cases and left elbow in 46 % of the cases. The most common admissions were in the spring season with 22 cases (40.0 %), mostly in May with 19 patients (30 %). Falls (in-house, out of house, and falls from height) were the most common injuries (96 %). All children first get a trial of closed reduction and pinning if the reduction is adequate. Only nine children were immediately taken for open reduction based on presentation nerve injury, vascular injury, fracture pattern displacement, excessive swelling, and previous bonesetter's bad intervened.

The majority of patients (75 %) were operated in the first 24 h. In 25 % of the cases, the time between injury and surgical intervention was more than 24 h, for various reasons. Five of all patients had accompanying injuries. Two had ipsilateral fractures of the distal radius, and the others had a first metacarpal basis fracture, a contralateral forearm both bone fractures, and a tibial spiral-oblique fracture. Four different incisions were preferred. Circulatory status of the skin, condition of the fracture fragments, and surgeons' preference has been effective in choice of the incision. Mean operation time was 45 (35–85) min. Average LHS was 2.9 (1–7) days. Average duration of splints was 3.5 (2–6) weeks, while the average removal period of the wires was 4.6 (3–8) weeks. Mean consolidation time was 4.6 weeks (3–8). Mean follow-up was 14.36 months. We have made radiological assessment including an AP and lateral X-ray of elbow for all of our patients at postoperative consolidation time and at the final follow-up. The Baumann angle was measured on AP radiographic view. Diaphysis-condylar angle was measured on lateral view. Mean HEW value was −0.43° at the average consolidation time and −1.23° at the last follow-up. The mean Baumann angle value was 71.9° (64°–82°) at the average consolidation time and 74.6° (64°–88°) at the last follow-up. The mean diaphysis-condylar angle was 42.3° at the average consolidation time 44.40 at the last follow-up. In clinical

findings for the average loss of mobility, loss of flexion was 1.6° and loss of extension was 0.8°.

Many scoring systems have been used for elbow disorders [12]. Our functional and cosmetic results performed by Flynn's Criteria. Flynn criteria are obtained measuring with goniometers the range of elbow movement and the carrying angle. Carrying angle difference among both elbows angle and loss in elbow motion is scored as follows: between 0 and 5°, excellent; 6–10°, good; 11–15°, fair; <15°, and poor. In our study, we performed 54 patients functional and cosmetic results. While 48 of the patients had satisfying results (excellent, good, or fair), six of them had unsatisfactory (poor) results.

In this study, we have detected power analysis follows: A sample size of 54 achieves 6 % power to detect an effect size (W) of 0.0677 using a 3° of freedom chi-square test with a significance level (alpha) of 0.05000.

Complications

Preoperative and postoperative complications were observed in seven patients. Complications were more frequent in patients with longer delay than 24 h between injury and surgical intervention. This was statistically significant ($p = 0.06$). Three (5.6 %), peripheral nerve lesions were seen in the first physical examinations at admission. Four superficial pin infections (7.4 %) were found at follow-up. These were treated with oral antibiotics and appropriate dressing. At the last controls, five (9.3 %) cubitus varus deformities were noted. The patient intervened by the bonesetter was one of these patients. Some examples of our patients have shown that they have been treated with different approaches and their various results are provided in Figs 1, 2, 3, and 4. The figures including anteroposterior (a–c) and lateral (e–f) view in preop., postop., and follow-up.

Discussion

Goals in the treatment of pediatric supracondylar humerus fractures are full recovery of elbow movements, achieving normal cosmetic view of elbow, protecting the patient from neurovascular complications that may occur. Supracondylar fractures of the humerus in children are more common under the age of 10. In particular, incidence peaks between the ages of 5–7 have been reported [4–6]. In our series, the age distribution is from 2 to 14. It has a peak incidence between 4 and 8 years of age (58.7 %), and the average age is 4.9. The mean age and the age range of peak incidence are consistent with the current literature. Supracondylar humerus fractures of childhood are more common in boys [4, 5, 13]. Archibeck et al. [14] have reported a rate of

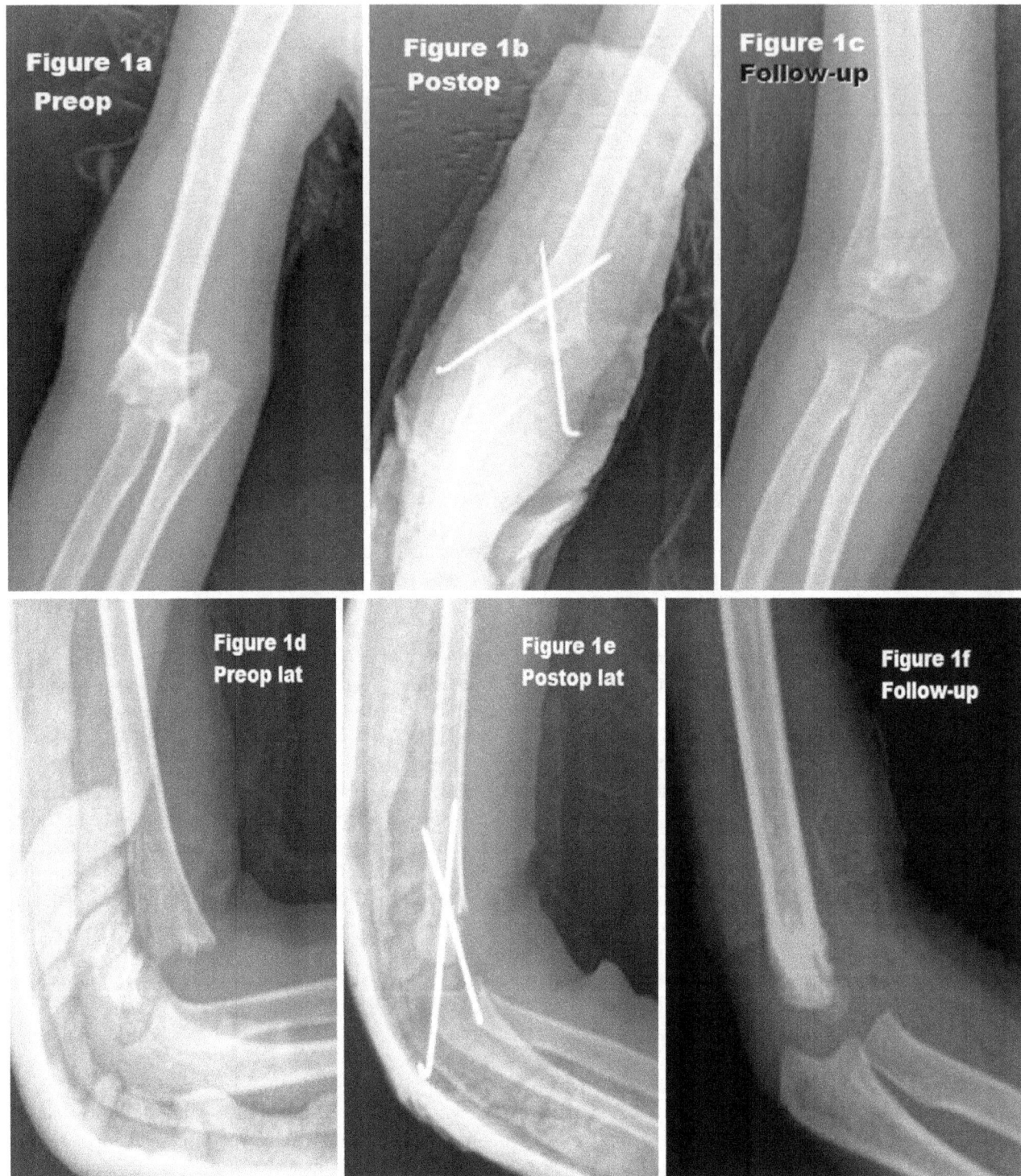

Fig. 1 Anteroposterior (**a–c**) and lateral (**d-f**) view in preop., postop., and follow-up. Four-year-old boy, anterior approach, poor result

57 % girls and 43 % boys in his series, Gosens and Bongers [15] have given the rate of 51 % female to 49 % male. In this study, 52 % were boys and 48 % were girls. Our data are consistent with the recent literature. These fractures are more frequent in boys. Boys are more active, and the games they play have a higher probability of injury.

Left elbow fractures were more common in previous studies [4, 13, 17]. Left arm handles a protective duty during a fall. In our study, right arm (54 %) was more commonly injured. There are studies with follow-up times up to 4.6 and 8.9 years [16–18]. Our study has a follow-up mean time of 14.36 months, and it may be considered

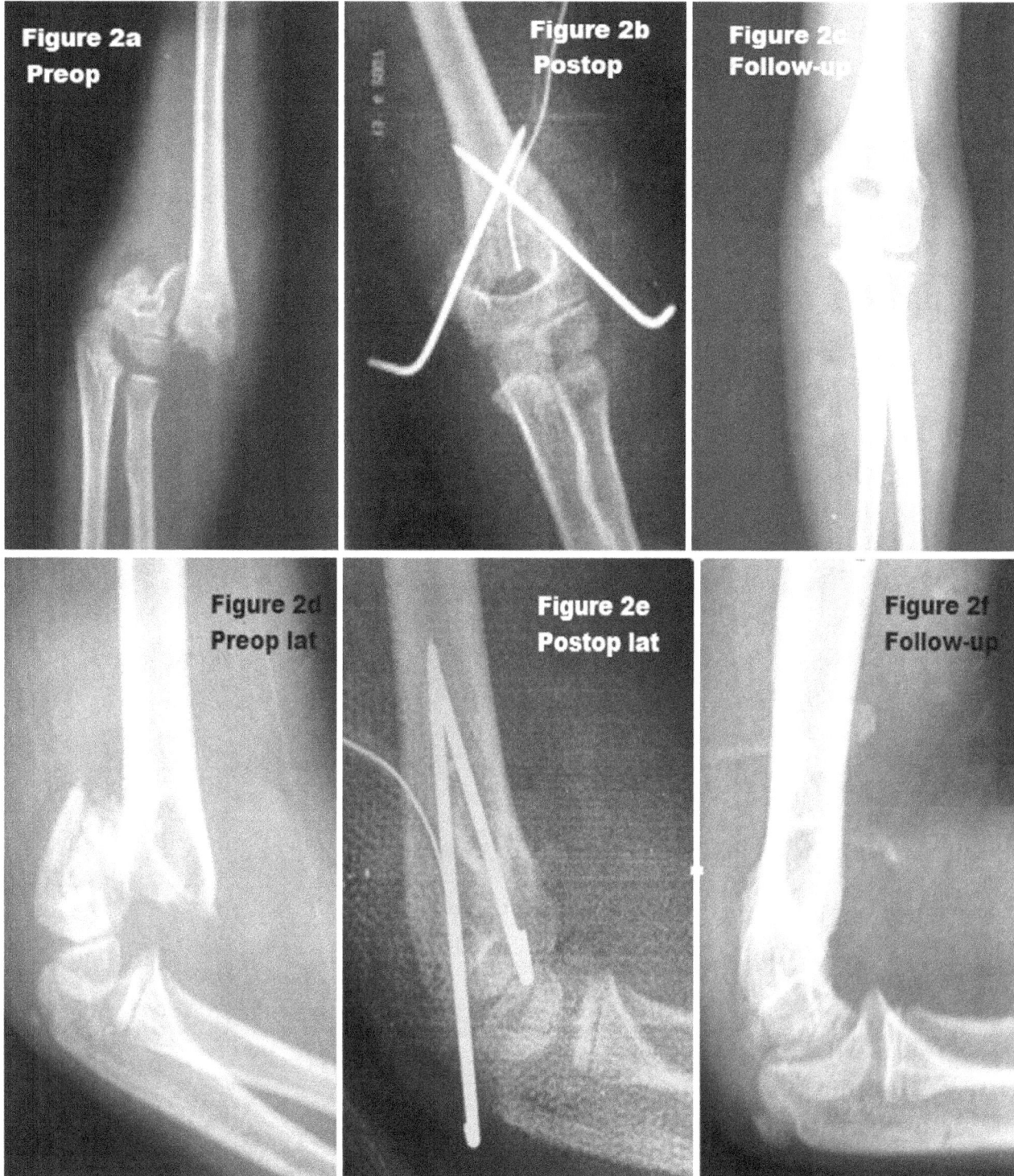

Fig. 2 Anteroposterior (**a–c**) and lateral (**d–f**) view in preop., postop., and follow-up. Twelve-year-old boy, lateral approach, fairy result

adequate for screening possible complications. These fractures may be associated with other fractures. Mazda et al. [13] reported seven (6 %) ipsilateral forearm fractures in their study of 116 patients. Gordon et al. [19] reported four ipsilateral forearms, one radial neck, one distal radius, one proximal end of the humerus fracture in their series of 138 cases. Pirone et al. [16] reported 20 (8.6 %) ipsilateral forearm fractures in their series. Our study included five patients with associated fractures. Two had ipsilateral fractures of the distal radius, and the others had first metacarpal basis fracture, contralateral forearm both bone fractures, and tibia spiral-oblique fracture. Additional

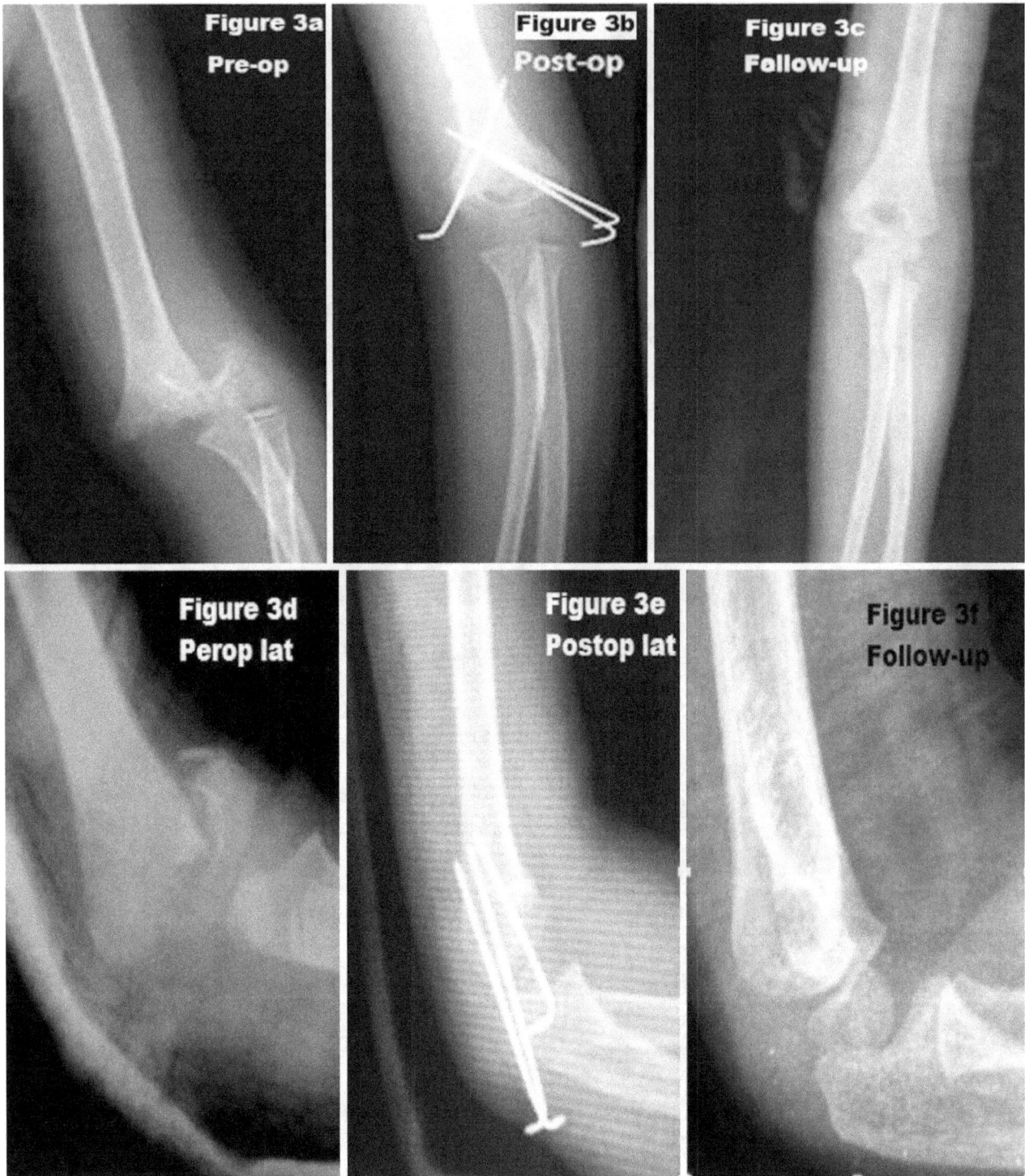

Fig. 3 Anteroposterior (**a–c**) and lateral (**d–f**) view in preop., postop., and follow-up. Five-year-old girl, medial approach, excellent result

trauma patients were treated in the same session. Mesherle et al. [17] reported the LHS as 1.6 days in their series of 36 patients. Mulhall et al. [18] reported LSH 2.5 days in their ORIF series. Karapinar et al. [20] reported a 3.01-day LSH for 236 cases. We had a mean LSH of 2.9 days. Extension-type fractures are more common in the literature [21, 22]. Pirone et al. [16] reported a rate of 38 % type 2 and 62 % type 3 fractures. Archibeck et al. [14] reported a rate of 22 % type 1, 16 % type 2, and 61 % type 3 fractures. Our results were similar with current studies, and all of our

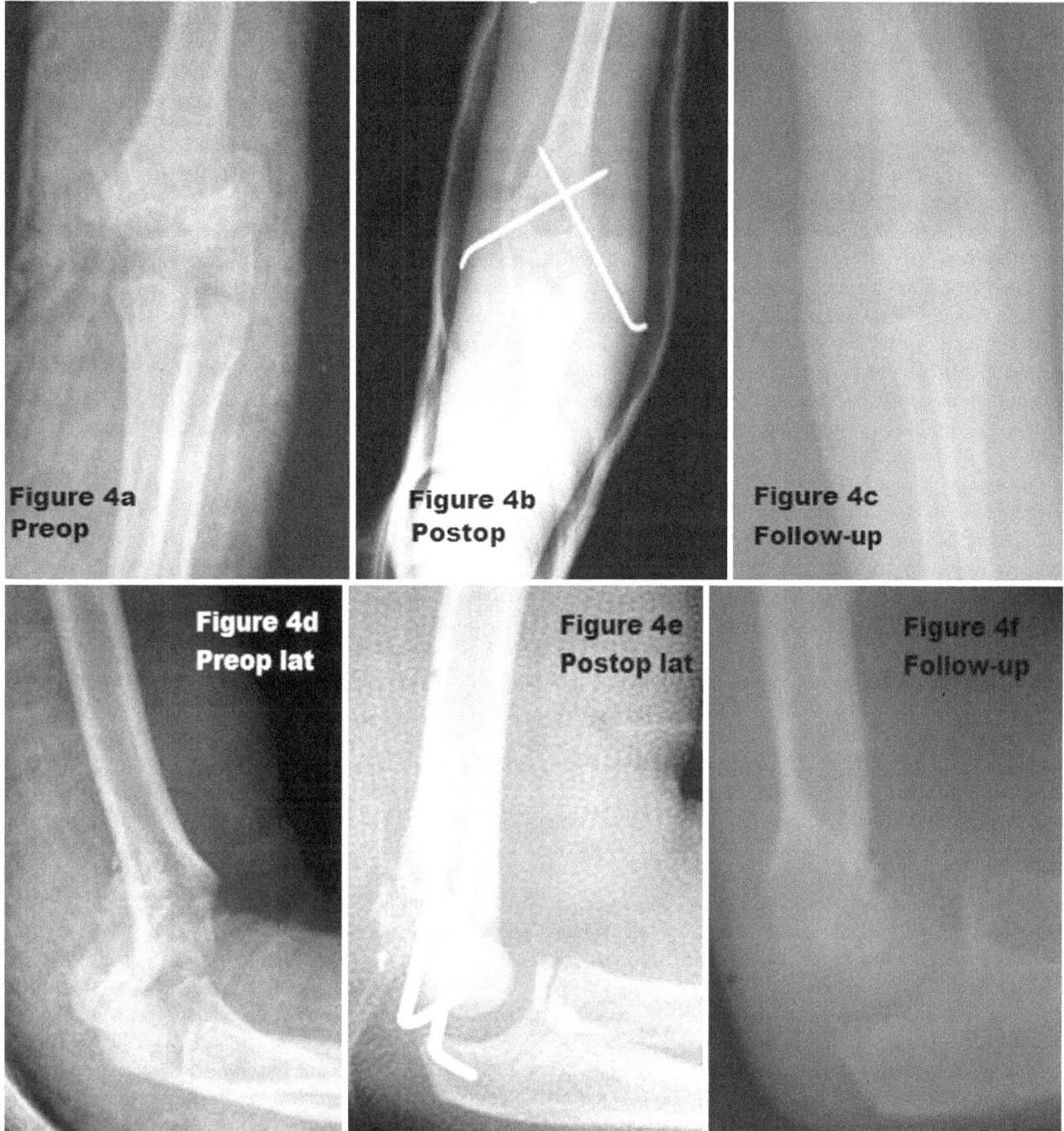

Fig. 4 Anteroposterior (**a–c**) and lateral (**d–f**) view in preop., postop., and follow-up. Nine-year-old boy, posterior approach, good result

patients had extension Gartland type 3 fractures. Supra-condylar humerus fractures in children are frequently associated with various complications such as neurovascular deficit and compartment syndrome. In total, 7–16.1 % neurological injuries are reported in the literature [3, 23, 24]. Anterior interosseous nerve injuries are the most common type of nerve injuries in extension fractures, and iatrogenic ulnar nerve injury is the most common type of nerve injury in flexion-type injuries [25]. These are commonly neuropraxia-type injuries in children and generally have a good prognosis. In particular,, type 3 fractures with late admission or excessive edema on the fracture increase the possibility of iatrogenic injury during manipulation and fixation. Nerve recovery is expected in 2–6-week period up to 3 months. Iatrogenic injuries are reported to improve in the first 6 months [5, 25, 26]. One median nerve and two radial nerve involvement were noted in our study. All these patients with neurological deficits were operated after 24 h. A bonesetter had intervened in one of these cases before hospital admission. Bonesetters intervene patients frequently in our society, and major sequels may occur in patients [27]. The patient intervened by a bonesetter was followed for one week due to edema and nerve injury. Only one case was intervened by a bonesetter in our study group. In the follow-up of this patient, 10° flexion loss deformity was observed. Also, no Volkman ischemic contractures or compartment syndromes were observed.

Closed reduction and percutaneous pinning have been accepted as the gold standard in reaching these goals by many authors [28]. If close reduction cannot be achieved, open reduction should be preferred in serious displaced fractures, flexion-type fractures, nerve injury after closed reduction, open fractures requiring irrigation and debridement, in posterolateral displaced fractures with a high risk of neurovascular injury [17, 29, 30]. On the other hand, Kazimoglu et al. [31] compared primarily open reduction and internal fixation versus closed reduction and percutaneous cross-pinning of Gartland type 3 extension supracondylar fractures in children. The study performed at two different centers was 80 cases included. They reported that according to Flynn's criteria, the outcomes of the open and closed reduction groups were not statistically significant. In conclusion, they say that closed reduction showed no superiority over open reduction. Kurer and Regan [32] evaluated open reduction of 259 cases reported by eight authors and revealed 63 % excellent, 21 % good, and 16 % poor results. In our study, the patients were treated only with surgery. While 48 of the patients had functionally satisfying results, six of them had bad results. And similarly, while 49 patients were satisfactory cosmetically, there were five poor results. In the literature, each method suggests better results than the others. We believe that the medial approach prevents iatrogenic ulnar nerve injuries, it gives a good vision ensuring the restoration of the medial column, and it is a method of the least incisional scar. The lateral approach is more secure because it is away from the neurovascular structures. The anterior approach is better in the assessment of the joint and neurovascular structures. The posterior approach is better than other approaches in manipulation of fracture fragments.

In management of these fractures, different pin configurations were also used, adding more heterogeneity to various studies in the literature [5–8]. Yousri et al. [4] as reported in the current systematic review article: There was no significant difference between crossed and lateral pinning in terms of loss reduction. Both configurations have similar stability. Also, the authors say that there is currently no level 1 evidence comparing the outcome of crossed pinning versus lateral entry pinning in extension-type Gartland III supracondylar fracture. Mostly, we used

crossed k-wires for fixation. But sometimes when it became risky for the ulnar nerve injury because of severe swelling and difficulty in pinning upon surgeon preference, two lateral pins were used.

Gennari et al. [33] reported that although the anterior approach is more technically demanding, it gives better functional results. A previous study showed that with lateral incision, postoperative range of motion was better than posterior incision. Ersan et al. [28] reported that a total of 46 patients were operated through anterior and 38 through lateral approach. According to Flynn's criteria [3], results were excellent in 19, good in 18, and fair in one in the lateral incision group, whereas in the anterior incision group, excellent results were obtained in 31 patients and good results in 15 of them. The authors say that anterior incision when open reduction is needed in pediatric supracondylar fractures offer the advantage of a smaller scar and easy access to structures that might be injured between the fractured fragments. In the study of Eren et al. [10], a total of 40 patients with type 3 supracondylar humeral fractures were divided equally into two groups as lateral or medial approach. They reported that in the lateral approach group, functional results were excellent in 18 patients (90 %), good in one patient (5 %), and fair in one patient, while cosmetic results were excellent in 19 patients (95 %) and good in one patient. In the medial approach group, 19 patients (95 %) had excellent and one patient (5 %) had good functional results, while all the patients had an excellent cosmetic result. Authors did not find significant differences between the groups. In a study comparing different approaches, Pretell Mazzini et al. [11] reported that a combined anteromedial approach could be the method which allows the achievement of better functional and cosmetic outcome according to Flynn's criteria. Whereas, in our study, while 48 of the patients have satisfying results, six of them have bad results at final follow-up functional assessment. There was no statistically significant difference between the four groups according to in terms of surgical approaches. And also cosmetic evaluation, while satisfactory of the 49 patients, the poor results were five and there was no statistically significant difference between the groups. In generally, K-wires can be removed 3–4 weeks after surgery in children under 10 years and in older children, it should be removed for 4–5 weeks [34]. Mean removal time of wires was 4.8 (3–8) weeks in our study. Although it is preferred to remove the K-wires until the end of 4th week, we generally removed the wires between 4th and 5th weeks. Our patients were generally coming from rural and distant areas to authors' hospitals. Usually, patient and family compliance and cooperation were moderate or poor. To prevent some postoperative complications such as losing reduction or refracture, authors have followed some more conservative approach.

Baumann angle is an important angle in control of the reduction. Normal range is between 64 and 81° [23]. In our study group, the mean Baumann angle was 74.6°. Body-condylar angle measured after the surgery shows flexion or extension displacement of the distal fracture fragment. This angle changes during skeletal maturation. Body-condylar angle changes are related with extension degrees of the elbow [35]. Normal range is 40–45°. In our study, we found this angle 44.4°. The most common complication of pediatric supracondylar fractures is cubitus varus (4–58 %). D'Ambrosia [36] revealed that cubitus varus is very rare after an adequate reduction and is related with medial angulation of the distal fragment. Ippolito et al. [22] state that varus deformity is due to the defect of the distal humeral epiphysis growth plate. Surgical intervention decreases the rate of varus deformity. Gosens and Bongers [15] reported a cubitus varus rate of 2.5 %. There were five cubitus varus cases in our study group. Cubitus valgus is not common, but associated with loss of extension and late ulnar nerve paralysis. Previous studies show a rate of 2.3 % about this complication [37]. In our study group, there was no cubitus valgus deformity. Early and delayed surgical intervention is controversial in supracondylar fractures [38]. Although the results of delayed surgical intervention are satisfactory in previous studies [39], complication rates were higher in our study group.

Limitations

Our study was retrospective, and the groups were not equal. All operations were performed by the authors randomly. Posterior and lateral approach patients were more than the others in our series. This was due to the fact that these two approaches are more popular. We also started using the anterior approach relatively more recently. We did not assess the results with respect to the implementation of two cross or lateral K-wires. Also performance of the operations by different surgeons may have influenced the results. We think that open reduction makes the pin placement some more difficult because of a desire to work within or around incisions. As can be seen in our cases pictures, there are some images where the pins are placed relatively high in the metaphysis, crossed at the fracture site, or the fracture is not completely reduced despite open treatment. These may be associated with many causes such as learning curve, the surgeon's experience, and surgical conditions.

Conclusion

The results of this study suggest that clinical results of surgical treatment of Gartland type 3 extension fractures were satisfactory. Also no difference between the results of different surgical approaches was found clinically. However, the delay in surgical treatment may cause a number of complications. The choice of surgical approach should be based on the characteristics of fracture and the experience of the surgeon in surgical treatment of displaced supracondylar fractures in children.

References

1. Hasler CC (2001) Supracondylar fractures of the humerus in children. Eur J Trauma 1:338–353
2. Cheng JC, Lam WY (1995) Closed reduction and percutaneous pinning for type 3 displaced supracondylar fractures of the humerus in children. J Orthop Trauma 9:511–515
3. Flynn JC, Matthews JG, Benoit RL (1974) Blind pinning of displaced supracondylar fractures of humerus in children. J Bone Joint Surg 56A:263–272
4. Yousri T, Tarassoli P, Whitehouse M, Monsell F, Khan WS (2012) Systematic review of randomized controlled trials comparing efficacy of crossed versus lateral K-wire fixation in extension type Gartland type III supracondylar fractures of the humerus in children. Ortop Traumatol Rehabil 14(5):397–405
5. Kasser JR, Beaty JH (2006). Supracondylar fractures of the distal humerus. In: Rockwood and Wilkins' fractures in children. 6th (ed.). Philadelphia, PA: Lippincott Williams & Wilkins. pp. 543–90
6. Pretell-Mazzini J, Rodriguez-Martin J, Auñon-Martin I et al (2011) Controversial topics in the management of displaced supracondylar humerus fractures in children. Strategies Trauma Limb Reconstr 6:43–50
7. Koudstaal MJ, De Ridder VA, De Lange S et al (2002) Pediatric supracondylar humerus fractures: the anterior approach. J Orthop Trauma 16:409–412
8. Kumar R, Malhotra R (2000) Medial approach for operative treatment of the widely displaced supracondylar fractures of the humerus in children. J Orthop Surg (Hong Kong) 8:13–18
9. Ay S, Akinci M, Kamiloglu S et al (2005) Open reduction of displaced pediatric supracondylar humeral fractures through the anterior cubital approach. J Pediatr Orthop 25:149–153
10. Eren A, Özkut AT, Altıntaş F et al (2005) Comparison between the lateral and medial approaches in terms of functional and cosmetic results in the surgical treatment of type III supracondylar humeral fractures in children. Acta Orthop Traumatol Turc 39:199–204
11. Pretell Mazzini J, Rodriguez Martin J, Andres Esteban EM (2010) Surgical approaches for open reduction and pinning in severely displaced supracondylar humerus fractures in children: a systematic review. J Child Orthop 4(2):52–143
12. Longo UG, Franceschi F, Loppini M, Maffulli N, Denaro V (2008) Rating systems for evaluation of the elbow. Br Med Bull 87:131–161
13. Mazda K, Boggione C, Fitoussi F et al (2001) Systematic pinning of displaced extension-type supracondylar fractures of the humerus in children. A prospective study of 116 consecutive patients. J Bone Joint Surg 83B:888–893
14. Arcibeck MJ, Scott SM, Peters CL (1997) Brachialis muscle entrapment in displaced supracondylar humerus fractures: a technique of closed reduction and report of initial results. J Pediatr Orthop 17:298–302
15. Gosens T, Bongers KJ (2003) Neurovascular complications and functional outcome in displaced supracondylar fractures of the humerus in children. Injury 34:267–273
16. Pirone AM, Graham HK, Krajbich JI (1988) Management of

displaced extension type supracondylar fractures of the humerus in children. J Bone Joint Surg 70A:641–650

17. Mehserle WL, Meehan PL (1991) Treatment of the displaced supracondylar fracture of the humerus (Type 3) with closed reduction and percutaneous cross-pin fixation. J Pediatr Orthop 11:705–711

18. Mulhall KJ, Abuzakuk T, Curtin W et al (2000) Displaced supracondylar fractures of the humerus in children. Int Orthop 24:221–223

19. Gordon JE, Patton CM, Luhmann SJ et al (2001) Fracture stability after pinning of displaced supracondylar distal humerus fractures in children. J Pediatr Orthop 21:313–318

20. Karapınar L, Öztürk H, Altay T et al (2005) Closed reduction and percutaneous pinning with three Kirschner wires in children with type III displaced supracondylar fractures of the humerus. Acta Orthop Traumatol Turc 39:23–29

21. Cekanauskas E, Degliüte R, Kalesinskas RJ (2003) Treatment of supracondylar humerus fractures in children, according to Gartland classification. Medicina 39:379–383

22. Ippolito E, Catenm R, Scola E (1986) Supracondylar fractures of the humerus in children. J Bone Joint Surg 68A:333–344

23. Aronson DD, Prager BI (1987) Supracondylar fractures of the humerus in children. Clin Orthop Relat Res 219:174–184

24. Piggot J, Graham HK, McCoy GF (1986) Supracondylar fractures of the humerus in children. J Bone Joint Surg 68B:577–583

25. Erdil M, İmren Y, Ceylan HH et al (2012) [Multiple neural injuries in a pediatric supracondylar humerus fracture]. J Clin Exp Invest 3:438–442

26. Otsuka NY, Kasser JR (1997) Supracondylar fractures of humerus in children. J Am Acad Orthop Surg 5:19–26

27. Sargın S, Ahmet Aslan, Konya MN, Atik A, Meriç G (2013) Bonesetter choice of Turkish society in musculoskeletal injuries and the affecting factors. JCEI 4(4):477–482

28. Ersan O, Gonen E, İlhan RD et al (2012) Comparison of anterior and lateral approaches in the treatment of extension-type supracondylar humerus fractures in children. J Pediatr Orthop B 21:121–126

29. Millis MB, Smger IJ, Hail JE (1984) Supracondylar fractures of the humerus in children. Clin Orthop 188:90–97

30. Ramsey RH, Gnz J (1973) Immediate open reduction and internal fixation of severely displaced supracondylar fractures of the humerus in children. Clin Orthop Relat Res 90:130–132

31. Kazimoglu C, Cetin M, Sener M, Aguş H, Kalanderer O (2009) Operative management of type III extension supracondylar fractures in children. Int Orthop 33(4):1089–1094

32. Kurer MHJ, Regan MW (1990) Completely displaced supracondylar fracture of the humerus in children. Clin Orthop Relat Res 256:205–214

33. Gennari JM, Merrot T, Piclet B et al (1998) Anterior approach versus posterior approach to surgical treatment of children's supracondylar fractures: comparative study of thirty cases in each series. J Pediatr Orthop B 7:307–313

34. Kabukçuoğlu Y, Öztürk L, Bulut G et al (1993) [The treatment of supracondylar fractures in children by open reduction]. Acta Orhop Traumatol Turc 27:243–247

35. Jones KG (1967) Percutaneous pin fixation of fractures of the lower end of the humerus. Clin Orthop Relat Res 50:53–69

36. D'ambrosıa RD (1972) Supracondylar fractures of humerus–prevention of cubitus varus. J Bone Joint Surg 54A:60–66

37. Ağuş H, Kalenderer Ö, Kayalı C (1999) Closed reduction and percutaneous pinning results in children with supracondylar humerus fractures. Acta Orhop Traumatol Turc 33:18–22

38. Yıldırım AO, Unal VS, Oken OF et al (2009) Timing of surgical treatment for type III supracondylar humerus fractures in pediatric patients. J Child Orthop 3:265–269

39. Tiwari A, Kanojia RK, Kapoor SK (2007) Surgical management for late presentation of supracondylar humeral fracture in children. J Orthop Surg (Hong Kong) 15:177–182

6

Efficacy of a compliant semicircular Ilizarov pin fixator module for treating infected nonunion of the femoral diaphysis

Ashraf A. Khanfour · Mohamed M. El-Sayed

Abstract Percutaneous transosseous Ilizarov wiring, whilst preferred in the tibia because of its unique properties, carries a high risk of complications in the femur. The aim of this work was to evaluate the efficacy of a more patient-friendly semicircular pin external fixator module built up from parts of the Ilizarov fixator components and its use in managing diaphyseal femoral nonunions. A group of 20 patients with infected diaphyseal nonunions of the femur after internal osteosynthesis were included in this study. The mean age of the patients at the time of surgery was 46 years (range 16–60, SD 15.6). The mean morbidity time since the original trauma was 10.2 months (range 6–15, SD 2.5). All the cases were fixed by the described external fixator module. Bony union with resolution of infection occurred in 18 (94.7 %) out of 19 cases after a mean period in the fixator of 11.2 months (range 8–18 SD 2.9). After a mean follow-up period of 3.5 years (range 2–9, SD 2.6), there were 14 excellent, 3 good, 1 fair and 1 poor results from radiological evaluation and 10 excellent, 7 good, 1 fair and 1 poor results from functional assessment. In conclusion, the described semi-circular pin fixator module is patient-friendly and effective in managing infected nonunions of the femoral diaphysis.

Keywords Femur · Ilizarov · External fixation · Infective nonunion · Compliant

A. A. Khanfour (✉)
Department of Orthopaedic Surgery, Damanhur National Medical Institute, Damanhur, Egypt
e-mail: Dr_ashrafkhanfour@hotmail.com

M. M. El-Sayed
Department of Orthopaedic Surgery, Tanta University, Tanta, Egypt

Introduction

A locked intramedullary nail is considered the method of choice for treating diaphyseal femoral fractures but is contraindicated in the presence of a concurrent or previous infection [1–5]. The percutaneously applied transosseous Ilizarov external fixator can be adopted for treating these cases, but there are disadvantages in patient compliance and interference with local anatomy [6]. These factors relate to a high risk of injury to the neurovascular structures during percutaneous transosseous wiring and tissue transfixation. Additionally, the application of the complete rings encircling the medial aspect of the patient's thigh causes a major hindrance to a patient's daily activities including personal hygiene [5, 7–13]. For these reasons, a classic Ilizarov fixator using tension wires in the proximal femoral segment is not popular [12, 14] leading to, in 1986, Italian surgeons Catagni and Cattaneo introducing the hybrid modification of using half-pins but maintaining all wires in the distal femur [11, 12]. This assembly has undergone many modifications including the introduction of concepts of a "dummy ring" and a more stable "delta" distal Schanz pin configuration (Fig. 1). Despite this, patient acceptance remains a major drawback [10, 12, 15–17].

This work evaluates the efficacy of a more patient-acceptable semicircular external fixator module built up from parts of the Ilizarov fixator components for managing diaphyseal femoral fractures.

Patients and methods

A consecutive cohort of 20 patients with infected diaphyseal nonunions of the femur (after previously unsuccessful internal osteosynthesis) was treated using the semicircular

Fig. 1 A hybrid Ilizarov external fixator of the femur with a dummy ring *(an empty ring without fixation to the bone. It is secured in the middle of the frame and acts as a force transmitter. It will effectively shorten the lengths of the rods and increases the stability of the frame)* and the distal delta configuration

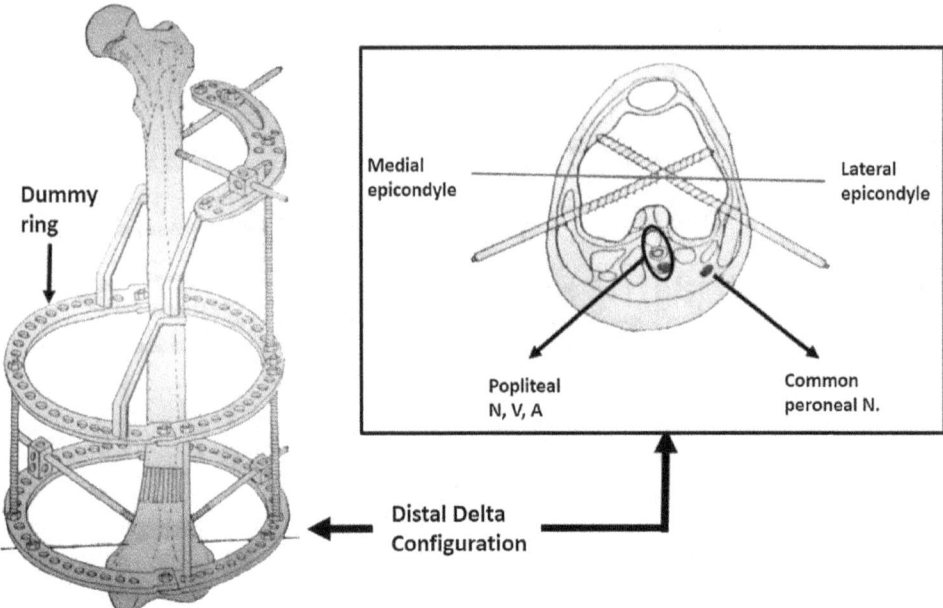

fixator. The patients presented between January 2003 and February 2010. The study was approved by the local ethical committee (General Organization of Teaching Hospitals and Institutes Research Ethical Committee) and was conducted in accordance with the Declaration of Helsinki and Ethical Guidelines for Epidemiological Research (2008). Informed written consent was obtained from all patients and their guardians before participation in the study.

The presence of a nonunion was established clinically: the ability to induce motion at the fracture site; deep tenderness; deformity; and inability to bear weight. Using radiographs, the diagnosis was supported by the presence of a radiolucent gap at the fracture site, sealing off of the medullary cavity, sclerosis of the fractured bone edges or absence of bridging callus after 6 months of the fracture event with evidence of loosening of the implant. The diagnosis was made also if the fracture showed no progressive radiological signs of healing on three successive months.

Infection was suspected clinically by the presence of local pain out of proportion to the nonunion, erythema, swelling and induration with or without chronic draining sinuses. Further evidence was obtained through investigations, which added to a high probability of sepsis: a raised CBC, ESR; the presence of sequestrum, involucrum, periosteal and endosteal new bone formation, cortical irregularities and visible resorption, especially around the osteosynthesis implant on X-rays.

The inclusion criteria were cases with an established infected nonunion of the femoral diaphysis after internal fixation. The exclusion criteria were very obese patients with a large thigh diameter rendering the half-pin offset to

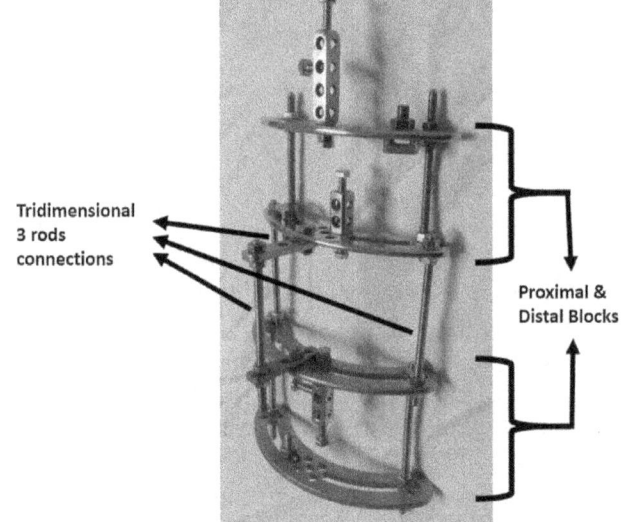

Fig. 2 The semicircular femoral Ilizarov pin fixator module used

be unacceptably long, an insensate limb and noncompliant patients.

The construct (Fig. 2)

The frame was composed of two blocks. Each block comprised two identical femoral arches connected as a pair and to which pin clamps or Rancho cubes were fixed as required. The two blocks were connected by three threaded rods in which the middle rod was lateralised by the aid of two straight plates connected orthogonally to the middle of these arches to add to the multiplanar stability of the frame (Fig. 2). The length of the entire fixator covered the whole

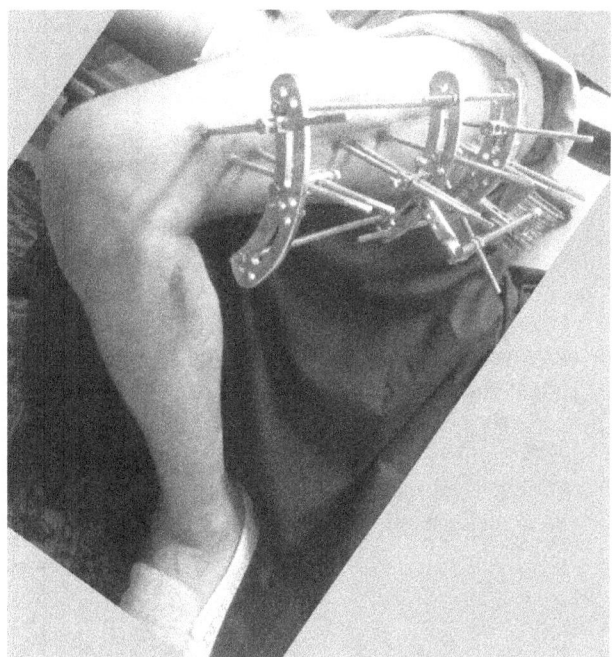

Fig. 3 This photograph shows the divergence and the spread of the pins across the femur. It also demonstrates the ability of the patient to bend his knee freely beyond 90°

length of the femur. Six millimetre diameter Schanz half-pins were used mainly with the smaller 5 mm pins for smaller diameter femurs.

Operative technique

The construct was assembled pre-operatively. A radiolucent table was used, and a pillow placed to support the ipsilateral buttock of the patient in the supine position. A first surgical strategy was to deal with the infected nonunion: a lateral approach, taking deep samples for culture and sensitivity, extraction of the implants and aggressive debridement of all devitalised soft tissue and bone. The bone ends were cut back square until punctate bleeding was clearly evident, and this followed by lavage with normal saline. The nonunion site was prepared for bone grafting by fish scaling (cortical flaps) and multiple drill holes. If the knee was mobile, the fixator was applied with the knee flexed to 90° at the end of a radiolucent operating table to ensure the quadriceps were transfixed in flexion by the pins. The fixator was applied orthogonally to the femur by first inserting a 6 mm diameter Schanz screw (5 mm in small diameter femurs) reference pin at the subtrochanteric level near the lesser trochanter, perpendicular to the bone and in the coronal plane. The pre-assembled proximal block was fixed to this reference pin, and further pins added to hold the proximal segment securely. With an assistant holding the reduction of the newly prepared bone ends,

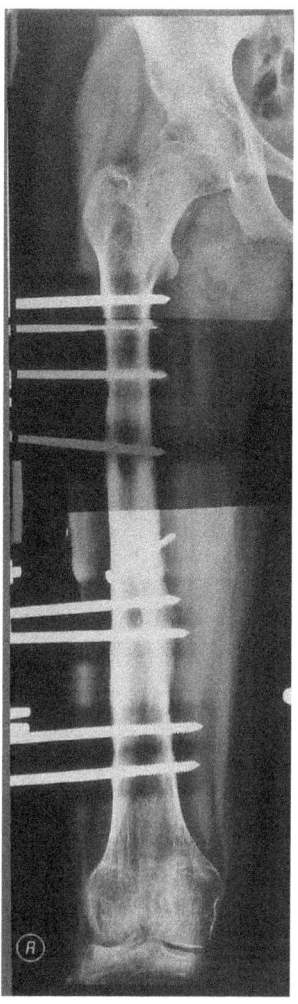

Fig. 4 Case no. 1 in table I. A-P view X-ray showing infected nonunion with a spiral fracture configuration at the mid shaft right femur fixed by the described semicircular Ilizarov pin fixator module augmented by an interfragmentary cortical screw

fixation of the distal fragment to the fixator was then carried out. At the completion of fixation, each segment had at least three to four pins in different planes with as much of a divergence angle in between as possible (Fig. 3). The fixation pins were at least 3 cm from the fracture site. Augmentative interfragmentary screw fixation was needed for one case (Fig. 4). Structural iliac bone grafts were used in seven cases that were fixed with a screw (Fig. 5). Iliac bone chips were used in two cases to stimulate healing. Two cases needed repeat bone grafting, one after 9 months and the other after 10 months to stimulate healing. In none of the cases was simultaneous bone lengthening performed.

The patient was discharged on the second or third postoperative day. Early assisted weight-bearing and continual knee exercises were encouraged. Antibiotics were prescribed according to culture and sensitivity results from deep samples submitted and were for 2 weeks after

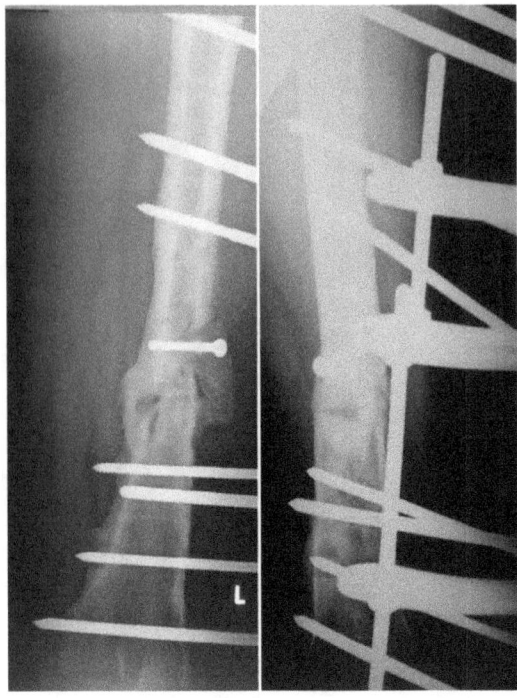

Fig. 5 Case no. 8 in table I. Illustrates an augmentative structural iliac bone graft that was securely fixed by a cortical screw. Union of the femoral fracture was achieved after incorporation of the strut graft

resolution of clinical signs of infection. Follow-up X-rays were obtained every month for the first 3 months, thereafter every 2 months until union and removal of the fixator. Frequent compression of the fracture site was needed if osteolysis at the fracture site was noted. Union was declared through observing bridging callus on anteroposterior, lateral and oblique views; this was confirmed clinically by dynamising the fixator and observing the ability of the patient to walk and perform a single-leg stance on the affected limb without pain, instability or deformation at the fracture site. The fixator was removed in the operating room under general anaesthesia.

Outcome was determined using a combination of radiological and functional criteria. The classification system by Paley and Maar [18, 19] was used. This is based on the presence or absence of each of these five criteria: union; infection; deformity in any plane $>5°$; limb length discrepancy >2.5 cm; and a weak cross-sectional area at the union site that requires long-term bracing or protection. An *excellent* bone result was assigned for those who achieved full union and resolution of infection with absence of the other three factors. A *good* bone result was as excellent with the presence of one of the other three criteria. A *fair* bone result was as excellent with the presence of two of the other criteria. A *poor* bone result was a persistent nonunion with or without persistent or recurrent bone infection.

Additional outcome reporting used a modification of the system derived from Paley and Maar in 2000 and Barbarossa V et al. in 2001 [19, 20]. This was based on five criteria: the ability for normal daily activities and a return to work; pain; the need for walking aids or braces; a loss of more than $20°$ of knee range of motion from the preoperative levels; and soft tissue dystrophy. An *excellent* result was assigned for those with full activity, and the other four criteria were absent. A *good* result was deemed if the patient was active with mild or no pain, and one of the other three criteria present. A *fair* result was declared if the patient was active with mild or no pain, and two of the other criteria present. A *poor* occurred if the patient had markedly limited activity regardless of the presence of other criteria, any patient with significant pain (requiring narcotics) or a patient with three of the other criteria.

Results

The mean age of patients at the time of surgery was 46 years (range 16–60, SD 15.6), 16 (80 %) were male and 4 (20 %) were females. The mean period since the original trauma was 10.2 months (range 6–15, SD 2.5). A history of road traffic accident was noted in 18 patients; one patient fractured after a fall (case no. 10), and one had a gunshot injury (case no. 7). Eighteen were initially closed fractures, and one was an open fracture grade II (Gustilo and Anderson Classification). The mean number of previous operative procedures was 3; these included repeated debridement, plating, intramedullary nailing, gentamicin bead implantation and external fixation. Four patients were diabetic and 1 positive for hepatitis C. One patient had ipsilateral anterior poliomyelitis of the lower limb.

Eleven patients presented with a stiff knee in extension. Eighteen had minor shortening <2 cm, whilst two patients presented with 3 and 2.5 cm shortening (cases no. 4 and 9), respectively. Five cases presented with >1/3 circumferential cortical defect (cases no. 2, 7–9, 13, 15, 18; Table 1).

The mean period spent in the fixator was 11 months (range 8–18, SD 2.9). After a mean follow-up period of 3.5 years (range 2–9, SD 2.6), bony union without recurrence of infection was noted in 18 out of 19 patients (94.7 %) who attended the final follow-up (Fig. 6). The patient lost to follow-up (case no. 12 in the table) was a 59-year-old diabetic male with an infected midshaft nonunion of the femur with two previous episodes of plate fixation. He was treated in the fixator for 8 months and then lost to follow-up.

Using the bony criteria, there were 14 excellent, 3 good, 1 fair and 1 poor result. Despite the inevitable shortening of the limb from freshening and squaring off the nonunion

Table 1 Patient demography

No.	Age (years)	Sex	Side	Presenting condition	General Comorbidity	Local Co-morbidity	No. of pre-op interferences	Period of nonunion (months)	Adjunctive synchronous procedure done	Further interference needed	Time spent in Ilizarov (M)	Union	Follow-up (years)
1	16	M	Rt	Infected non union with plate fixation	–	Stiff knee in extension	plating	7	Augmentative interfragmental screw	–	9	+	2
2	17	M	Rt	Infected non union with plate fixation	–	Stiff knee in extension	Plating. 2 time depridement	8	Strut Iliac bone graft	Re-grafting after 9 m	18	+	2
3	42	M	Rt	Infected non union with plate fixation	–	Stiff knee in extension	Plating. 3 time depridement	14	–	–	10	+	4
4	58	M	Rt	Infected non union with ILN fixation	Diabetic	Stiff knee in extension	ILN 10 time depridement. 1 time septobal beeds insertion.	12	–	–	9	+	2
5	58	M	Lt	Infected non union with plate fixation	–	–	plating	10	–	–	10	+	9
6	60	F	Lt	Infected non union with ILN fixation)	–	Stiff knee in extension	Plating. 3 time depridement	8	Iliac bone graft	–	9	+	3
7	46	M	Rt	Infected nonunion with Ilizarov hybrid fixation with intramedullary Ruch pin	–	Stiff knee in extension	Interlocking nail, that was extracted after 6 m	13	Strut Iliac bone graft	–	11	+	3
8	55	F	Lt	Infected nonunion with plating	–	–	Plating. 2 time depridement	9	Strut Iliac bone graft that was fixed by a screw	–	9	+	4
9	18	M	Rt	Infected nonunion with IMN	–	Stiff knee in extension	IMN. Orthofix for 3 m	13	Strut Iliac bone graft	–	9	+	2
10	58	M	Lt	Infected nonunion with a long DHS	Diabetic	–	DHS. 2 times depridement.	10	–	–	8	+	7
11	59	M	Lt	Infected nonunion with Orthofix fixation	Diabetic	Stiff knee in extension	Orthofix	10	–	–	13	+	4
12	59	M	Rt	Infected nonunion with plating	Diabetic	–	Plating	15	–	–	??	Missed	–

Table 1 continued

No.	Age (years)	Sex	Side	Presenting condition	General Comorbidity	Local Co-morbidity	No. of pre-op interferences	Period of nonunion (months)	Adjunctive synchronous procedure done	Further interference needed	Time spent in Ilizarov (M)	Union	Follow-up (years)
13	48	M	Rt	Infected nonunion with plating	Ipsilateral poliomyelitis	Stiff knee in extension	2times plating	8	Strut Iliac bone graft	–	11	+	3
14	58	M	Lt	Infected nonunion with plating	–	–	plating	6	–	–	11	+	9
15	55	F	Rt	Infected nonunion with plating	–	–	Plating. 4 time depridement	8	Strut Iliac bone graft	–	10	+	5
16	55	M	Rt	Infected nonunion with plating	Hepatitis C positive	Stiff knee in extension	Plate femur 4 time depridement	9	–	–	9	Not united	–
17	45	M	Lt	Infected nonunion with ILN	–	–	Interlocking nail. 4 time depridement	11	Iliac graft bone chips	–	13	+	6
18	53	M	Lt	Infected nonunion with ILN	–	–	ILN 3 time depridement.	9	Strut Iliac bone graft -	–	14	+	2
19	39	M	Rt	Infected nonunion with plating	–	–	Plating.	13	–	Re-grafting after 10 m	17	+	3
20	21	F	Lt	Infected nonunion with ILN	–	Stiff knee in extension	ILN	11	–	–	11	+	4

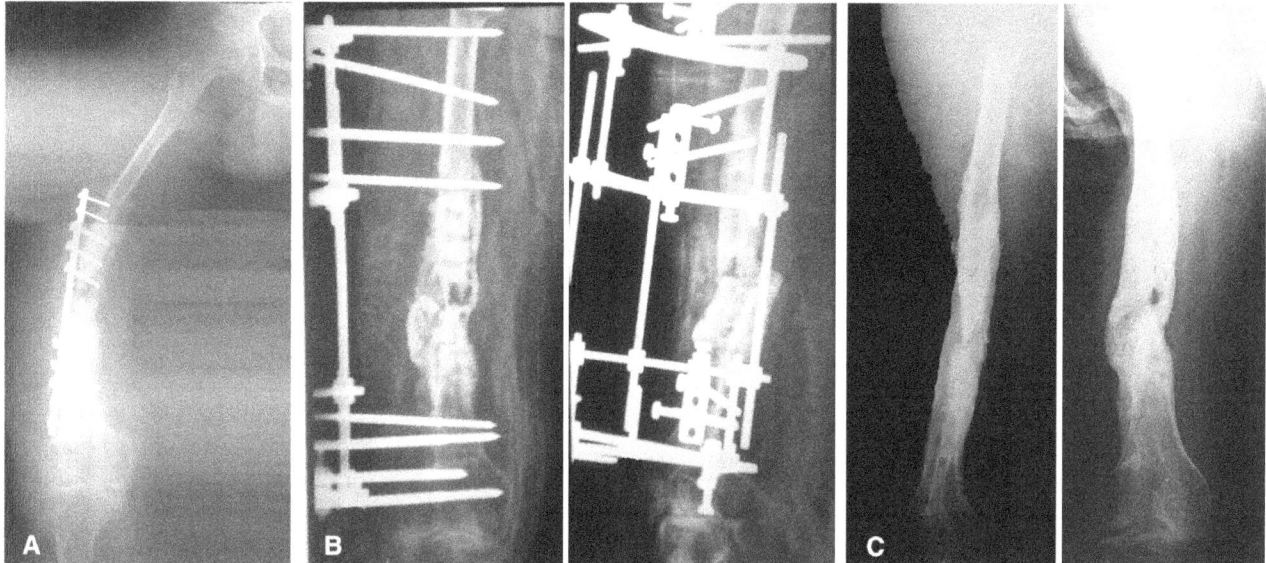

Fig. 6 a–c Case no. 13 in table I. **a** A-P view of showing infected nonunion of the midshaft femur with periosteal and endosteal new bone formation, cortical irregularities and visible resorption, especially around the plate and screws with loosening of the fixation. **b** Postoperative A-P and lateral X-rays with the fixator. **c** Follow-up X-rays after 3 years. This was classed an excellent result from both bony and functional outcomes

bone ends, only two patients showed significant shortening >2.5 cm (cases no. 4 and 9 with 5 and 4 cm, respectively) but were also the cases who presented initially with 3 and 2.5 cm shortening. The poor result (case no. 16 in the table) was a 55-year-old male with infected nonunion fracture of the upper to mid third right femoral shaft after previous plating. He was positive for hepatitis C infection with a stiff knee in extension. After 9 months in the fixator, he refused to continue with treatment and asked for removal of the fixator and substitution with an ischial weight-bearing orthosis. Using functional criteria, there were 10 excellent, 7 good, 1 fair and 1 poor result (Table 2).

During the period of external fixation, patients noted easier compliance with this fixator in carrying out their physiological daily activities, personal hygiene, sitting or lying down. All patients had one or more pin track infections that were resolved by local dressing and systemic antibiotics. There were bouts of pain, oedema and reactive depression, all of which resolved after completion of treatment. A refracture occurred in one patient 2 years after completion of treatment following new trauma and was managed by the same fixator; this united after 8 months. Of the eleven patients who presented with stiff knees in extension, none showed any noticeable improvement at the end of follow-up. For those patients who developed loss of knee motion during the period of fixation, this was noted to improve by the end of follow-up with the exception of three cases (Table 2).

Discussion

When external fixation is indicated, a balance between the desirable characteristics of the fixator assembly and patient tolerability is important [7, 21]. Biomechanically and in the femur, unilateral fixators are weaker in bending, axial and torsional stability. In contrast, ring fixators give excellent three-dimensional stability but at the expense of the patient comfort. Even in a hybrid fixator, the distal transfixing wires (apart from being difficult to tolerate) are not sufficiently rigid against bending forces in the sagittal plane as the permitted safe corridor for insertion is narrow and located mainly in the frontal plane [7, 22].

Factors which determine the stiffness of a fixator construct depend on its two main constituents: the device material and configuration on one hand and the pins on the other. Fixator rigidity is directly proportion to pin stiffness that is increased by: firstly improving material properties; secondly by increasing pin diameter—but not to exceed one-third of the bone diameter—and thirdly a decreased pin offset (the free bending length of pins which is the distance between the bone surface and the external pin clamp). Other pin factors that add to fixator rigidity are increased pin spread (length of the fractured bone involved in fixation), increased pin numbers and levels and lastly, increased pin divergent angle in the axial plane [7, 11, 21–25]. Considering the aforementioned factors, the design of the external fixator used in this study can be considered as a modification of the Catagni and Cattaneo module in 1986

Table 2 Bone and functional results

No.	Bone results	Functional results
1	G (Frontal plane varus 8°)	E
2	F (Weak union site cross-sectional area that necessitates long bracing for 9 months)	F (Soft tissue dystrophy and need walking brace for 9 months)
3	E	G (Soft tissue dystrophy)
4	G (LLD 5 cm)	E
5	E	E
6	E	G (Soft tissue dystrophy)
7	E	E
8	E	E
9	G (LLD 4 cm)	G (Need walking brace for 10 months)
10	E	E
11	E	G (Loss of >20° knee ROM from the presenting range)
12	Missed case	
13	E	E
14	E	E
15	E	G (Loss of >20° knee ROM from the presenting range)
16	P (Nonunion)	P (Marked limitation of daily activity)
17	E	E
18	E	G (Need for walking aid)
19	E	E
20	E	G (Loss of >20° knee ROM from the presenting range)

E excellent result, *G* good result, *F* fair result, *P* poor result

[11, 12] but where the distal rings are replaced by femoral arches.

From a patient's perspective of fixator tolerability and comfort, this fixator conveniently spares encircling the medial aspect of the patient's thigh with bulky rings. From a biomechanical point of view, it is a versatile semicircular multiplanar device. It allows for frequent compression of the fracture site postoperatively when fracture site resorption is observed. The mechanical axis of the femur lies outside the bone itself and medial to its anatomical axis. Axial loading on the femoral head will create compression forces on its medial side and a tensile force on the lateral side. Consequently, stable fixation of a femoral diaphyseal fracture is accomplished if, provided that inherent bone stability (through fracture site bone contact) was obtained first, a sufficiently rigid external fixator is applied laterally and is sufficient to act as a tension band fixation [5, 10, 26–28].

Inherent bone stability and bone contact, especially of the medial cortex, are of utmost importance for fixation stability that enables the patient to weight bear early. Bone contact increases the effective diameter of the fracture to obtain a good cross-sectional area of bone at the future union site [5, 22, 29]. This was achieved using different ways of squaring off the bone ends and occasional use of supplemental minimal osteosynthesis (interfragmentary screws) to stabilise unstable oblique fractures or with structural grafts to fill a partial circumferential bone defect if this was >1/3 diameter of the femur.

Concomitant bone lengthening for cases with infected nonunion of the femur has been reported to carry significant complications [20, 30]. These findings were also reported again by Blum et al. in 2010 [30]. This suggests deferring lengthening—if required—to a second stage after achieving full fracture consolidation and recovery of the patient's physical, functional and psychological status. It should be reserved for those who are able to cope with the strenuous combined treatment protocols of external fixation and lengthening. Fortunately, it has been reported that patients may tolerate shortening well up to 2 cm without the need for a shoe lift and, for those with up to 4 cm shortening, comply well with a shoe lift of 2 cm [31, 32].

The final results presented in this consecutive series are comparable with those from similar studies [2–4, 20, 33]. The mean time in the fixator was 11.2 months and is comparable to other published works [2–4, 20]. The prevalence of knee stiffness is not always a complication of the use external fixation but is related to other factors such as the fracture location, the extent of soft tissue damage, pre-exiting stiffness and the severity and duration of infection [3]. The limitations of this study include the absence of a control group and the small cohort of patients but this attributable to the restriction in the inclusion criteria to preserve group homogeneity.

Conclusion

A semi-circular external fixator module which is entirely half-pin based is described, which is shown to be patient tolerable and effective for managing infected nonunion of the femoral diaphysis.

References

1. Ricci WM, Gallagher B, Haidukewych GJ (2009) Intramedullary nailing of femoral shaft fractures: current concepts. J Am Acad Orthop Surg 17(5):296–305
2. Krishnan A, Pamecha C, Patwa JJ (2006) Modified Ilizarov technique for infected nonunion of the femur: the principle of distraction-compression osteogenesis. J Orthop Surg (Hong Kong) 14(3):265–272
3. Ueng SW, Wei FC, Shih CH (1999) Management of femoral diaphyseal infected nonunion with antibiotic beads local therapy, external skeletal fixation, and staged bone grafting. J Trauma 46(1):97–103

4. Saridis A, Panagiotopoulos E, Tyllianakis M, Matzaroglou C, Vandoros N, Lambiris E (2006) The use of the Ilizarov method as a salvage procedure in infected nonunion of the distal femur with bone loss. J Bone Jt Surg [Br] 88-B:232–237

5. Khanfour AA, Zakzouk SA (2012) Distal femur non-union after interlocked intramedullary nailing. Successful augmentation with wave plate and strut graft. Acta Orthop Belg 78(4):492–499

6. Grivas TB, Magnissalis EA (2011) The use of twin-ring Ilizarov external fixator constructs: application and biomechanical proof-of-principle with possible clinical indications. J Orthop Surg Res 6:41

7. Moss DP, Tejwani NC (2007) Biomechanics of external fixation: a review of the literature. Bull NYU Hosp Jt Dis 65(4):294–299

8. Fenton P, Phillips J, Royston S (2007) The use of Ilizarov frames in the treatment of pathological fracture of the femur secondary to osteomyelitis: a review of three cases. Injury 38(2):240–244

9. Kishan S, Sabharwal S, Behrens F, Reilly M, Sirkin M (2002) External fixation of the femur: basic concepts. Tech Orthop 17(2):239–244

10. Fragomen AT, Rozbruch SR (2007) The mechanics of external fixation. HSS J 3(1):13–29

11. Green SA, Harris NL, Wall DM, Ishkanian J, Marinow H (1992) The Rancho mounting technique for the Ilizarov method. A preliminary report. Clin Orthop Relat Res 280:104–116

12. Belhan O, Ekinci A, Karakurt L, Yılmaz E, Serin E (2008) The treatment of femoral shaft fractures in adults with hybrid Ilizarov external fixator. Jt Dis Rel Surg 19(2):50–54

13. Cavusoglu AT, Ozsoy MH, Dincel VE, Sakaogullari A, Basarir K, Ugurlu M (2009) The use of a low-profile Ilizarov external fixator in the treatment of complex fractures and non-unions of the distal femur. Acta Orthop Belg 75:209–218

14. Benedetti GB, Argnani F (1991) Group. ASAMI. Fractures of the femur. In: Maiocchi AB, Aronson J (eds) Operative principles of Ilizarov fracture treatment—nonunion—osteotomies—lengthening—deformity correction. Williams and Wilkins, Baltimore, Hong Cong, London, Sydney, pp 125–145

15. Baran O, Havitcioglu H, Tatari H, Cecen B (2008) The stiffness characteristics of hybrid Ilizarov fixators. J Biomech 41(14):2960–2963

16. Mahran MA, Elgebeily MA, Ghaly NA, Thakeb MF, Hefny HM (2011) Pelvic support osteotomy by Ilizarov's concept: is it a valuable option in managing neglected hip problems in adolescents and young adults? Strateg Trauma Limb Reconstr 6(1):13–20

17. Catagni MA (2003) Atlas for the insertion of transosseous wires and half-pins Ilizarov method. 2nd. ed. Melan-Italy: Il quadratinoItaly; p. 23–29

18. Paley D, Catagni MA, Argnani F, Villa A, Benedetti GB, Cattaneo R (1989) Ilizarov treatment of tibial nonunions with bone loss. Clin Orthop Relat Res 241:146–165

19. Paley D, Maar DC (2000) Ilizarov bone transport treatment for tibial defects. J Orthop Trauma 14(2):76–85

20. Barbarossa V, Matkovic BR, Vucic N, Bielen M, Gluhinic M (2001) Treatment of osteomyelitis and infected non-union of the femur by a modified Ilizarov technique: follow-up study. Croat Med J 42(6):634–641

21. Bronson DG, Samchukov ML, Birch JG, Browne RH, Ashman RB (1998) Stability of external circular fixation: a multi-variable biomechanical analysis. Clin Biomech (Bristol, Avon) 13(6):441–448

22. Karaharju EO, Aalto K (1983) The deformation of external fixation devices during loading. Int Orthop 7(3):179–183

23. Willie B, Adkins K, Zheng X, Simon U, Claes L (2008) Mechanical characterization of external fixator stiffness for a rat femoral fracture model. J Orthop Res 27:687–693

24. Pugh KJ, Wolinsky PR, Pienkowski D, Banit D, Dawson JM (1999) Comparative biomechanics of hybrid external fixation. J Orthop Trauma 13(6):418–425

25. Lenarz C, Bledsoe G, Watson J (2008) Circular External Fixation Frames with Divergent Half Pins. A Pilot Biomechanical Study. Clin Orthop Relat Res 466:2933–2939

26. Baruah RK (2007) Ilizarov methodology for infected non union of the Tibia: classic circular transfixion wire assembly vs. hybrid assembly. Indian J Orthop 41(3):198–203

27. Sabharwal S, Kishan S, Behrens F (2005) Principles of external fixation of the femur. Am J Orthop 34(5):218–223

28. Sabharwal S (2005) Role of Ilizarov external fixator in the management of proximal/distal metadiaphyseal pediatric femur fractures. J Orthop Trauma 19(8):563–569

29. Khalily C, Voor M, David S (1998) Fracture Site Motion with Ilizarov and "Hybrid" external fixation. J Orthop Trauma 12(1):21–26

30. Blum AL, BongioVanni JC, Morgan SJ, Flierl MA, dos Reis FB (2010) Complications associated with distraction osteogenesis for infected nonunion of the femoral shaft in the presence of a bone defect: a retrospective series. J Bone Jt Surg Br 92(4):565–570

31. Rose R (2009) Complications of Femoral Lengthening using the Ilizarov Fixator. Internet J Orthopedic Surg 15(1):1–6

32. Benedetti M, Catani F, Benedetti E, Berti L, Gioia A, Giannini S (2010) To what extent does leg length discrepancy impair motor activity in patients after total hip arthroplasty? Int Orthop 34:1115–1121

33. Struijs PA, Poolman RW, Bhandari M (2007) Infected nonunion of the long bones. J Orthop Trauma 21(7):507–511

7

Adjuvant treatment of chronic osteomyelitis of the tibia following exogenous trauma using OSTEOSET®-T: a review of 21 patients in a regional trauma centre

Gemma Humm · Saqib Noor · Philippa Bridgeman ·
Michael David · Deepa Bose

Abstract Surgical debridement and prolonged systemic antibiotic therapy are an established management strategy for infection after tibial fractures. Local antibiotic delivery via cement beads has shown improved outcome but requires further surgery for extraction of beads. OSTEO-SET®-T is a resorbable bone void filler composed of calcium sulphate and 4 % tobramycin that is packed easily into bone defects. This is a review of the outcomes of 21 patients treated with OSTEOSET®-T for osteomyelitis of the tibia. This is a retrospective case note and clinical review. In all cases, the strategy was debridement, with removal of any implants, with excision back to bleeding bone. OSTEOSET®-T pellets were packed into any contained defects or the intra-medullary canal with further bony stabilisation ($n = 9$) and soft tissue reconstruction ($n = 7$) undertaken as required. Intravenous vancomycin and meropenem were administered after sampling with substitution to targeted antibiotic therapy for between 6 weeks and 6 months. The average follow-up was 15 months. Union rate after tibial reconstruction was 100 %. Wound complications were encountered in 52 %: a wound discharge in the early post-operative period was noted in seven patients (33 %) independent of site of pellet placement. In the 14 cases without a wound leak, five developed wound complications ($p = 0.06$, Fisher's exact test) either from delayed wound-healing or pin-site

infections. One patient developed a transient acute kidney injury and one refractory osteomyelitis. OSTEOSET®-T is an effective adjunct in the treatment of chronic tibial osteomyelitis following trauma based on the low incidence of relapse of infection within the period of follow-up in this study, but significant wound complications and one transient nephrotoxic event were also recorded.

Keywords Osteomyelitis · Tibia · Trauma · Osteoset · Antibiotic

Introduction

Antibiotics are an important part of the strategy in treating infection after tibial fractures. In established osteomyelitis, surgical debridement is followed with systemic and, sometimes, local antibiotic delivery. Antibiotic-impregnated cement beads are frequently used as an adjunct to delivery of antibiotics but often require a further surgical procedure for removal.

The ability to treat chronic osteomyelitis with single-stage surgery potentially reduces the risk and morbidity associated with repeated operative procedures and general anaesthetic. Reduction in theatre time and length of in-patient stay are added economic benefits. Despite single-stage surgery showing reasonable success in achieving union in infected non-union of long bones, persistent infection and subsequent revision surgery may be needed [1].

Calcium sulphate has been used successfully in the treatment of non-union and is an osteo-conductive void filler that is resorbed at a rate similar to that of bone formation [2, 3]. OSTEOSET®-T (Wright Medical Technology Inc. Arlington TN USA) comes pre-packaged in small pellets to allow easy packing into bone. It comes preloaded

G. Humm · S. Noor · P. Bridgeman · M. David · D. Bose
Queen Elizabeth Hospital, University Hospitals Birmingham
NHS Foundation Trust, Mindelsohn Way,
Birmingham B15 2GW, UK

G. Humm (✉)
East and North Hertfordshire NHS Trust, Lister Hospital,
Coreys Mill Lane, Stevenage SG1 4AB, UK
e-mail: gemmahumm@hotmail.co.uk

with 4 % tobramycin, and drug elution profiles have shown levels up to 10,000 times the minimum inhibitory concentration for most strains of *Staphylococcus* [4]. No further surgery is required to remove the resorbable pellets. Animal studies have demonstrated that its use prevents intramedullary and post-operative wound infection following the treatment of open, contaminated long-bone fractures [5, 6].

OSTEOSET®-T has been used as a bone graft substitute with success in the management of infected non-union of the tibia. Management involves radical debridement of infected bone and placement of gentamicin-impregnated beads, prior to definitive fixation and the use of OSTEOSET®-T [7]. Union was achieved without the need for autologous bone graft and without recurrence of infection. A retrospective comparison of the use of OSTEOSET®-T with debridement versus debridement alone has supported the use of OS-TEOSET®-T in single-stage surgery in the treatment of adult osteomyelitis. Chang et al. [8] have described the use of vancomycin with OSTEOSET®-T for cases of tobramycin resistance. However, it has been associated with wound complications, e.g. in the development of sinuses draining a sterile effluent, but this was found to be self-limiting and resolved after the complete absorption of OSTEOSET®-T and without recurrence of infection [9, 10].

The aminoglycosides used in the treatment of bone infections belong to the protein synthesis inhibitor family of antibiotics, binding to the bacterial ribosomal 30S subunit to achieve a bacteriostatic effect through transcription errors during cell division [11]. An additional ability to disrupt bacterial cell membranes accounts for its bactericidal properties [12]. They have a broad spectrum and are effective against both gram-positive and gram-negative organisms [13]. *Pseudomonas aeruginosa*, *Staphylococcus aureus* and *Enterobacteriaceae* are sensitive to tobramycin which has a lower side-effect profile than gentamicin [14].

This case series reports on the outcome of 21 patients with chronic osteomyelitis managed by single-stage surgery and using OSTEOSET®-T as an adjunct to intravenous antimicrobial therapy.

Materials and Methods

Twenty-one cases of chronic tibial osteomyelitis in which treatment involved the use of OSTEOSET®-T as a space filler and local antibiotic delivery system were identified by a retrospective review over a 30-month period from 2010 to 2012. Data were collected using a proforma and included demographics, record of the intra-operative procedure, relevant microbiology, renal function, complications relating to recurrent infection and wound healing, the presence of a wound leak and repeat surgeries. A wound leak was defined

subjectively as a serous leakage considered a potential risk to normal wound healing [15]. A standardised surgical protocol and antibiotic regime based on guidance from our local microbiology department were followed.

In all cases, surgery was directed at excising infected tissue and sinuses; a radical debridement was performed, guided by pre-operative magnetic resonance imaging, until bleeding confirmed on residual bone. Metalwork, if present, was removed. Once complete, OSTEOSET®-T pellets were packed into any defects or into the intra-medullary canal in those cases where an intramedullary nail had been removed. Further, tibial stabilisation and soft tissue cover were carried out as deemed necessary. The protocol involved taking a minimum of five tissue samples from deep tissues using fresh instruments for each sample. Empiric intravenous vancomycin and meropenem were administered after samples were taken. Meropenem was discontinued after 3 days in the absence of gram-negative growth, and vancomycin continued until the 7-day culture results became available. Thereafter, targeted antibiotic therapy was continued for a period of 6 weeks to 6 months, or empiric ciprofloxacin and rifampicin if no growth was seen. This approach is based on the probability of involvement of a *Staphylococcus* bacterium species contraposed to local antibiotic resistance patterns and the previous published literature on the effectiveness of combination of dual therapy [15–17].

Data analysis and parametric tests were performed using Microsoft Excel for Mac 2011, while nonparametric statistical tests done with GraphPad QuickCalcs (2013 GraphPad Software, Inc.). Statistical significance was set at *p* value of ≤0.05.

Results

There were 18 males and 3 females with a mean age of 49 (range 26–88) and follow-up of 16 months (range 6–25). Six patients were classified as Cierney-Mader grade 3A, one patient as grade 3B, 13 patients grade 4A, and one patient grade 4B. In situ metal work was removed (Fig. 1).

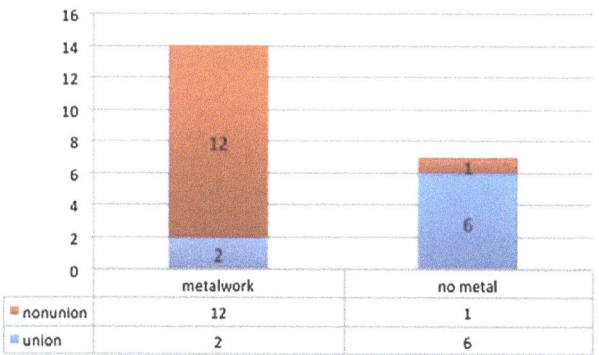

Fig. 1 Cases of non-union and the presence of metal work

Table 1 Causative organisms involved

Organism	Cases	%
Polymicrobial	4	19
Coagulase-negative *Staphylococci*	4	19
Staphylococcus aureus	4	19
Negative cultures	3	14
Other organisms	6	29
Serratia sp.	2	
Corynebacterium sp.	1	
Enterococcus sp.	1	
Mixed anaerobes	1	
Propionibacterium	1	

Nine cases required fixation: eight with circular external fixators and one with a monolateral external fixator. Seven cases required reconstructive soft tissue cover provided by our resident plastic surgical team: there were four local flaps and three free vascularised flaps.

Microbiological analysis of the samples revealed 38 % of the infections were caused by a strain of *Staphylococcus* species. A significant number either had mixed growth or no identified growth. This is summarised in Table 1. Renal function was assessed in all cases. One case was complicated by a transient post-operative acute kidney injury which resolved after 1 week without the need for renal support. This patient had pre-existing comorbidities of obesity and essential hypertension.

Seven cases were complicated by wound leakage; the location of OSTEOSET®-T pellets in either a closed intramedullary cavity or an open cortical defect did not relate to its incidence (Fig. 2). Three-quarters of these cases with a wound leak went on to have problems with wound healing as compared to just one-third of the cases without a leak. A serous leak appears to double the relative risk of wound-healing problems (Fig. 3).

Successful eradication of infection, as determined in the time of follow-up in this series, was achieved in 20 cases.

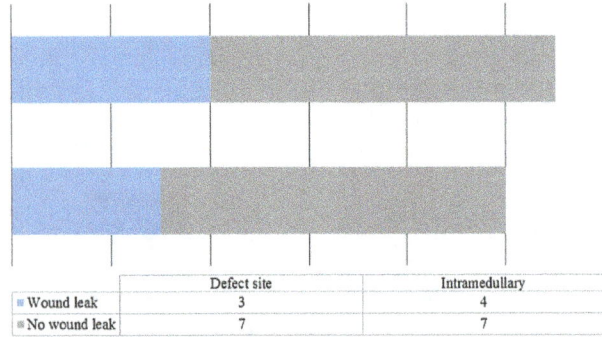

	Defect site	Intramedullary
Wound leak	3	4
No wound leak	7	7

Fig. 2 Impact of site of placement of OSTEOSET®-T placement and the presence of a post-operative wound leak ($p = 1.0$, Fisher's exact test)

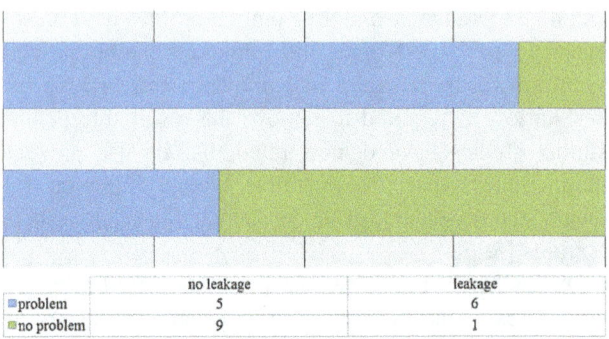

	no leakage	leakage
problem	5	6
no problem	9	1

Fig. 3 Impact of wound leakage on healing ($p = 0.06$, Fisher's exact test)

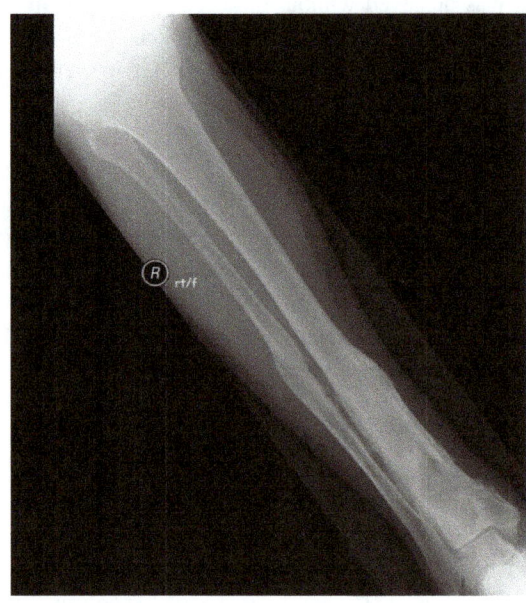

Fig. 4 Pre-operative plain radiograph of the right distal tibial in a 57 year old male with chronic post-traumatic osteomyelitis distal tibia

Only one patient required further debridement and soft tissue coverage and remained free of continuing infection at latest follow-up. One patient required further surgery for the correction of residual deformity.

Figures 4, 5, 6, 7 and 8 show the successful management of a 57 year old man with post traumatic chronic tibial osteomyelitis using OSTEOSET®-T as an adjunct to surgical debridement.

Discussion

This case series included a sample of patients with chronic osteomyelitis of the tibia secondary to trauma. The use of OSTEOSET®-T was an effective adjunct with eradication of infection in all of our cases in the period of follow-up, although one patient required a further surgical debridement owing to an unhealthy appearance of the wound and suspected

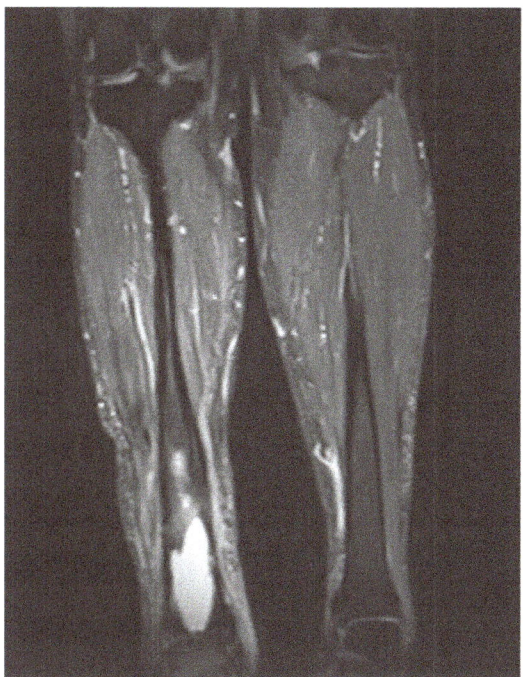

Fig. 5 MRI appearances of chronic osteomyelitis of the right distal tibia

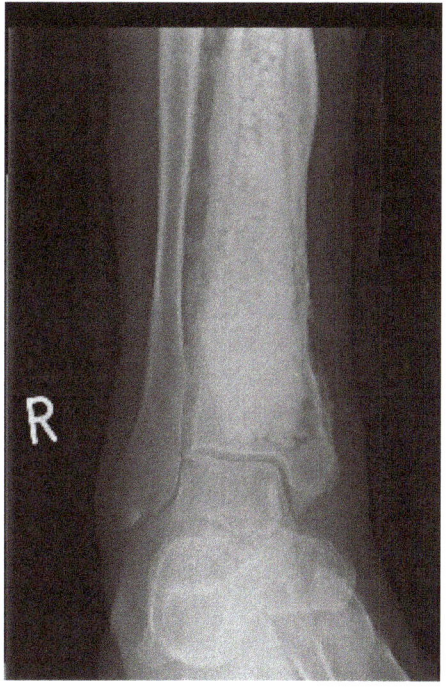

Fig. 7 Post-operative plain radiograph of right distal tibia packed with OSTEOSET®-T

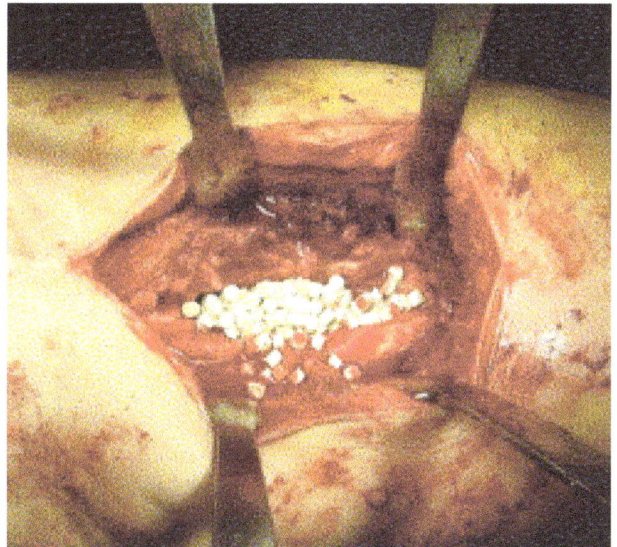

Fig. 6 Intra-operative use of OSTEOSET®-T

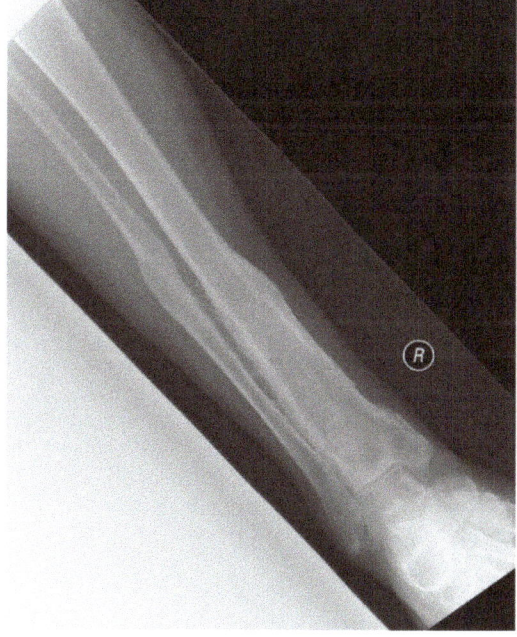

Fig. 8 Plain radiograph of the right distal tibia following second stage bone grafting

persistent infection. The occurrence of a sterile effluent was a significant complication, as was its associated risk of impaired wound healing. Reported concerns over acute kidney injury (potential nephrotoxic side-effect of high local concentrations of aminoglycosides) were unfounded in our series; the one incident of transient acute kidney injury seen was thought to have occurred from the intravenous antimicrobial therapy in a patient with a background of hypertensive nephropathy.

This case series is limited by the following: the absence of a control group, small numbers and the minimum follow-up period of 6 months. A retrospective case–control study, which contained a mixed group of long-bone infections, found favour in the use of OSTEOSET®-T [8]. Prospective data on OSTEOSET®-T are limited, with published work concentrating on post-traumatic osteomyelitis in long bones but without comparison with controls [9].

Conclusion

This case series supports continued use of OSTEOSET®-T as an *adjunct* in the treatment of chronic osteomyelitis of the tibia following trauma but highlights potential issues with wound problems. Further prospective and controlled studies are needed to evaluate the role of local antibiotic delivery systems in the treatment of chronic osteomyelitis.

Acknowledgments No financial support was received for this study.

References

1. Struijs PA, Poolman RW, Bhandari M (2007) Infected nonunion of the long bones. J Orthop Trauma 21(7):507–511
2. Wright Medical Technology Inc (2006) OSTEOSET®-T: medicated bone graft substitute technical monograph. http://www.ossano.se/Produkter/Bensubstitut/Osteoset/651-1097%20R5.06%20OSTEOSET%20T%20Tech%20Monograph.pdf. Accessed 15 Dec 2014
3. Tay BK, Patel VV, Bradford DS (1999) Calcium sulfate- and calcium phosphate-based bone substitutes. Mimicry of the mineral phase of bone. Orthop Clin North Am 30(4):615–623
4. Wahl P, Livio F, Jocobi M, Gautier E, Buclin T (2011) Systemic exposure to tobramycin after local antibiotic treatment with calcium sulphate as carrier material. Arch Orthop Trauma Surg 131:657–662
5. Beardmore AA, Brooks DE, Wenke JC, Thomas DB (2005) Effectiveness of local antibiotic delivery with an osteoinductive and osteoconductive bone-graft substitute. J Bone Joint Surg Am 87(1):107–112
6. Thomas BD, Brooks DE, Bice TG, DeJong ES, Lonergan KT, Wenke JC (2005) Tobramycin-impregnated calcium sulfate prevents infection in contaminated wounds. Clin Orthop Relat Res 441:366–371
7. Tsai YH, Tsung-Jen H, Shih HN, Hsu RW (2004) Treatment of infected tibial nonunion with tobramycin-impregnated calcium sulfate: report of two cases. Chang Gung Med J 27(7):542–547
8. Chang W, Colangell M, Colangell S, Di Bella C, Gozzi E, Donati D (2007) Adult osteomyelitis: debridement versus debridement plus Osteoset T® pellets. Acta Orthop Belg 73(2):238–243
9. McKee M, Wild LM, Schemitsch EH, Waddell JP (2002) The use of an antibiotic-impregnated osteoconductive, bioabsorbable bone substitute in the treatment of infected long bone defects: early results of a prospective trial. J Orthopt Trauma 16(9):622–627
10. Wright Medical Technology Inc (2011) OSTEOSET®: resorbable mini-bead kit. http://www.ossano.com/Produkter/Bensubstitut/Osteoset/SK409-511.pdf. Accessed 15 Dec 2014
11. Rang HP, Dale MM, Ritter JM (1999) Rang, Dale and Ritter's pharmacology, 4th edn. Churchill Livingstone, New York
12. Shakil S, Khan R, Zarrilli R, Khan A (2007) Aminoglycosides versus bacteria—a description of the action, resistance mechanism, and nosocomial battleground. J Biomed Sci 15(1):5–14
13. Edson RS, Terrell CL (1999) The aminoglycosides. Mayo Clin Proc 74(5):519–528
14. Bendush CL, Weber R (1976) Tobramycin sulfate: a summary of worldwide experience from clinical trials. J Infect Dis 134(Suppl):S219–S234
15. Vuolo J (2004) Current options for managing the problem of excess wound exudate. Prof Nurse 19(9):487–491
16. Zimmerli W, Widmer AF, Blatter M, Frei R, Ochsner PE (1998) Role of rifampin for treatment of orthopedic implant-related *Staphylococcal* infections: a randomized controlled trial. Foreign-Body Infection (FBI) Study Group. JAMA 279:1537–1541
17. Spellberg B, Lipsky B (2012) Systemic antibiotic therapy for chronic osteomyelitis in adults. Clin Infect Dis 54(3):393–407

8

The effect of the timing of antibiotics and surgical treatment on infection rates in open long-bone fractures: a 6-year prospective study after a change in policy

Andreas Leonidou · Zoltan Kiraly ·
Hristifor Gality · Shane Apperley ·
Sean Vanstone · David A. Woods

Abstract Our current protocol in treating open long-bone fractures includes early administration of intravenous antibiotics and surgery on a scheduled trauma list. This represents a change from a previous protocol where treatment as soon as possible after injury was carried out. This review reports the infection rates in the period 6 years after the start of this protocol. Two hundred and twenty open long-bone fractures were reviewed. Data collected included time of administration of antibiotics, time to theatre and seniority of surgeon involved. The patients were followed up until clinical or radiological union occurred or until a secondary procedure for non-union or infection was performed. Clinical, radiological and haematological signs of infection were documented. If present, infection was classified as deep or superficial. Surgical debridement was performed within 6 h of injury in 45 % of cases and after 6 h in 55 % of cases. Overall infection rates were 11 and 15.7 %, respectively ($p = 0.49$). The overall deep infection rate was 4.3 %. There was also no statistically significant difference in the subgroups of deep ($p = 0.46$) and superficial ($p = 0.78$) infection. Intravenous antibiotics were administered within 3 h of injury in 80 % of cases and after 3 h in 20 % of cases. The infection rates were 14 and 12.5 %, respectively ($p = 1.0$). There was no statistically significant difference in the subgroups of deep ($p = 0.62$) and superficial ($p = 0.73$) infection. Further statistical analysis did not reveal a significant difference in infection rates for any combination of timing of antibiotics and surgical debridement. Infection rates where the most senior surgeon present was a consultant were 9.5 % as opposed to 16 % with the consultant not present, but this trend was not statistically significant. These results suggest that the change in policy may have contributed to an improvement of the deep infection rate to 4.3 % from the previous figure of 8.5 % although this decrease is not statistically significant. Surgeons may have had concerns that delaying theatre may lead to an increased infection rate, but these results do not substantiate this concern.

Keywords Open long-bone fracture · Time to theatre · Grade of surgeon · Infection rate

Introduction

Infection is a recognized complication of open fractures. Surgical debridement of open fractures has been conducted usually within 6 h of injury based on studies conducted by Leopold Freidrich that showed an increase in the growth of microbiological colonies after 6 h in a guinea pig model. In recent years, the validity of the 6-h rule has been questioned by studies showing no statistically significant increase in infection rates beyond 6 h providing that there is prompt administration of antibiotics and the wound is not overtly contaminated [1–3].

In 2009, the British Orthopaedic Association (BOA) in conjunction with the British Association of Plastic Reconstructive and Aesthetic Surgeons (BAPRAS) produced guidelines on the management of open long-bone fractures. Within the guidance, it is advocated that surgical debridement should be carried out by a senior orthopaedic surgeon within 24 h of injury unless contamination, compartment syndrome, vascular compromise or the open

A. Leonidou (✉) · Z. Kiraly · H. Gality · S. Apperley ·
S. Vanstone · D. A. Woods
Department of Trauma and Orthopaedic Surgery, Great Western
Hospitals NHS Foundation Trust, Marlborough Road,
Swindon SN3 6BB, UK
e-mail: leonidou@doctors.org.uk

fracture being a part of multiple injuries necessitated earlier surgical intervention [4].

A change in the protocol to reflect the need for early administration of intravenous antibiotics (within 3 h of admission) as well as aiming to perform surgical debridement once the patient and surgical team were fully optimized, typically at the next consultant-led trauma list was instituted. This study reviews the infection rates since the protocol change in 2006 and asks whether early antibiotic administration and senior surgical care reduce infection in open long-bone fractures.

Patients and method

All open long-bone fractures managed in our department from 1 January 2006 to 31 December 2011 were identified from records and studied. This is a prospective cohort study of a series of consecutive patients.

The initial management was aimed at providing:

1. A senior orthopaedic surgeon (registrar or above) involved in the care of the patient from the outset.
2. Wounds superficially cleaned, photographed and covered with an antiseptic-soaked dressing.
3. Fracture splintage.
4. Intravenous antibiotics within 3 h of the time of injury.
5. Anti-tetanus prophylaxis if indicated.
6. Urgent transfer to a level 1 trauma centre if a neurovascular injury or significant tissue loss requiring plastic surgical input was evident.

Patients not in the category above were added to the next available trauma theatre list for surgical wound debridement and initial or definitive fracture stabilization. This included patients with significant tissue loss (GA IIIB) that did not get transferred urgently to a level 1 trauma centre. In these cases, a wound debridement and application of external fixation were performed prior to the subsequent transfer to a tertiary centre for definitive management and appropriate coverage of soft tissue defects as required.

Specifically, there were no cases where the open fracture underwent internal fixation without prior soft tissue cover nor were any wounds left open for gradual spontaneous closure with granulation tissue.

There were 220 consecutive open long-bone fractures in 212 patients included in the study. Choice of intravenous antibiotic was as per trust protocol which had changed from Cefuroxime and Metronidazole to Augmentin as of September 2008. The fractures were stabilized using a variety of techniques depending on individual fracture patterns and the treating surgeon's preference. The wounds were either closed primarily where appropriate or left open,

and the patients were re-operated at 48 h for secondary debridement or closure.

Patients who died within 3 months of injury were excluded from the study. There was insufficient time from injury to death for the outcome of infection to be known. Patients who required transfer to a specialist unit for definitive treatment of the bony injury were excluded; this group included patients with more severe injuries (GA IIIB and IIIC) and patients who required treatment for both the bony and soft tissue injuries out with facilities of this hospital.

Follow-up was continued until clinical or radiological union, or a secondary procedure for non-union or infection was performed. The diagnosis of deep infection was made along the criteria set by Horan et al. [5]. More specifically, these were: purulent drainage from the deep incision; deep abscess formation; fascial dehiscence either by the infection or during reoperation; or deep infection in the presence of a metallic implant around bone [5]. Additionally, the diagnosis of deep or superficial infection was also based on radiological evidence and cultures obtained either at the time of a secondary procedure to treat infection or non-union, or from discharging wounds. All patients with a diagnosis of superficial wound infection were treated with oral antibiotics and the infection resolved.

The data on all open fractures were recorded in regular weekly audit meetings, attended by the duty trauma consultant, junior staff and members of the departmental clinical audit team. In each case, in addition to the age and gender of the patient, the following were recorded: (1) the site and severity of the fracture using the Gustilo Anderson classification (confirmed in theatre after debridement); (2) the time of admission to the emergency department or time from injury when possible; (3) the time of administration of antibiotics (> or <3 h); (4) the time to surgery (> or <6 h); (5) the grade of the most senior surgeon present in surgery; and (6) whether or not infection (deep vs. superficial) subsequently developed.

The collected data were statistically analysed using the two-tailed Fisher's exact test with the significance level set at $p = 0.05$.

Results

Two hundred and twenty fractures were identified. Two patients died within 3 months of the injury. A further 57 fractures were excluded from the study. Of these, 27 patients (47 %) were transferred to a tertiary hospital for plastic surgical care, 17 patients (30 %) were lost to follow-up (mostly due to living out of our area) and 13 patients (23 %) were excluded because of errors in data collection. As a result, the 161 remaining fractures in 75

Table 1 Infection in open long-bone fractures in relation to timing of antibiotics and time to theatre from the injury

	Timing of antibiotics (h)		Timing of theatres (h)	
	<3	>3	<6	>6
No infection	111	28	64	75
	18 (14 %)	4 (12.5 %)	8 (11 %)	14 (15.7 %)
Infection				
Deep infection	5 (4 %)	2 (6.25 %)	2 (2.7 %)	5 (5.7 %)
Superficial infection	13 (10 %)	2 (6.25)	6 (8.3 %)	9 (10 %)

female and 86 male patients were included in the study. The mean age of the patients was 45 years (range 8–92 years). According to the Gustilo Anderson Classification, 59 fractures were type I, 32 fractures type II, 40 fractures type IIIA and 30 fractures type IIIB (subsequently transferred).

The overall infection rate in the study group was 13.6 %, with 4.3 % deep infections and 9.3 % superficial. The number of infections in relation to timing of initial antibiotics and first surgery is shown in Table 1.

Surgical debridement was performed within 6 h of injury in 45 % of cases and after 6 h in 55 % of cases. Overall infection rates were 11 and 15.7 %, respectively, and was not statistically significant ($p = 0.49$). The deep infection rate in the patients operated within 6 h was 2.7 % and in the patients operated after 6 h 5.7 %. The superficial infection rate in the patients operated within 6 h was 8.3 % and in the patients operated after 6 h 10 %. There was no statistically significant difference in the subgroups of deep ($p = 0.46$) and superficial ($p = 0.78$) infection.

Intravenous antibiotics were administered as per protocol within 3 h of injury in 80 % of cases and after 3 h in 20 % of cases. Overall infection rates were 14 and 12.5 %, respectively, and was not statistically significant ($p = 1$). The deep infection rate in the patients with administered antibiotics within 3 h of injury was 4 % and in those after 3 h from injury 6.25 %. The superficial infection rate in the patients with administered antibiotics within 3 h of injury was 10 % and in those after 3 h from injury 6.25 %. There was no statistically significant difference in the subgroups of deep ($p = 0.62$) and superficial ($p = 0.73$) infection.

Further statistical analysis did not reveal any significant difference in infection rates for any combination of timing of antibiotics and time to first surgical debridement.

In 63 cases, the most senior surgeon present at the operation was a consultant and in the remaining 98 cases a non-consultant middle grade surgeon. Overall infection rates were 9.5 and 16 %, respectively, but this was not statistically significant ($p = 0.24$). The deep infection rate in the patients operated with a consultant present was 4.7 % and in the patients operated with a middle grade present 4 %. The superficial infection rate in the patients operated with a consultant present was 4.8 % and in the patients

Table 2 Comparative data between the previous and current antibiotic policy

	Previous policy (cefuroxime + metronidazole)	Current policy (co-amoxiclav)
Number of cases	93	68
Deep infection	5 (5.3 %)	2 (3.1 %)
Superficial infection	12 (12.9 %)	3 (4.4 %)
Overall infection	17 (18.2 %)	5 (7.3 %)

operated with a middle grade present 11 %. There was also no statistically significant difference in the subgroups of deep ($p = 1$) and superficial ($p = 0.16$) infection.

Our protocol for antibiotics in open long-bone fractures changed in September 2008 from intravenous Cefuroxime and Metronidazole to intravenous Co-amoxiclav. The overall infection rate before and after the implementation of the new policy was 18.2 and 7.3 %, respectively, and was not statistically significant ($p = 0.06$). There was also no statistically significant difference in the subgroups of deep ($p = 0.7$) and superficial ($p = 0.09$) infection. The detailed comparative data are presented in Table 2.

The previously published data from our department before the change in the policy included 248 open long-bone fractures with a deep infection rate of 8.5 % [3]. From these patients, 62 % were operated within 6 h of injury and 38 % after 6 h [3]. The overall deep infection rate in our current study was 4.3 % which is lower but not statistically significant in comparison with our previous data ($p = 0.16$). A comparative presentation of the data before and after the change in policy is shown in Table 3.

The isolated organisms in the cases of deep and superficial infection are shown in Table 4.

In order for the difference in deep infection rate to have been statistically significant and the study to have had a power of 0.80, our sample size should have been 834.

Discussion

The results of the present study on the less severely injured open long-bone fractures demonstrate that following the

Table 3 Comparative data before and after the change in the policy for managing open long-bone fractures in 2006

	Before the change	After the change
Number of cases	248	161
Time to theatre <6 h	154 (62 %)	94 (38 %)
Time to theatre >6 h	72 (45 %)	89 (55 %)
Deep infection cases	21 (8.5 %)	7 (4.3 %)

Table 4 Isolated organisms in cases of deep and superficial infection and number of cases

Deep infection	Superficial infection
Coagulase negative *Staphylococcus* [3]	*Staphylococcus aureus* [7]
Staphylococcus aureus [3]	*Enterococcus* [4]
Methilicinne resistant *Staphylococcus aureus* [2]	Mixed Coliform Bacilli [3]
Mixed Coliform Bacilli [3]	Diphtheroids [4]
Enterococcus [1]	Non-haemolytic *Streptococcus* [1]
Diphtheroids [1]	
Escherichia coli [1]	
Pseudomonas [1]	
Enterobacter cloacae [1]	
Mixed anaerobes [1]	

change in our policy of early administration of antibiotics and operative management in the next organized trauma list, the deep infection rate has not increased; on the contrary, it has decreased although not to a statistically significant degree. Furthermore, timing of antibiotics and timing to theatre are not statistically correlated with the development of either deep or superficial infection. The grade of surgeon showed a trend of decreased infection rates with a consultant present; nevertheless, this was not statistically confirmed. It must be emphasized at the beginning of this discussion that we are not advocating delaying surgery in all cases. The most severe open long-bone fractures with associated neurovascular injury or tissue loss still remain a surgical emergency, and the current policy in the UK is to send all of these patients to a level 1 trauma centre.

The findings of this review are in agreement with our previously published results in 2007 where the conclusion of there being no significant correlation between the operation time (within or more than 6 h of injury) and the development of deep infection in patients with open long-bone fractures is held [3]. Several recent published studies convey the same conclusion. Crowley et al. [6] in their review paper commented on the lack of scientific evidence supportive of early surgery in open fractures, particularly with relation to the historical 6 h rule. Furthermore, Pollak

et al. [2] on their prospective study of 315 patients with open fractures concluded that time from injury to operative debridement is not a significant independent predictor of the risk of infection. Additionally, Sungaran et al. [7] recommended delaying surgery on open tibia fractures until optimal operating environment can be provided. This was on the basis of their study in which 161 open tibia fractures were divided into three groups depending on the time to theatre. Interestingly, five infections occurred in the early operated (within 6 h) group, whereas only one infection occurred in the 6–12 h group and none in the 12–24 h group [7].

A recent meta-analysis by Schenker et al. [8] did not identify an association between delayed debridement of open long-bone fractures and the post-operative development of either deep or superficial infection. In addition to the aforementioned studies where time to theatre has been shown not to correlate with infective complications, several authors have studied the effect of after-hours surgery on patient's morbidity and surgical outcome. More specifically, it has been suggested that after-hours surgery results in increased surgical complications, technical errors as well as increased reoperation rates [9–11]. Sleep deprivation and the subsequent decreased mental alertness and manual dexterity have been hypothesized to be responsible for these worse surgical outcomes during out-of-hours operating [10, 11].

The previously published data from our unit led to a change in our policy of managing open long-bone fractures. This change was in line with the most recent BOA/BAPRAS guidelines and reflected the need for early administration of intravenous antibiotics (within 3 h of admission) as well as performing surgical exploration and debridement only once the patient and surgical team were fully optimized, typically at the next consultant-led trauma list [4]. Comparing the results of the present study to our previously published data, it is of note that the deep infection rate has improved following the change in policy. More specifically, the deep infection rate in our previous study was found to be 8.5 % [3]. In the present study, the overall infection rate is 13.6 % with 4.3 % of infections being classified as deep. An improvement of 4.2 % in the deep infection rate occurred. It is of note that the change in the antibiotic policy resulted in a decrease in superficial infection rates but did not affect the deep infection rates as shown in Table 2. It is therefore suggested that the decrease in deep infection rates is not a result of the change in the administered antibiotic regime.

In cases where the most senior surgeon present was a consultant, the overall infection rates were 9.5 % as opposed to 16 % when the most senior surgeon was a non-consultant middle grade surgeon. Nevertheless, this trend was not statistically confirmed and was probably due to small number of patients in the sample. Harrison et al. [12] have recently investigated the effect of the grade of the surgeon in the development of deep infections following hip fracture surgery. The authors concluded that operations performed by a consultant or a hip fracture specialist had half the rate of the infection in comparison with non-consultant grades, and this was statistically confirmed [12]. Furthermore, Edwards et al. [13] have shown that more experienced surgeons have lower grade of infection in hip fracture surgery, but this was not statistically confirmed.

The strength of our study is that it is a retrospective review of a consecutive series on a large number of open long-bone fractures. The main limitation was that our study was underpowered as the desirable sample size to elicit a statistically significant difference at the deep infection rates was 834 fractures. We continue to collect data and may in future be able to statistically confirm any difference with larger numbers of patients. There are also many confounding factors which render the analysis of the reasons for any change in outcome difficult, such as age, patient co-morbidities, fracture configuration, mechanism of injury and surgical technique. Finally, 59 patients were lost to follow-up because of errors in data collection but most importantly because of transfer to a major trauma centre for further treatment. These cases transferred to a specialist unit were in the majority high-energy injuries with high Gustilo and Anderson grade.

Conclusion

We have investigated the infection rate in open long-bone fractures not associated with neurovascular injury or severe tissue loss following a change in our management policy from treating these injuries as soon as possible to treat them on the next available trauma list when appropriately trained nursing and medical staffs are available. The overall infection rate was 13.6 %, with 4.3 % deep infections and 9.3 % superficial. The deep infection rate before the change in the policy was 8.5 %. The improvement in the deep infections rate was not affected by the change in the antibiotics policy. We have not yet analysed our data for other outcomes, such as ultimate healing of the fracture, number of subsequent operations or outcome for the limb, but we are able to suggest that delaying the surgery in order to maximize the whole operative team has not resulted in an increased deep infection rate and would support continued application of the BOA/BAPRAS guidelines.

Acknowledgments No financial support was received for this study.

References

1. Charalambous CP, Siddique I, Zenios M, Roberts S, Samarji R, Paul A et al (2005) Early versus delayed surgical treatment of open tibial fractures: effect on the rates of infection and need of secondary surgical procedures to promote bone union. Injury 36(5):656–661 Epub 2005/04/14
2. Pollak AN, Jones AL, Castillo RC, Bosse MJ, MacKenzie EJ (2010) The relationship between time to surgical debridement and incidence of infection after open high-energy lower extremity trauma. J Bone Joint Surg Am. 92(1):7–15 Epub 2010/01/06
3. Al-Arabi YB, Nader M, Hamidian-Jahromi AR, Woods DA (2007) The effect of the timing of antibiotics and surgical treatment on infection rates in open long-bone fractures: a 9-year prospective study from a district general hospital. Injury. 38(8):900–905 Epub 2007/06/23
4. Nanchahal J, Nayagam S, Khan U, Moran C, Barrett S, Sanderson F, Pallister I (2009) Standards for the management of open fractures of the lower limb. A Short Guide. BOA/BAPRAS. ISBN: 978-1-85315-911-4
5. Horan TC, Gaynes RP, Martone WJ, Jarvis WR, Emori TG (1992) CDC definitions of nosocomial surgical site infections, 1992: a modification of CDC definitions of surgical wound infections. Infect Control Hosp Epidemiol 13(10):606–608 Epub 1992/10/01
6. Crowley DJ, Kanakaris NK, Giannoudis PV (2007) Debridement and wound closure of open fractures: the impact of the time factor on infection rates. Injury 38(8):879–889 Epub 2007/05/29
7. Sungaran J, Harris I, Mourad M (2007) The effect of time to theatre on infection rate for open tibia fractures. ANZ J Surg 77(10):886–888 Epub 2007/09/07
8. Schenker ML, Yannascoli S, Baldwin KD, Ahn J, Mehta S (2012) Does timing to operative debridement affect infectious complications in open long-bone fractures? A systematic review. J Bone Joint Surg Am 94(12):1057–1064 Epub 2012/05/11
9. Henriques JP, Haasdijk AP, Zijlstra F (2003) Outcome of primary angioplasty for acute myocardial infarction during routine duty hours versus during off-hours. J Am Coll Cardiol 41(12):2138–2142 Epub 2003/06/25
10. Taffinder NJ, McManus IC, Gul Y, Russell RC, Darzi A (1998) Effect of sleep deprivation on surgeons' dexterity on laparoscopy simulator. Lancet 352(9135):1191 Epub 1998/10/20
11. Ricci WM, Gallagher B, Brandt A, Schwappach J, Tucker M, Leighton R (2009) Is after-hours orthopaedic surgery associated with adverse outcomes? A prospective comparative study. J Bone Joint Surg Am 91(9):2067–2072 Epub 2009/09/03
12. Harrison T, Robinson P, Cook A, Parker MJ (2012) Factors affecting the incidence of deep wound infection after hip fracture surgery. J Bone Joint Surg Br 94(2):237–240
13. Edwards C, Counsell A, Boulton C, Moran CG (2008) Early infection after hip fracture surgery: risk factors, costs and outcome. J Bone Joint Surg Br 90(6):770–777 Epub 2008/06/10

9

The incidence of deep vein thrombosis and pulmonary embolism with the elective use of external fixators

David J. S. Roberts[1] · Anna Panagiotidou[2] · Matthew Sewell[3] · Peter Calder[3] · David Goodier[3]

Abstract Little evidence exists about the incidence of deep vein thrombosis (DVT) and pulmonary embolism (PE) with the use of external fixators. We investigated this in a cohort of 207 consecutive patients undergoing 258 elective frame applications by case note review. Case notes were obtained for 84 % of the sample population. The type of surgery, demographic data, thromboembolic risk factors and the incidence of DVT/PE were recorded. One patient experienced DVT (0.39 %) and one a PE (0.39 %). Both were of high risk and had received mechanical and chemical thromboprophylaxis during their inpatient stay. These complications were identified at least 3 months postoperatively. These findings help to more accurately counsel patients undergoing elective frame surgery on the risks of DVT/PE and also contribute to the discussion between surgeons about whether or not extended course chemical thromboprophylaxis would be of overall benefit.

✉ David J. S. Roberts
djsroberts@hotmail.com

Anna Panagiotidou
panagiotidou@btinternet.com

Matthew Sewell
matbuzz1@hotmail.com

Peter Calder
Peter.Calder@rnoh.nhs.uk

David Goodier
David.Goodier@rnoh.nhs.uk

[1] London North West Healthcare NHS Trust, Harrow, UK

[2] UCL Institute of Biomedical Engineering, London, UK

[3] The Royal National Orthopaedic Hospital, Stanmore, Stanmore, UK

Keywords Thrombosis · Prophylaxis · Frame · Elective · Incidence

Introduction

Deep vein thrombosis (DVT) and pulmonary embolism (PE) are potential complications of lower limb orthopaedic surgery, and reported rates vary widely (DVT 0.33–0.40 %, PE 0.04–0.22 %) [1, 2, 5, 7]. Little evidence exists about the incidence of DVT and PE with the use of external fixators. Sems et al. [3] reported that 3 of 143 (2.1 %) patients screened with duplex ultrasonography following frame application for the temporary stabilisation of complex lower limb fractures were found to have a DVT.

The National Institute of Health and Clinical Excellence (NICE) provides guidance for thromboprophylaxis in orthopaedic surgery with specific recommendations for hip and knee arthroplasty and for hip fractures. Chemical thromboprophylaxis is recommended for 28–35 days for hip arthroplasty and following hip fracture surgery and 10–14 days following knee replacement. For other forms of orthopaedic surgery besides hip and knee arthroplasty and hip fracture surgery NICE recommends that individual patients should be assessed for thrombotic risk factors and chemical thromboprophylaxis given if risk factors for DVT/PE are present [4].

No published work exists regarding DVT/PE incidence with the elective use of external fixators. The aim of this work is to establish the rate of DVT/PE in those undergoing elective treatment with external fixators in our practice.

Materials and methods

At the Royal National Orthopaedic Hospital, Stanmore, external fixators are used for elective surgery such as paediatric, adolescent and adult deformity correction and for treatment of fracture non-union. Thromboprophylaxis use is guided by the risk of thromboembolism and risk of bleeding in these cases with chemical thromboprophylaxis used only for individuals considered to be at high risk of thrombosis.

A database of individuals undergoing external fixator application by the senior authors is maintained prospectively. Information from this database and case notes were examined for consecutive patients from March 2005 to June 2011.

Occurrences of post-operative DVT or PE detected by ultrasound or CT angiogram were recorded. Risk factors for thromboembolism, type of thromboprophylaxis and time from end surgery to first dose of chemical thromboprophylaxis were also noted. Patient demographics (age, weight and height), indication for surgery, operation performed and length of operation were recorded. The length of operation was calculated as the period between the first incision of the surgeon and the time the patient left the operating theatre, both noted on the perioperative care record by theatre nursing staff. Although the time of surgeon completing the operation was not recorded, we considered our measure of length of operation time to be an acceptable estimate as the time between completion of surgery and the patient leaving operating theatre is typically five minutes or less.

Patients are counselled in clinic pre-operatively by a specialist nurse about practical and social aspects of undergoing treatment with an external fixator. The use of thromboprophylaxis in all cases was decided on individual risk factor assessment balanced with risk of bleeding. Where appropriate, a compression stocking and an intra-operative calf pump were used on the contralateral leg before, during and after surgery. Long surgical time as an isolated risk factor is not considered an indication for using chemical thromboprophylaxis by a senior author (PC). Mobilisation was commenced the morning after surgery and the majority of patients were permitted to bear weight fully as symptoms allowed.

The application of the external fixator was performed under general anaesthetic and fluoroscopic guidance without use of a tourniquet. Osteotomies, where needed, were made through small open incisions with multiple drill holes and completed in a controlled manner with an osteotome.

Results

Two hundred and seven patients underwent 258 consecutive primary applications of an Ilizarov, Taylor Spatial Frame (TSF) or monolateral fixator by one of the senior authors

(PC) in the study period. Data including the age of patient, indication for surgery, bone to which the frame was applied and type of fixator were available for all patients from the electronic database (Figs. 1, 2, 3, 4). Case notes were obtained for 176 individuals (84 %), representing 217 frame applications (85 %). In nine cases frames for correction of clubfoot deformity involved pins or wires in the foot with a frame bridging and immobilising the ankle. If an individual had bilateral application of external fixators under the same anaesthetic it was considered as two separate frame application events. We found no bleeding complications.

Two individuals were affected by DVT or PE. One had a DVT and one a PE, an overall isolated DVT rate of 1/258 (0.39 %) and PE rate of 1/258 (0.39 %). Considering only individuals aged 16 and older, the DVT rate was 1/183 (0.55 %) and PE 1/183 (0.55 %). In both cases, mechanical and chemical prophylaxis had been used.

Case 1

A 43-year-old male smoker was diagnosed with non-union of a femoral shaft fracture. The fracture was sustained in July 2008 and managed with intramedullary nail fixation. For the non-union he had an unsuccessful revision nailing and subsequent drilling with bone marrow injection. In February 2009 the nail was removed and plate fixation with formal bone autograft in May 2009 resulted in bony union.

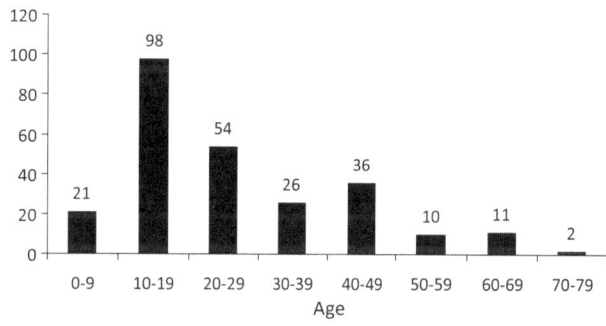

Fig. 1 Ages of those undergoing frame application

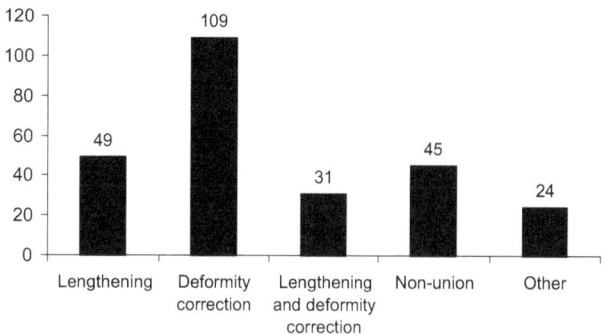

Fig. 2 Indications for surgery

Implants were removed and a unilateral external fixator was applied in January 2011 to correct shortening of the femur. He developed a DVT in April 2011 while the fixator was still in situ. He subsequently developed some symptoms of a post-phlebitic limb.

Case 2

A 44-year-old male smoker of high BMI with a diagnosis of recurrent adamantinoma underwent excision of the

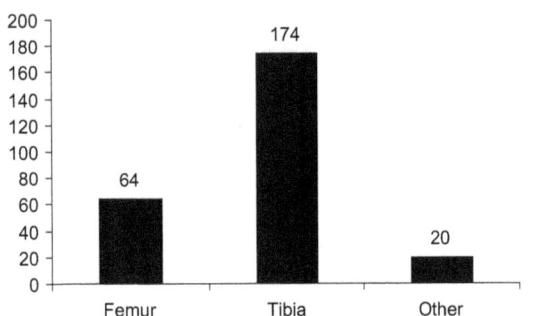

Fig. 3 Bone to which frame applied

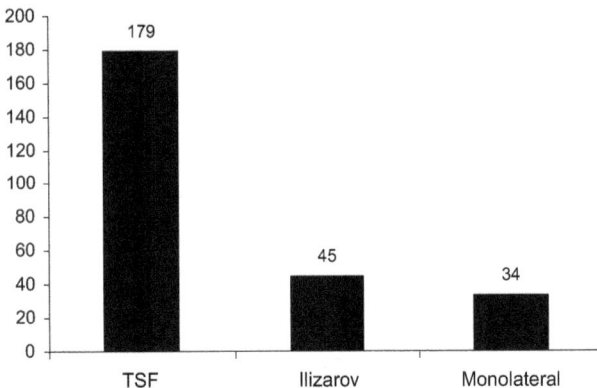

Fig. 4 Type of external fixator

Fig. 5 Length of procedure

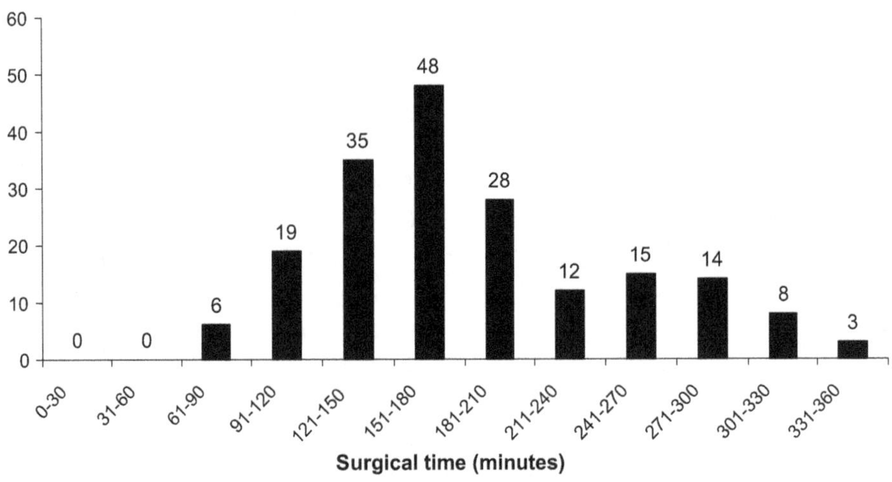

lateral tibial cortex tumour and medullary curettage in April 2010. Due to a recurrence in November 2010, a segmental diaphyseal excision and application of a TSF was performed for bone transport. In the last month of a 4-month course of frame treatment he experienced a PE with symptoms of mild shortness of breath which fully resolved. Of note, this man was resident overseas and throughout the course of his frame treatment made several flights of over 3 h between the UK and his home.

Other than surgical time (Fig. 5), 47 individuals had one risk factor, six had two, and three patients had three. Risk factors are summarised in Table 1.

Of the procedures for which records were obtained, patients received post-operative prophylactic dose low molecular weight heparin (LMWH) for 71 procedures. Forty of those who received LMWH had identifiable risk factors on review of case notes. Of the 31 without an identified risk factor, we have postulated the potential reason for the use of chemical thromboprophylaxis which is summarised in Table 2. If the first dose of chemical prophylaxis was more than 36 h post-operatively, the use of LMWH was thought to be due to prolonged immobility. For those with insufficient data to calculate a BMI, it was surmised that this was the risk factor for which LMWH was used. One individual had polio and another who underwent simultaneous application of an ipsilateral femoral and tibial frame may have been considered to be risks of thromboembolism.

Twenty patients were found to have risk factors for thrombosis but were not treated with chemical thromboprophylaxis, summarised in Table 3. Of 12 adults with high BMI, only three had a BMI over 40; four whose only risk factor was age > 60 were aged between 62 and 66. These cases of patients with a BMI and age close to the threshold of a risk of thrombotic event may not have had their risk status noted on clinical assessment.

Table 1 Risk factors for DVT/PE in our population

Risk factor	Incidence
Obesity (BMI > 30)	48
Previous DVT/PE	4
Recent travel over 2 h	1
Age 60 or greater	12
Thrombophilia	1
Recent/active cancer	2

Table 2 Summary of risk factors in patients treated with low molecular weight heparin (LMWH)

Those with thrombotic risk factors treated with LMWH	40
Those with no thrombotic risk factors treated with LMWH	31
Postulated[a] reason for LMWH treatment in those with no recorded risk factors	
Prolonged post-operative immobility	9
High BMI	10
Polio	1
No reason identified	11

[a] Following review of patient records

Table 3 Those individuals with risk factors for thrombosis not treated with LMWH

High BMI	12
High BMI, under 16 years old	3
Age over 60	4
High BMI and age over 60	1
Total	20

Subsequent to this study population, there have been two further cases of DVT/PE in patients treated with external fixators by the senior authors. These cases were not included in the above data, but their histories are included below (Cases 3 and 4) to help inform further discussion.

Case 3

A 53-year-old man with knee osteoarthritis secondary to malunion of a proximal tibial fracture sustained at age 26 underwent application of a Taylor Spatial Frame for deformity correction in November 2012. The frame was removed in March 2013. Three weeks after frame removal, calf swelling prompted an investigation and a DVT was found. Following a course of anticoagulant treatment he has no residual symptoms.

Case 4

A 30-year-old male smoker was treated with a unilateral fixator to lengthen a malunited femoral shaft fracture,

which had been sustained with other injuries in a traffic collision in August 2011. He developed multiple pulmonary emboli and respiratory symptoms for 3 days following osteotomy and application of fixator in October 2012. His symptoms fully resolved. It was noted that he had reduced mobility due to his accompanying injuries.

Discussion

The incidence of clinically significant DVT has been reported from 0.33 to 40 % with fatal PE 0.04–0.22 % in hip and knee arthroplasty [1, 2, 5, 6]. The incidence of DVT detected by screening with venogram or duplex ultrasound has been reported between 30 and 56 % [7, 8]. The work by Sems et al. [3] involved investigating all patients with duplex ultrasound following application of an external fixator as a temporary measure (2–3 weeks) in severe lower limb fractures. They found that 3 of 143 (2.1 %) patients screened with duplex ultrasonography following frame application were found to have a DVT. No bleeding complications from chemical thromboprophylaxis were experienced. This information has limited applicability to elective practice as external fixators were used in short-term stabilisation compared with the significantly longer-term use in elective surgical practice. Furthermore, trauma results in additional prothrombotic risks such as a high-energy insult to the limb, haemodynamic changes with its effect on coagulation and greater short-term immobility due to other injuries.

Efforts continue at our hospital to optimise thromboprophylaxis including optimal patient hydration, the use of mechanical thromboprophylaxis and optimal post-operative pain control to enable early mobilisation. One limitation of mechanical thromboprophylaxis in this group of patients is that the use of TEDS or intermittent compression stockings is impossible on the operated leg. Towards the end of our study period, a local Thromboprophylaxis Risk Assessment Prescribing Guide came into use and alternative tools for adolescents and children have been developed and are now used.

Limitations of this study are the retrospective collection of a significant proportion of the data, resulting in some cases of missing data. Of particular note, our postulated reasons for using chemical prophylaxis in the absence of identifiable risk factors as well as for not prescribing it for those with risk factors contribute to weakness of our data and analysis. Further confounding was from the chemical thromboprophylaxis prescription guided by individual patient factors, with some individuals given low molecular weight heparin and others not. Even so, there remains a lack of strong evidence for the routine use of chemical thromboprophylaxis in orthopaedic practice with a lack of consensus [4, 9, 10]. The aim of this work was to provide information in elective external fixator surgery to allow surgeons to inform patients of the risks of DVT and PE in this surgery and to highlight the need for further research and discussion between clinicians about appropriate thromboprophylactic regimes.

The two patients in our study population did not become symptomatic with DVT or PE until 3 months post-operatively although it is not possible to know when the clots began, whether at the time of surgery or months after discharge from hospital. One of the two additional presented cases outside our study population (Case 3) also experienced such a delay in presentation. Therefore, if an extended course chemical thromboprophylaxis was to be used in high-risk patients, these findings suggest that it would be required for at least 3 months. Although the number of patients in our study means it is one of the largest studies of DVT and PE in elective frame surgery, these numbers are insufficient for it to provide conclusive guidance on extended course. Larger studies are required.

Conclusion

A thromboembolic event was identified in two patients from a sample of 258 fixator applications in 207 patients. This produces an incidence of approximately 1 % of patients undergoing fixator surgery. Due to the heterogeneous manner in which prophylaxis was used, no specific conclusions can be made over the protection given by chemical or mechanical thromboprophylaxis.

Informed consent For this type of study formal patient consent is not required.

References

1. Clayton RAE, Gaston P, Watts AC, Howie CR (2009) Thromboembolic disease after total knee replacement: experience of 5100 cases. Knee 16:18–21
2. Howie C, Hughes H, Watts AC (2005) Venous thromboembolism associates with hip and knee replacement over a ten-year period. J Bone Joint Surg [Br] 87-B(12):1675–1680
3. Sems SA, Levy BA, Dajani K, Herrera DA, Templeman DC (2009) Incidence of deep venous thrombosis after temporary joint spanning external fixation for complex lower extremity injuries. J Trauma 66:1164–1166
4. No authors listed. Venous thromboembolism: reducing the risk: Reducing the risk of venous thromboembolism (deep vein thrombosis and pulmonary embolism) in patients admitted to hospital (CG92). http://publications.nice.org.uk/venous-thromboembolism-reducing-the-risk-cg92. Last accessed 29 September 2013
5. Murray DW, Britton AR, Bulstrode CJK (1996) Thromboprophylaxis and death after total hip replacement. J Bone Joint Surg [Br] 78-B(6):863–870
6. Imperiale TF, Speroff T (1994) A meta-analysis of methods to prevent venous thromboembolism following total hip replacement. JAMA 271:1780–1785
7. Maynard MJ, Sculco TP, Ghelman B (1991) Progression and regression of deep vein thrombosis after total knee arthroplasty. Clin Orthop 273:125–130
8. Kim YH, Oh SH, Kim JS (2003) Incidence and natural history of deep vein thrombosis after total hip arthroplasty. J Bone Joint Surg [Br] 85-B(5):661–665
9. http://www.aaos.org/Research/guidelines/VTE/VTE_summary_of_recs.pdf
10. Bozic KJ, Vail TP, Pekow PS, Maselli JH, Lindenauer PK, Auerbach AD (2010) Does aspirin have a role in venous thromboembolism prophylaxis in total knee arthroplasty patients? J Arthroplasty 25(7):1053–1060

10

Bone transport through an induced membrane in the management of tibial bone defects resulting from chronic osteomyelitis

Leonard Charles Marais[1] · Nando Ferreira[1]

Abstract Wide resection of infected bone improves the odds of achieving remission of infection in patients with chronic osteomyelitis. Aggressive debridement is followed by the creation of large bone defects. The use of antibiotic-impregnated PMMA spacers, as a customized dead space management tool, has grown in popularity. In addition to certain biological advantages, the spacer offers a therapeutic benefit by serving as a vehicle for delivery of local adjuvant antibiotics. In this study, we investigate the efficacy of physician-directed antibiotic-impregnated PMMA spacers in achieving remission of chronic tibial osteomyelitis. This retrospective case series involves eight patients with chronic osteomyelitis of the tibial diaphysis managed with bone transport through an induced membrane using circular external fixation. All patients were treated according to a standardized treatment protocol. A review of the anatomical nature of the disease, the physiological status of the host and the outcome of treatment in terms of remission of infection, time to union and the complications that occurred was carried out. Seven patients, with a mean bone defect of 7 cm (range 5–8 cm), were included in the study. At a mean follow-up of 28 months (range 18–45 months), clinical eradication of osteomyelitis was achieved in all patients without the need for further reoperation. The mean total external fixation time was 77 weeks (range 52–104 weeks), which equated to a mean external fixation index of 81 days/cm (range 45–107). Failure of the skeletal reconstruction occurred in one patient who was not prepared to continue with further reconstructive surgery and requested amputation. Four major and four minor complications occurred. The temporary insertion of antibiotic-impregnated PMMA appears to be a useful dead space management technique in the treatment of post-infective tibial bone defects. Although the technique does not appear to offer an advantage in terms of the external fixation index, it may serve as a useful adjunct in order to achieve resolution of infection.

Keywords Chronic osteomyelitis · Bone transport · Distraction osteogenesis · Induced membrane · Masquelet technique · Circular external fixation

Introduction

Wide resection of infected bone improves the odds of relapse-free periods in patients with chronic osteomyelitis. Aggressive debridement creates segmental bone defects. While small defects may be managed with acute shortening or cancellous bone grafting, larger segmental bone defects typically require bone transport with regeneration of the deficient bone segment through distraction osteogenesis [1]. The size of critical bone defect which by definition cannot be managed with cancellous bone graft remains controversial. Tiemann et al. [2] recommended 2 cm as the maximum size of a segmental diaphyseal tibial defect that should be managed with autologous cancellous grafting alone.

The induced membrane (Masquelet) technique, involving the placement of a polymethylmethacrylate (PMMA) spacer in the defect with subsequent bone grafting, has emerged as a useful adjunct in the management of large

✉ Leonard Charles Marais
Leonard.Marais@kznhealth.gov.za

[1] Tumor, Sepsis and Reconstruction Unit, Department of Orthopaedic Surgery, Greys Hospital, University of KwaZulu-Natal, Private bag X9001, Pietermaritzburg 3201, South Africa

defects. The induced membrane is highly vascularized and secretes several growth factors, including VEGF and BMP-2 [3]. Furthermore, extracts from the membrane have been shown to stimulate bone marrow cell proliferation and differentiation of progenitor cells to the osteoblast lineage [4]. These factors combine to facilitate successful consolidation of cancellous bone graft within an induced membrane in segmental tibial defects of up to 25 cm in length [5].

Distraction osteogenesis remains a method of choice for the management of bone defects in excess of 4 cm [6, 7]. The procedure offers several advantages in the scenario of post-osteomyelitis skeletal reconstruction, including the increase in regional blood flow for a period up to 17 weeks following the corticotomy [8]. Although bone transport can be achieved with various devices, circular external fixation in accordance with Ilizarov principles remains foremost due to its reliability, modularity and safety in the presence of infection.

The use of antibiotic-impregnated PMMA spacers, as a customized dead space management tool after debridement for chronic osteomyelitis, has grown in popularity [9, 10]. Apart from the biological advantages illustrated by Masquelet et al., the spacer offers potential therapeutic benefit as a vehicle for delivery of local adjuvant antibiotics. Physician-directed antibiotic-impregnated PMMA spacers have been shown to effectively elute antibiotics at the site of infection for up to several months following implantation [11]. This characteristic has been used to good effect in periprosthetic infections where staged reconstruction has been shown to be safe after removal of the spacer [12]. The biological, mechanical and therapeutic advantages offered by the Masquelet technique have prompted the use of antibiotic-impregnated PMMA spacers in larger segmental defects requiring bone transport.

The aim of this study was to determine whether the use of antibiotic-impregnated PMMA spacers followed by bone transport with circular external fixation is effective in achieving remission of infection following segmental resection in chronic tibial osteomyelitis. A secondary objective was to determine the external fixation index of these cases and to compare it to those of other authors using traditional Ilizarov methods.

Materials and methods

A retrospective review was conducted of all patients treated by bone transport through an induced membrane at our tertiary level limb reconstruction unit over a 4-year period between June 2009 and June 2013. All adult patients treated for a diaphyseal tibial bone defect by bone transport were included in the study. Patients were excluded if the standard treatment protocol was not completed. The subjects' charts were reviewed and data extracted in order to describe the patient demographics, cause of the bone defect, physiological status of the host in accordance with the Cierny and Mader classification system, relevant local and systemic risk factors, the number and nature of surgical procedures performed, time to union and, finally, the complications that occurred.

All patients were treated according to a standardized treatment protocol. Following comprehensive clinical, biochemical and radiological evaluation, patients were classified according to the Cierny and Mader classification system [13]. The initial surgical procedure included a wide resection of all necrotic and ischemic tissue to a well-perfused margin, insertion of an antibiotic-impregnated PMMA spacers in the resulting bone defect, reconstruction of the soft tissue defect with a local flap and application of a standard five ring circular fine wire external fixator capable of effecting bone transport (Fig. 1). The PMMA spacers were constructed from Palacos R+G® bone cement (Heraeus Medical, Hanau, Germany) containing 500 mg gentamicin per 40 mg of PMMA powder, mixed with 2 g of vancomycin powder per 40 mg of PMMA. In the majority of cases, the spacer was shaped outside the body and only inserted into the defect once it had hardened and most of the heat had dissipated. In later cases, the PMMA spacer was inserted before the cement had completely hardened, in order to allow the ends of the cement to overlap the bone ends.

Post-operatively, all patients were treated with generic parenteral antibiotics, in the form of vancomycin and meropenem, until results from 7-day microscopy, cultures and microbial antibiotic sensitivity (MCS) became available. Oral antibiotic therapy, tailored according to the results of culture and sensitivity, was then commenced and continued for a period of 6 weeks. During this initial period, the patient was allowed to mobilize partial weight-bearing in order to curtail disuse osteopenia. The second-stage procedure was performed after a minimum of 6 weeks from the index procedure and only if there was no clinical or biochemical evidence of ongoing infection as indicated by normal white blood cell count, C-reactive protein and erythrocyte sedimentation rate. The second-stage procedure involved removal of the spacer through an incision at the edge of the flap, debridement of the bone edges, as well as suturing of the incision made in the induced membrane. At the same sitting, a metaphyseal osteotomy was performed, according to the technique described by De Bastiani, in preparation for bone transport [14]. A latency period of 7 days was observed prior to commencement of bone transport which was performed according to standard Ilizarov principles of 0.25 mm distraction increments, four times per day [15]. During this

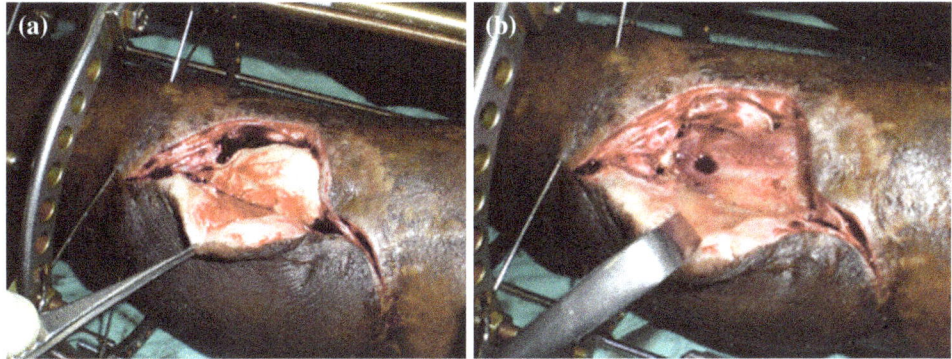

Fig. 1 **a** Antibiotic-impregnated PMMA spacer, which was inserted into the bone defect prior to soft tissue cover and stabilization. **b** Induced membrane at time of removal of the spacer

stage of the treatment protocol, full weight-bearing, with no more than a single crutch, was advocated.

Once the bone ends were brought into close apposition through bone transport, a formal docking procedure was performed in the form of a cancellous and Phemister-type bone graft [16]. No internal fixation of docking sites or regenerated segments was performed. Pin track care was performed according to a previously published protocol [17]. When three out of the four cortices of the regenerate were judged well formed on AP and lateral X-rays and the docking site had united, the circular fixator was removed. The external fixation index was defined as the total time of external fixation per centimetre of bone transport.

Ethical approval was obtained from the relevant ethics review board prior to commencement, and the study was performed in accordance with the pertinent ethical guidelines.

Results

The records of eight patients, who were referred to our unit with Cierny and Mader anatomical type IV chronic osteomyelitis of the tibial diaphysis, were reviewed. One patient, who did not complete the standard treatment protocol, was excluded from the study. The follow-up period for this case was <18 months. Of the remaining seven patients, chronic osteomyelitis occurred after treatment for open tibia fractures in six and the final patient developed contiguous osteomyelitis following an open reduction and intramedullary nail for failed non-operative management of a closed fracture of the tibia shaft.

The mean age of patients was 29 years (range 28–44 years), and the mean time from injury to referral to our unit was 3 months (ranging from 1 to 14 months). Systemic risk factors, namely hypoalbuminemia, substance-induced psychiatric disorder and cigarette smoking, were identified in five of the patients (Table 1). The mean

follow-up period in this series of patients was 28 months (range 18–45 months). The mean interval between the index (first stage) procedure and removal of the spacer and tibial osteotomy (second stage) was 12 weeks (range 9–28 weeks), and the mean time from the second-stage procedure to bone grafting of the docking site was 17 weeks (8–39 weeks).

Clinical resolution of infection was achieved in all patients as indicated by normal clinical and biochemical findings at last follow-up. The mean magnitude of the bone defect following debridement was 7 cm (range 5–8 cm). Leg length was restored to within 1 cm of the contralateral side in all of the cases. Union of the docking site and consolidation of the regenerated segment was achieved in all but one of the cases. This patient was poorly compliant with the follow-up, rehabilitation and circular fixator care programs; he requested an amputation 17 months after presentation. The median value of the total time spent in the circular external fixator was 77 weeks (ranging from 52 to 104 weeks), and the mean external fixation index was 81 days/cm (range 45–107).

Complications were common and occurred in six of the seven cases. Unplanned additional surgeries were required in two patients, and the circular external fixator of one patient was revised at the time of the formal docking procedure in order to create the optimal biomechanical environment for union at the docking site (Table 1). Four major complications occurred. Despite the fact that all soft tissue flaps were performed by a plastic surgeon, flap dehiscence occurred in two cases. A flexion contracture of the knee combined with an equinus contracture of the ankle occurred in one patient (who had an associated substance-induced psychotic disorder). These deformities necessitated extension of the circular external fixator frame across the knee and ankle joints to allow gradual correction (Fig. 2). In one patient, a fracture of the docking site occurred 1 year following removal of the circular fixator. This fracture was treated successfully with a second

Table 1 Risk factors, magnitude of bone defect, treatment intervals, follow-up duration and complications

Patient	Age	Systemic risk factors	Post-debridement bone defect (cm)	First to second stage (weeks)	Time in frame (weeks)	Fixator index (days/cm)	Follow-up period (months)	Complications
1	30	Substance-induced psychotic disorder	8	14	52	45	28	Knee flexion and ankle equinus contractures requiring unplanned reoperation
2	28	Hypoalbuminemia	5	28	77	107	30	Flap dehiscence, fracture of docking site requiring second external fixator
3	28	Smoking	7	11	104	104	45	Pin track sepsis necessitating removal of one wire (Checketts and Otterburn grade 3), 5° equinus contracture
4	39	None	8	13	80	70	41	None
5	29	None	6	12	58	67	21	New circular fixator with acute compression of docking site at formal docking
6	44	Poor compliance, smoking	8	n/a	n/a	n/a	21	Flap dehiscence, pin track sepsis (Checketts and Otterburn grade 2), patient eventually requested amputation
7	30	Smoking	5	9	58	81	18	Pin track sepsis (Checketts and Otterburn grade 2)

circular fixator combined with a fibula osteotomy; union occurred after 21 weeks in external fixation.

Four minor complications occurred. A functional range of motion of the adjacent joints was achieved in all but one patient with a residual equinus contracture of five degrees. Minor pin track infection (Checketts and Otterburn grade 2 and 3) was experienced in three cases and necessitated the removal of the offending wire in one of these patients [18]. The incidence of pin track sepsis did not appear to differ from a previous study involving circular fixation [19].

Discussion

Surgical resection of avascular bone should be considered a mainstay of treatment when embarking on a curative treatment strategy aimed at eradication of infection in patients with chronic osteomyelitis [6]. Systemic and local antibiotic therapy is considered to play an adjunctive role in this setting. The resection margin, which can be thought of in oncological terms as being either marginal or wide, has been shown to affect the outcome. Wide resection margins, in comparison with marginal resection, have been shown to decrease the recurrence of infection and improve cure rates [20–22]. Wide resection of all avascular bone creates large bone defects and necessitates the implementation of an appropriate dead space management strategy [23].

The management of post-infective bone defects is dependent on several factors including the host's physiological status, the size of the defect, duration of the defect (i.e. acute or chronic), quality of the surrounding soft tissue, the presence of deformity, joint contracture/instability or limb length discrepancy, as well as the experience of the surgeon. Smaller defects may be treated by autologous bone graft [24]. The size of a segmental bone defect that should be considered critical, and thus not suitable for autologous cancellous bone grafting, remains controversial. Traditionally, 4 cm has been recommended as the cut-off point [1, 25]. The main concern with cancellous bone grafting of larger bone defects is its dependence on the surrounding soft tissues for incorporation. Large grafts may undergo central necrosis in the absence of an excellent soft tissue envelope [2]. Secondly, the regenerated segment may be weak and prone to fracture as a result of partial graft resorption [26]. As a result, it has been recommended that the length of a segmental diaphyseal tibial defect that can be managed with autologous cancellous grafting should not exceed 2 cm [14].

Masquelet et al. redefined the role of cancellous bone grafting in limb reconstruction by taking advantage of the mechanical and biological characteristics of the induced membrane. They reported the successful use of this technique in 35 cases, with defects ranging from 4 to 25 cm [3]. These results appear to be reproducible, with others reporting 90 % union rates of large defects (average size 5.8 cm) through the use of reamer–irrigation–aspiration graft [27]. Richards et al. [28] also utilized a modification of this technique in the management of bone loss following open fractures. Through the use of form-fitting spacers and

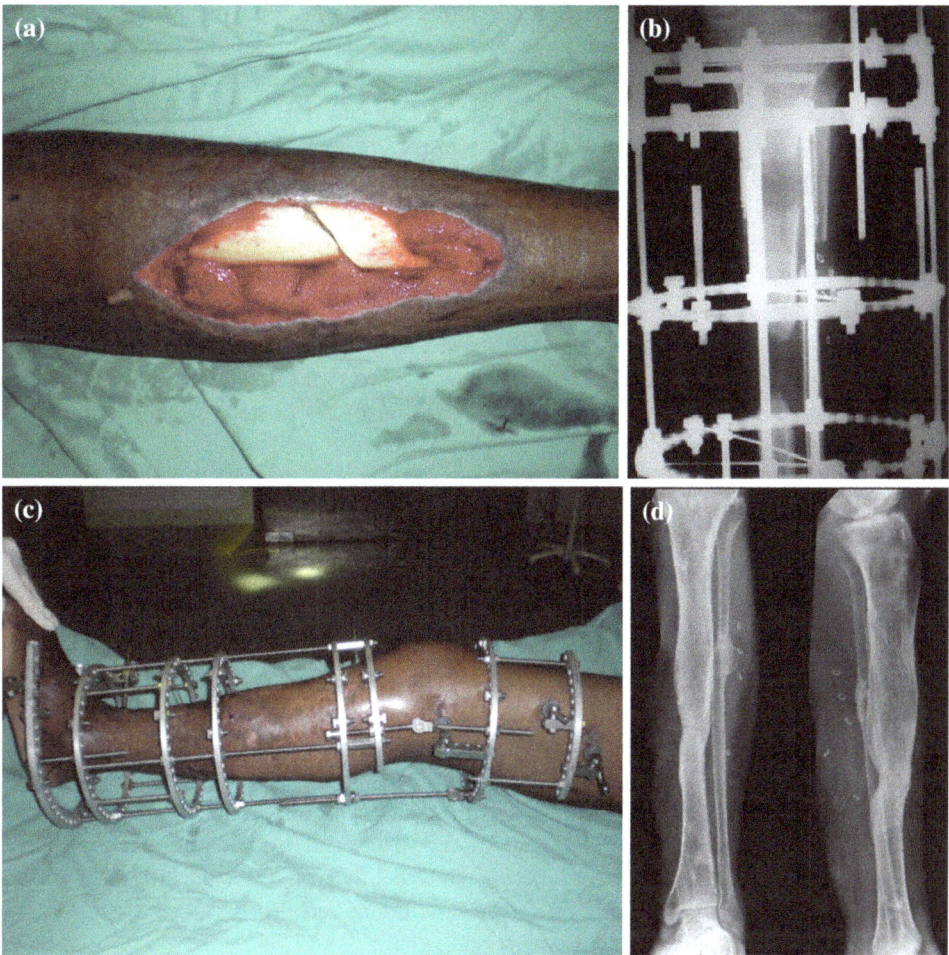

Fig. 2 Clinical and radiological features of a case complicated by knee flexion and equinus contractures. **a** Wound dehiscence following open reduction and intramedullary nailing of a neglected tibia fracture. **b** Distraction osteogenesis following removal of the PMMA spacer. **c** Gradual correction of the knee and ankle deformities. **d** Final radiographs showing satisfactory consolidation of the regenerate and union at docking site

subsequent autogenous bone grafting, the authors were able to achieve union in 18 out of 18 patients with bone defects involving a minimum of 50 % of the circumference of the tibia, ranging in size from 2 to 16 cm (average 4 cm).

Although the induced membrane technique offers several theoretical and practical advantages, caution should be applied in the use of cancellous bone graft in defects exceeding 4 cm [14]. Furthermore, the classic Masquelet technique, involving cancellous grafting onto the induced membrane, appears to deliver more predictable results in the presence of pre-existing periosteal new bone formation at the margins of the defect. In their original series, Masquelet et al. [3] reported that some of the patients required repeated bone grafts and that fracture occurred in four of the 35 cases. In their subsequent, prospective series that involved the adjunctive use of BMP-7, three of the eight patients with segmental defects developed deformities and another patient required amputation. Although Stafford et al. reported a high union rate, 80 % of their patients received BMP in addition to bone graft, only nail or plate fixation was used and seventeen of the 25 defects were ≤4 cm in size [18]. Richards et al. reported excellent results with the use of form-fitting spacers in the management of post-traumatic bone loss, but only two of their eighteen patients had circumferential bone loss and all fractures were treated with nail and plate fixation.

PMMA spacers offer several potential advantages in the setting of post-infective reconstruction. Bone transport through scar tissue, using more traditional Ilizarov techniques, can be particularly problematic. The use of temporary PMMA spacers prevents soft tissue impingement between the leading edge of the transport segment and the target segment. As illustrated in an animal model, the induced membrane prevents protrusion of adjacent soft tissue and neurovascular structures into the defect and adheres to the resected bone edges without collapse despite removal of the spacer, thus delineating a cavity corresponding to the volume of the retrieved cement spacer [6, 29]. This so-called spacer effect can be utilized in the reconstruction of bone defects where the resulting cylindrical cavity forms a stable envelope through which a bone segment may be transported.

As a result of the biological, therapeutic and mechanical advantages offered, and supported by the positive results reported in periprosthetic infections, antibiotic-impregnated PMMA spacers appear to be an attractive option in the management of other Cierny and Mader anatomical type IV infections associated with a bone defect. A case report where a similar technique, involving the use of a PMMA spacer with subsequent distraction osteogenesis, was used in the management of an infected open fracture is published [10]. The authors made use of a monolateral external fixator for bone transport. Circular external fixation was preferred in our series due to its modularity, minimally invasive nature and ability to effect bone transport and deformity correction (as illustrated in the case which developed joint contractures). The attributes of fine wire external fixators may also offer theoretical advantages in terms of bone healing. This stems from the three-dimensional stability combined with the low axial stiffness exhibited by fine wire circular external fixators [30, 31]. In addition, meta-analysis has shown that the Ilizarov method of distraction osteogenesis significantly reduces the risk of deep infection in infected osseous lesions [32].

Spiegl et al. [9] have published a series of cases where segmental bone defects as a result of chronic tibial osteitis were managed with PMMA spacers and subsequent distraction osteogenesis. The authors report an average overall treatment time of 93 weeks. Complications were common, and infection requiring reoperation occurred in 28 % of cases at 2-year follow-up. In our series of cases, the technique of bone transport through an induced membrane was confirmed to be a useful option for reconstruction of post-infective tibial defects in excess of 4 cm. Remission of infection was achieved in all cases without the need for reoperation for infection. This is, however, also a function of patient selection, and only Cierny and Mader type A and B hosts were considered suitable candidates for this procedure. The improved cure rates in our series may be the result of judicious patient selection rather than technical prowess. Union of the docking site and consolidation of the regenerated segment was achieved in all but one of the cases (who elected to have an amputation). Traditional Ilizarov methods, involving monofocal strategies without spacers, have been noted to produce external fixation indices of up to 50 days/cm [33, 34]. Considering the high external fixation index in our series (mean 81 days/cm), as well as the 57 days/cm reported by Speigl et al. [9], it appears that the use of PMMA spacers necessitate an increased period of external fixation. This may partly be explained by the time spent awaiting the formation of the induced membrane prior to initiation of bone transport.

There was a high rate of complications in our series. Spiegl et al. [9] had a similar experience with this technique, reporting 22 minor and 13 major complications (including one amputation) in their series of 19 cases. Interestingly, internal fixation of the docking site was performed in 16 of their 25 patients. The authors emphasized the challenging nature of the technique and stated that the procedure places considerable physical and emotional stress on the patient. The frequency of complications may be a reflection of the complexity of the cases involved but may also be related to the technical demands of the procedure.

There are several limitations to this study: its retrospective nature; a small sample size and short follow-up period; as well as the lack of a control group involving traditional Ilizarov-type bone transport. The Masquelet technique is still relatively new and many questions remain. Further investigation is required regarding the possibility of improved union at the docking site related to the biological advantages offered by the induced membrane. This will require a control group of cases managed without PMMA spacers. Our knowledge of certain technical aspects is still evolving. The optimal time for removal of the spacer and initiation of bone transport remains unclear. Internal fixation of the docking site may possibly also offer additional benefit [9].

Conclusion

The temporary insertion of a PMMA appears to be a useful dead space management technique in the treatment of post-infective tibial bone defects. Although the technique does not appear to offer an advantage in terms of the external fixation index, it may serve as a useful adjunct in achieving resolution of infection. Patient selection, however, appears to be a crucial step in ensuring a remission of tibial osteomyelitis.

Acknowledgments The corresponding author has received a research Grant from the South African Orthopaedic Association for research in the field of chronic osteomyelitis.

References

1. Lasanianos NG, Kanakaris NK, Giannoudis PV (2009) Current management of long bone large segmental defects. Orthop Trauma 24(2):149–163
2. Tiemann AH, Schmidt HGK, Braunschweig R, Hofmann GO (2009) Strategies for the analysis of osteitic bone defects at the diaphysis of long bones. Strateg Trauma Limb Reconstr 4:13–18

3. Masquelet AC, Begue T (2010) The concept of induced membrane for reconstruction of long bone defects. Orthop Clin N Am 41:27–37

4. Viateau V, Bensidhoum M, Guillemin G et al (2010) Use of the induced membrane technique for bone tissue engineering purposes: animal studies. Orthop Clin N Am 41:49–56

5. Masquelet AC, Fitoussi F, Begue T, Muller GP (2000) Reconstruction of the long bones by the induced membrane and spongy autograft. Ann Chir Plast Esthet 45(3):346–353

6. Rodner CM, Browner BD, Pestani E (2002) Chronic osteomyelitis. In: Browner B (ed) Skeletal trauma, 1st edn. Saunders, Philadelphia, pp 483–506

7. El-Gammal TA, Shiha AE, El-Deen MA, El-Sayed A, Kotb MM, Addosooki AI et al (2008) Management of traumatic tibial defects using free vascularized fibula or Ilizarov bone transport: a comparative study. Microsurgery 28:339–346

8. Aronson J (1994) Temporal increases in blood flow during distraction osteogenesis. Clin Orthop 301:124–131

9. Spiegl U, Pätzold R, Friederichs J, Hungerer S, Militz M, Bühren V (2013) Clinical course, complication rate and outcome of segmental resection and distraction osteogenesis after chronic tibial osteitis. Injury 44:1049–1056

10. Uzel A-P, Lemonne F, Casoli V (2010) Tibial segmental bone defect reconstruction by Ilizarov type bone transport in an induced membrane. Orthop Traumatol Surg Res 96:194–198

11. Anagnostakos K, Kelm J, Regitz T et al (2005) In vitro evaluation of antibiotic release from and bacteria growth inhibition by antibiotic-loaded acrylic bone cement spacers. J Biomed Mater Res B Appl Biomater 72(2):373–378

12. Anagnostakos K, Fürst O, Kelm J (2006) Antibiotic-impregnated PMMA hip spacers. Acta Orthop 77(4):628–637

13. Cierny G, Mader JT, Penninck JJ (1985) A clinical staging system for adult Osteomyelitis. Contemp Orthop 10:17–37

14. De Bastiani G, Aldegheri R, Renzi-Brivio L, Trivella G (1987) Limb lengthening by callus distraction (callotasis). J Pediatr Orthop 7:129–134

15. Shortt N, Keenan GF (2006) Ilizarov and trauma reconstruction. Curr Orthop 20:59–71

16. Phemister D (1947) Treatment of ununited fractures by onlay bone grafts without screw or tie fixation and without breaking down the fibrous union. J Bone Joint Surg Am 29(4):946–960

17. Ferreira N, Marais LC (2012) Prevention and management of external fixator pin tract sepsis. Strateg Trauma Limb Reconstr 7:67–72

18. Checketts RG, MacEachern AG, Otterburn M (2000) Pin track infection and the principles of pin site care. In: Goldberg A, De Bastiani A, Graham Apley A (eds) Orthofix external fixation in trauma and orthopaedics. Springer, Berlin, pp 97–103

19. Ferreira N, Marais LC (2012) Pin tract sepsis: incidence with the use of circular fixators in a limb reconstruction unit. SA Orthop J 11(1):10–18

20. Spellberg B, Lipsky BA (2012) Systemic antibiotic therapy for chronic osteomyelitis in adults. Clin Infect Dis 54(3):393–407

21. Simpson AH, Deakin M, Latham JM (2001) Chronic osteomyelitis. The effect of the extent of surgical resection on infection-free survival. J Bone Joint Surg Br 83:403–407

22. Atway S, Nerone VS, Springer KD, Woodruff DM (2012) Rate of residual osteomyelitis after partial foot amputation in diabetic patients: a standardized method for evaluating bone margins with intraoperative culture. J Foot Ankle Surg 51:749–752

23. Cierny G (2011) Surgical treatment of osteomyelitis. Plast Reconstr Surg 127(Suppl 1):190S–204S

24. Roa N, Ziran BH, Lipsky BA (2011) Treating osteomyelitis: antibiotics and surgery. Plast Reconstr Surg 127(Suppl):177S–187S

25. Tiemann AH, Hofmann GO (2009) Principles of the therapy of bone infection in adult extremities. Strateg Trauma Limb Reconstr 4:57–64

26. Masquelet AC (2003) Muscle reconstruction in reconstructive surgery: soft tissue repair and long bone reconstruction. Langenbecks Arch Surg 388:344–346

27. Stafford PR, Norris BL (2010) Reamer–irrigator–aspirator bone graft and bi Masquelet technique for segmental bone defect nonunions: a review of 25 cases. Injury 41(Suppl 2):S72–S77

28. Richard MJ, Creevy WR, Tornetta P (2012) The use of solid form-fitting antibiotic cement spacers in bone loss of the lower extremity. Curr Orthop Prac 23(5):453–457

29. Viateau V, Guillemin G, Yang YC et al (2004) A technique for creating critical-size defects in the metatarsus of sheep for use in investigation of healing of long-bone defects. Am J Vet Res 65:1653–1657

30. Cunningham JL (2001) The biomechanics of fracture fixation. Curr Orthop 15:457–464

31. Roberts CS, Antoci V, Antovi V Jr, Voor MJ (2005) The effect of transfixion wire crossing angle on the stiffness of fine wire external fixation: a biomechanical study. Injury 36:1107–1112

32. Papakostidis C, Bhandari M, Giannoudis PV (2013) Distraction osteogenesis in the treatment of long bone defects of the lower limbs. Effectiveness, complications and clinical results; a systematic review and meta-analysis. Bone Joint J 95-B:1673–1680

33. Paley D (1990) Problems, obstacles and complications of limb lengthening by Ilizarov technique. Clin Orthop 250:81–104

34. Kristiansen LP, Steen H (2001) Reduced lengthening index by use of bifocal osteotomy in the tibia. Acta Orthop Scan 73(1):92–97

11

Retrospective analysis of extra-articular distal humerus shaft fractures treated with the use of pre-contoured lateral column metaphyseal LCP by triceps-sparing posterolateral approach

Yatinder Kharbanda[1] · Yashwant Singh Tanwar[1] · Vishal Srivastava[2] ·
Vikas Birla[1] · Ashok Rajput[2] · Ramsagar Pandit[1]

Abstract Management of extra-articular distal humerus fractures presents a challenge to the treating surgeon due to the complex anatomy of the distal part of the humerus and complicated fracture morphology. Although surgical treatment has shown to provide a more stable reduction and alignment and predictable return to function, it has been associated with complications like iatrogenic radial nerve palsy, infection, non-union and Implant failure. We in the present series retrospectively analysed 20 patients with extra-articular distal humerus shaft fractures surgically treated using the extra-articular distal humeral locking plate approached by the triceps-sparing posterolateral approach. The outcome was assessed using the DASH score, range of motion at the elbow and the time to union. The mean time to radiographic fracture union was 12 weeks.

Keywords Distal humerus fracture · Extra-articular distal humerus LCP · Posterolateral approach humerus

Introduction

Extra-articular fractures of the distal humeral shaft are relatively rare injuries and have been in the limelight owing to a higher incidence of radial nerve injuries, as well as the dilemmas surrounding their management [1, 2]. Both conservative and surgical treatment options exist for these fractures, with the ideal treatment still being debatable. Bracing has been an acceptable option for humeral shaft fractures; however, in the distal third of the humerus in adults it can cause problems owing to difficulty in controlling angulation. Sarmiento reported his results of functional bracing for comminuted extra-articular fractures of the distal third humerus. There was varus deformity averaging 9 degrees in 81% of patients, but loss of range of movement was minimal and functional results were good [3]. However, O'Driscoll et al. [4] showed that cubitus varus deformity secondary to supracondylar malunion or congenital deformity of the distal part of the humerus may not always be a benign condition and may have important long-term clinical implications including tardy posterolateral instability.

Although surgical treatment seems to provide a more reliable and predictable alignment and potentially quicker return of function, iatrogenic radial nerve palsy is a cause of major concern [5]. If the decision to proceed to surgical intervention has been made, then plate osteosynthesis is the usual standard option [6]. The classical teaching for fixation of a humeral shaft fracture has been with a narrow/broad 4.5 mm low-contact dynamic compression plate, purchasing a minimum of eight cortices (i.e. 4 screws) on either side of the fracture zone or at least six cortices (3 screws) on either side if a lag screw has been used [6]. This, however, becomes difficult to achieve in distal humeral shaft fractures owing to the limited space available distally, as well as the curved shape of the distal humerus when approaching anteriorly and the presence of the olecranon fossa posteriorly (Fig. 1). Double-column plating using two 3.5-mm plates in orthogonal or parallel patterns is another

✉ Yashwant Singh Tanwar
tanwar_yashwant@yahoo.co.in

[1] Department of Orthopedics, Apollo Hospital, HNo299, Pocket B, DDA Flats, Sarita Vihar, New Delhi, Delhi 110076, India

[2] Department of Orthopedics, Dr. RML Hospital and PGIMER, New Delhi, Delhi 110001, India

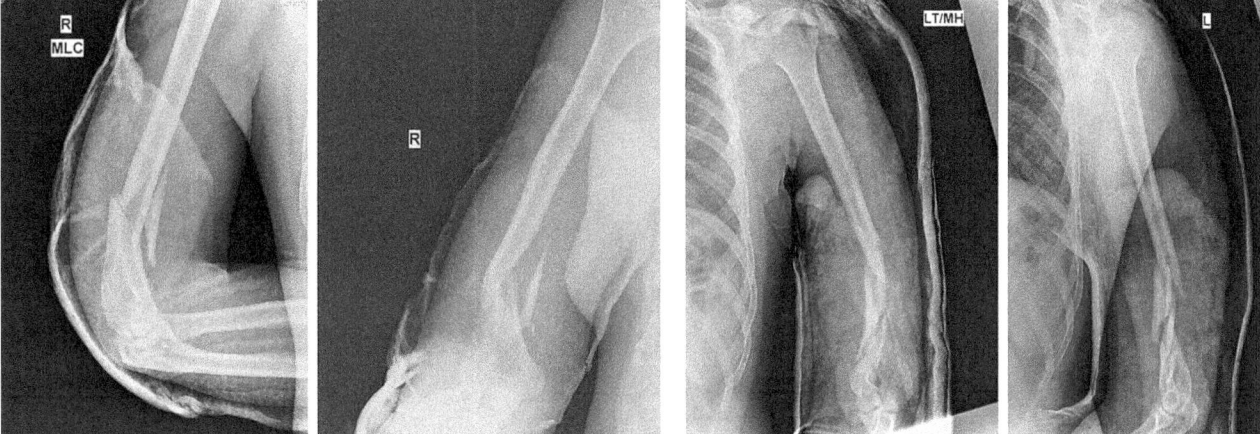

Fig. 1 Showing AP and lateral views of X-rays with low distal humeral "extra articular" fracture

option [7], but it requires greater soft tissue stripping and exposure, leading to a potentially higher non-union and infection rate and elbow stiffness reported in some series [5, 8].

In the present retrospective case series, we present our clinical experience with use of a single column pre-contoured extra-articular distal humeral locking compression plate (J plate Synthes, Solothurn, Switzerland) for treatment of extra-articular distal humeral fractures. It was a retrospective study aimed to evaluate the clinical and radiographic results after fixation of fractures of the distal humerus shaft with this single column system.

Materials and methods

Implant

3.5-mm LCP (Locking Compression Plate) extra-articular distal humerus plate (AO Synthes) is an anatomically shaped and angular stable fixation system for extra-articular fractures of the distal humerus. Distally, the plate accepts five 3.5-mm locking screws and is tapered to minimize soft tissue irritation and the screw hole density is greater to allow larger number of screws to be placed in the distal fragment (Fig. 2). The two most distal screw holes are angled towards the capitellum and trochlea, which allows longer locking screws to be placed distally. Proximally, the thickness of the plate is based on LCP 4.5/5.0, narrow and has combi-holes. Locking screws create a fixed-angle construct, providing angular stability, whereas the combi-holes can be used to provide inter-fragmentary or dynamic axial compression. As the plates are anatomically contoured, there are different plates for the right and left sides and it is available from 4 hole (122 mm) to 14 (302 mm) hole length.

Patients

Between Sept 2010 to Feb 2013, 20 patients with metaphyseal extra-articular distal humerus fractures—AO Type 12 A/B/C—were treated at our institution using the EADHP (Table 1). Inclusion criteria for the patients were: fractures of the distal humeral shaft which could not be fixed with conventional LCDCP's with minimum of six/eight cortices distally, age >18 years, closed fractures of the distal humeral shaft, with or without radial nerve palsy, recent fractures and non-unions. Patients who did not satisfy these inclusion criteria were not included in the study. All the surgeries were performed by the same senior author (YK) at one institution only.

Clinical outcome was assessed using Disabilities of the Arm, Shoulder and Hand (DASH) score and the range of motion of the elbow joint for each patient. The union was assessed clinically and radiologically; clinically by absence of pain and tenderness on palpation and range of motion at elbow joint, ability to perform activities of daily living without pain. Anteroposterior and lateral radiographs were done, and the healing progress of the distal humerus fracture was assessed. Union was defined by the absence of fracture line or bridging of the fracture site on at least 3 of the 4 cortices and the absence of implant loosening or failure.

Surgical technique

Patient is placed in the lateral position under general anaesthesia, with the arm hanging by the side. A triceps-reflecting posterolateral approach of Gerwin et al. [9] is utilized to expose the fracture site. After performing a midline skin incision on the posterior aspect of arm, full thickness flaps are developed on the lateral side (Fig. 3). On the lateral side, using blunt dissection, the lower lateral

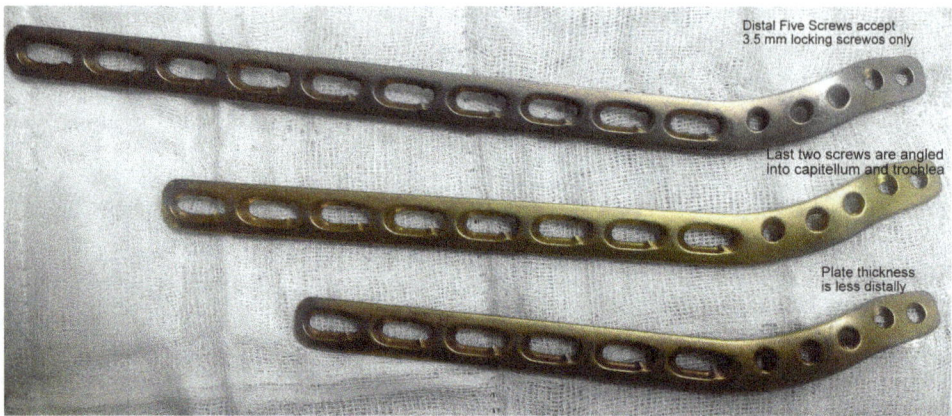

Fig. 2 Extra-articular distal humerus plate

cutaneous nerve of the arm is identified and its origin traced to the radial nerve (Fig. 4). The triceps is elevated from the lateral inter-muscular septum and the lateral supracondylar ridge, and the radial nerve is then carefully dissected (Fig. 5). After adequate fracture visualization, reduction clamps are used to reduce the fracture fragments. Provisional fixation is achieved with K wires, and lag screws are used wherever possible to increase the strength of the construct and achieve adequate compression in spiral fractures (Fig. 6). Finally, the Synthes TM extra-articular distal humerus plate is applied over the posterior surface of humeral shaft and fixed with locking screws distally and a combination of cortical and locking screws proximally. The plate is positioned so that its shaft portion is located centrally on the posterior aspect of the humerus, while the distal end curved along the posterior aspect of the lateral column (Fig. 7). Plate bending is required in some cases for better seating of the plate to the bone surface. Postoperatively, the patient is placed in a soft dressing and arm pouch sling and early range of motion of the elbow, wrist and shoulder is started.

Results

It was retrospective study of 20 patients with extra-articular distal humeral shaft fractures who were operated using the EADHP system from Sept 2011 to May 2014. Patients age, sex, mode of injury, interval between injury and surgery, status of radial nerve, associated injuries, time to union and elbow range of motion were noted. The final DASH score was measured at 1 year. Additional support in the form of elbow brace/plaster-of-paris cast/slab was not used in any of the patients. The average age of the patients at the time of surgery was 44 years (range 31–56 years) with 13 males and 7 females. The most common mode of injury was road traffic accidents (11 patients), followed by fall from height

(9 patients) and 2 had non-union. Two patients had associated radial nerve palsy, but intra-operatively the nerve was found to be intact in both the cases and nerve function recovered with time (Fig. 8). Three patients sustained additional injuries; two had an ipsilateral radial fracture, while one had an ipsilateral tibial shaft fracture. Eighteen patients were operated within 5 days of injury, whereas the other two had non-union following conservative management and were operated at 3 and 4 month interval, respectively.

The mean time to radiographic fracture union was 12 weeks (range 10–18 weeks) (Fig. 9). ROM and DASH scores are presented in Table 1. At final follow-up, the mean flexion was 125° and only one patient had a flexion deformity of 5°. The mean DASH score at 1 year was 17.6 ranging from 13.3 to 38.3 points. The normal DASH score in the general population has been reported to be around 10 with a standard deviation of 14.68 [10]. There were no patients with secondary loss of reduction at the fracture site, non-union, ulnar nerve problems, superficial or deep infection. The most common fracture pattern was spiral: AO type 12 A1 (simple spiral): three cases; B1 (wedge spiral): nine cases; C1 (comminuted spiral): three cases. Lag screws (ranging from 1 to 5) were used in all the cases. Eight hole plate length was used in the majority of the cases (18 out of 20), and in the rest ten hole plate was used. A total of 3–4 screws were used for proximal fixation, and 5–6 were used for distal fixation (Fig. 9).

Discussion

Open reduction and internal fixation of distal humeral shaft fractures is increasingly becoming an acceptable treatment modality. [5, 11–14] Options for internal fixation include intramedullary nailing and plate osteosynthesis either with double-column plating or a single column plate applied on

Table 1 Showing the different variables which were observed

Sr no.	Age	Sex	Mode of injury	Radial nerve	Time interval between injury and surgery in days	Associated injuries	Follow-up duration in months	Dash score at 1 year	Time to union in weeks	Elbow flexion	Elbow pronation supination	AO type	Number of lag screws	Plate length combi-holes	Proximal fixation	Distal fixation
1	31	F	Fall	Intact	1	Nil	24	14.2	12	0–130	85/85	12B2	2	8 Hole	3	5
2	42	M	Fall	Intact	2	Nil	15	13.3	16	0–140	80/80	12 A2	1	8 Hole	3	3
3	38	M	RTA	Intact	1	Ipsilateral shaft radius and ulna	18	15	16	0–120	80/75	12C1	3	8 Hole	3	5
4	56	F	RTA	Intact	4	Nil	38	18.3	18	0–135	90/85	12C1	3	10 Hole	3	5
5	62	M	Fall	Intact	2	Ipsilateral radius fracture	30	23.3	15	0–125	80/85	12B1	3	8 Hole	4	5
6	50	M	Fall	Neuropraxia	1	Nil	22	30	12	5–120	75/80	12C1	5	10 Hole	4	6
7	44	M	RTA	Intact	120	Nil	29	18.3	16	0–130	75/75	12B1	2	8 Hole	3	5
8	48	F	RTA	Intact	3	Nil	40	17.5	12	0–135	80/80	12B1	3	8 Hole	4	5
9	39	M	Fall	Intact	5	Ipsilateral tibia fracture	12	18.3	12	0–120	80/85	12A1	2	8 Hole	3	5
10	54	F	RTA	Intact	2	Nil	20	20	12	0–120	85/90	12C1	3	8 Hole	3	5
11	49	F	RTA	Intact	1	Nil	17	19.2	16	0–115	85/85	12B1	2	8 Hole	3	5
12	56	M	RTA	Neuropraxia	1	Nil	28	31.7	16	0–110	75/80	12B1	3	8 hole	3	6
13	37	M	Fall	Intact	2	Nil	33	15.8	10	0–130	90/90	12A1	3	8 Hole	3	5
14	33	M	RTA	Intact	2	Nil	42	15	12	0–130	90/90	12B1	2	8 Hole	3	5
15	52	M	Fall	Intact	1	Nil	22	14.2	18	0–120	85/90	12B1	3	8 Hole	3	5
16	46	M	Fall	Intact	2	Nil	21	12.5	12	0–125	90/90	12B2	2	8 Hole	3	5
17	40	F	RTA	Intact	90	Nil	18	16.7	16	0–115	85/85	12B1	3	10 Hole	4	5
18	35	F	RTA	Intact	2	Nil	32	15	12	0–130	90/90	12A1	2	8 Hole	3	5
19	37	M	Fall	Intact	1	Nil	36	11.7	12	0–135	90/90	12A2	1	8 Hole	3	5
20	32	M	RTA	Intact	1	Nil	15	12.5	12	0–125	85/80	12B1	2	8 Hole	4	5

the posterior or posterolateral side. Biomechanical studies have shown superior bending properties of humeral fractures fixed with a plate and screw system versus intramedullary devices. Also, the distal fragment is short and the medullary canal is narrow, rendering it difficult to perform nail osteosynthesis in distal third fractures [15].

Dual plating although offers a better biomechanical strength [16] does so at the expense of greater soft tissue

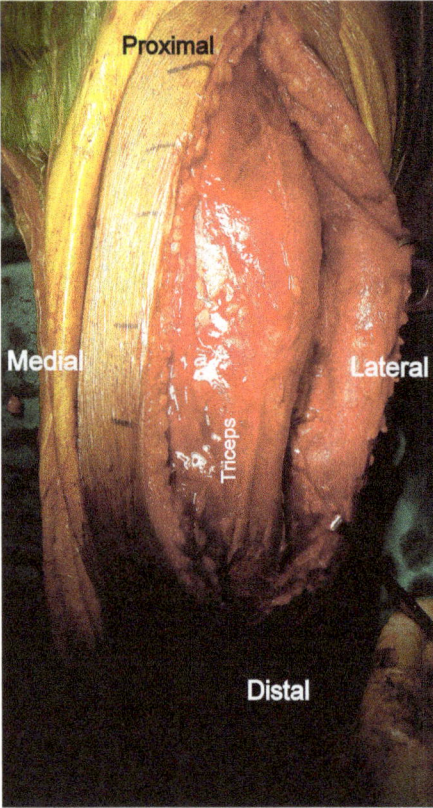

Fig. 3 Midline skin incision and elevation of full thickness lateral flap

dissection. It requires almost circumferential exposure of both the medial and lateral column. Such an enormous soft tissue dissection and exposure although justifiable for intraarticular fractures seems unreasonable for extra-articular shaft fractures. Preservation of the soft tissue envelope is an important aspect in fracture healing, and it has led to the change in the earlier concept of anatomic reduction and rigid fixation [17]. This concept is no longer valid for most of the extra-articular fractures with complex fracture patterns, where minimal soft tissue dissection and stable fixation has shown to have better results and is now the standard principle [18]. Although there have been no comparative studies of dual column vs. single column fixation for distal humerus fractures, we believe and suggest that the higher infection and non-union rates quoted in many series of distal humerus fractures may in part be due to greater soft tissue dissection and a longer operative time required for dual column plating [5, 8].

Yang et al. [18] also suggested that the excessive soft tissue dissection required for dual plating may be responsible for the increased incidence of iatrogenic radial nerve palsy reported in some series. Placement of implant over the distal medial aspect of humerus which has a scant soft tissue cover also leads to a high incidence of implant-related complications such as ulnar neuropathy [19]. To circumvent these problems, single column plating has been suggested by many to be the answer. Standard single column plating techniques fail to achieve adequate stabilization owing to many factors; the most important being inadequate distal purchase. Levy et al. [20] used modified Synthes Lateral Tibial Head Buttress Plate (Synthes, Paoli, PA) that allowed for a centrally placed posterior plating of the humeral shaft that angled anatomically along the lateral column to treat far distal humeral shaft fractures.

The advent of modern locking plates has allowed improved fixation of the peri-articular fractures. Numerous

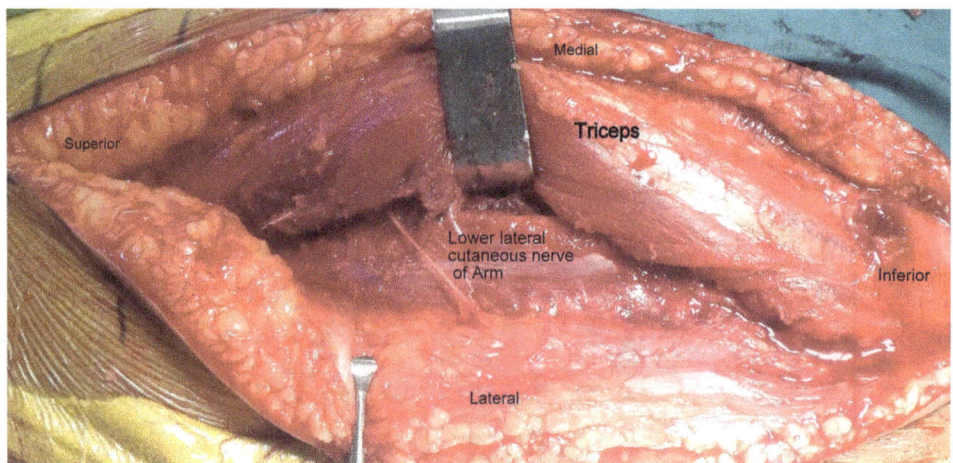

Fig. 4 Lower lateral cutaneous nerve of the arm which can be traced proximally to the radial nerve

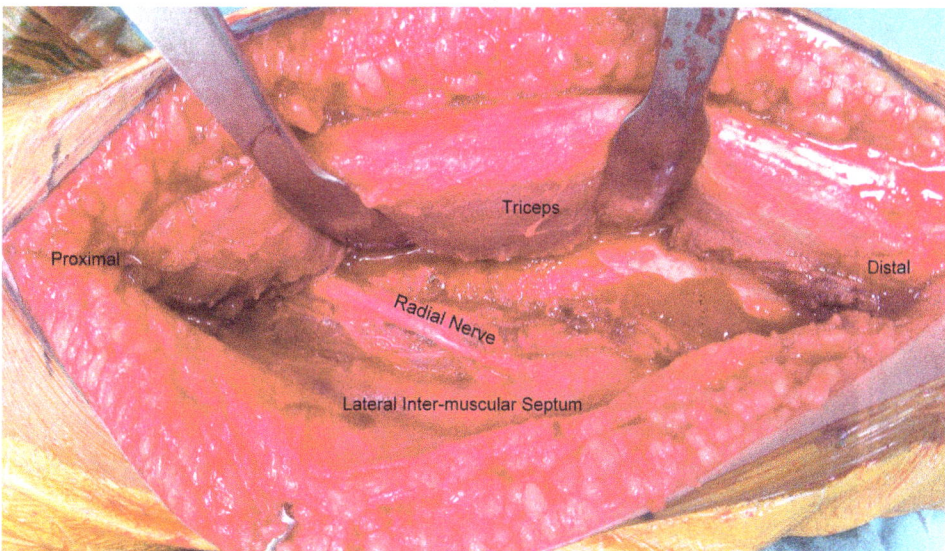

Fig. 5 Elevation of the triceps from the lateral inter-muscular septum and radial nerve dissection

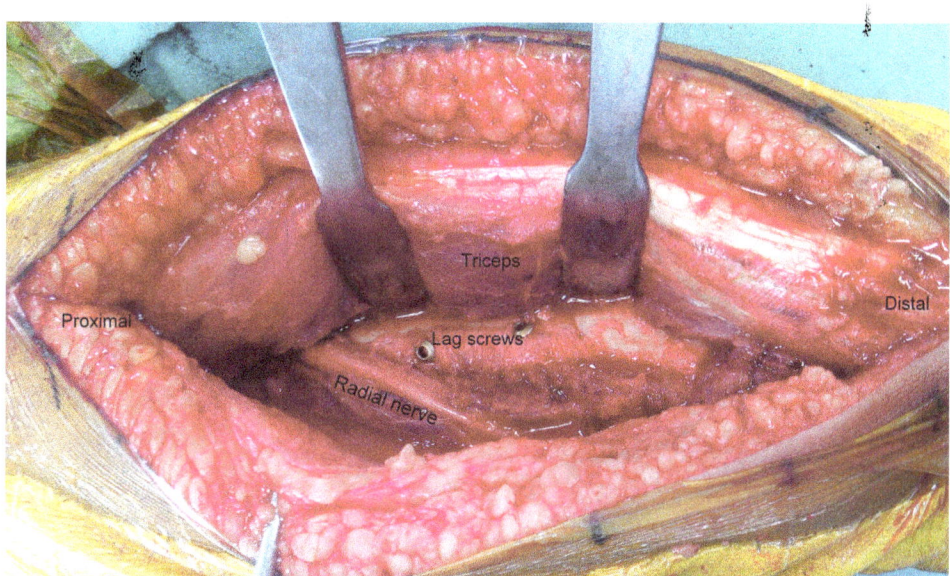

Fig. 6 Lag screw fixation

studies have demonstrated and confirmed the increased stability provided by locking plates at the distal femur, proximal tibia, calcaneum, distal radius and proximal humerus [21–25]. This increased strength of fixation has in some cases obviated the need for dual column fixation. Several studies have demonstrated that the mechanical stability and overall stiffness of a laterally placed locked plate in the proximal tibia is equivalent to the control of historical dual plating [26–28].

The extra-articular distal humeral locking plate is based on a similar concept of single column plating. Owing to greater screw hole density distally, it allows the placement of adequate number of screws in the distal fragment and the locking construct increases the stability. Since only the lateral column is exposed, it decreases both the soft tissue dissection and the surgical time. As compared to the trochlea, the posterior aspect of the lateral column is non-articular and allows for posterior placement of implant without risk of injury to the cartilage or risk of impingement with flexion and extension. We in the present series used the posterolateral approach of Gerwin et al. [9] which has several advantages over the traditional triceps splitting approach. Sparing the triceps muscle limits the formation of intramuscular adhesions and scar formation and theoretically reduces the chances of elbow contracture and improves post-operative triceps function. The exposure can

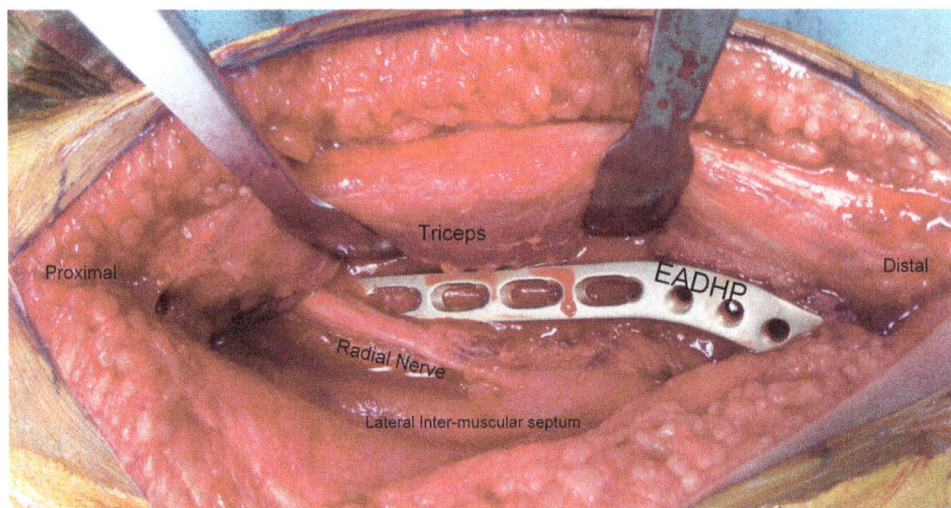

Fig. 7 Placement of plate over lateral column, note that the medial column is not dissected at all

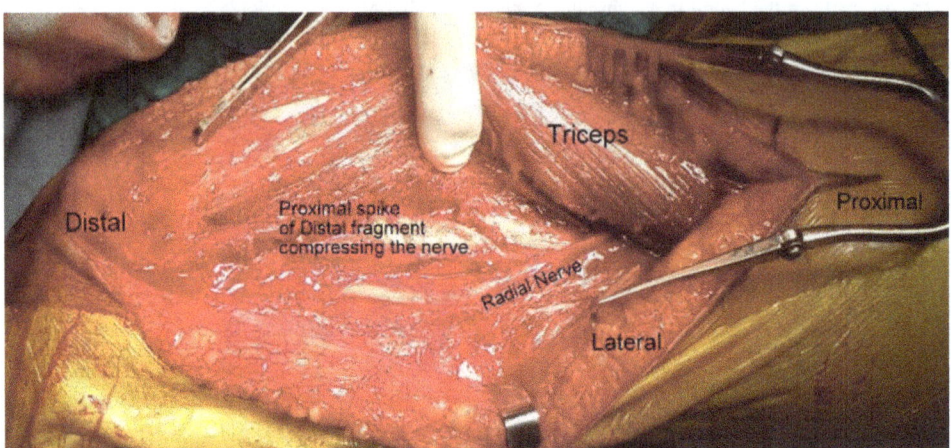

Fig. 8 Compression of the radial nerve by proximal spike of the distal fragment

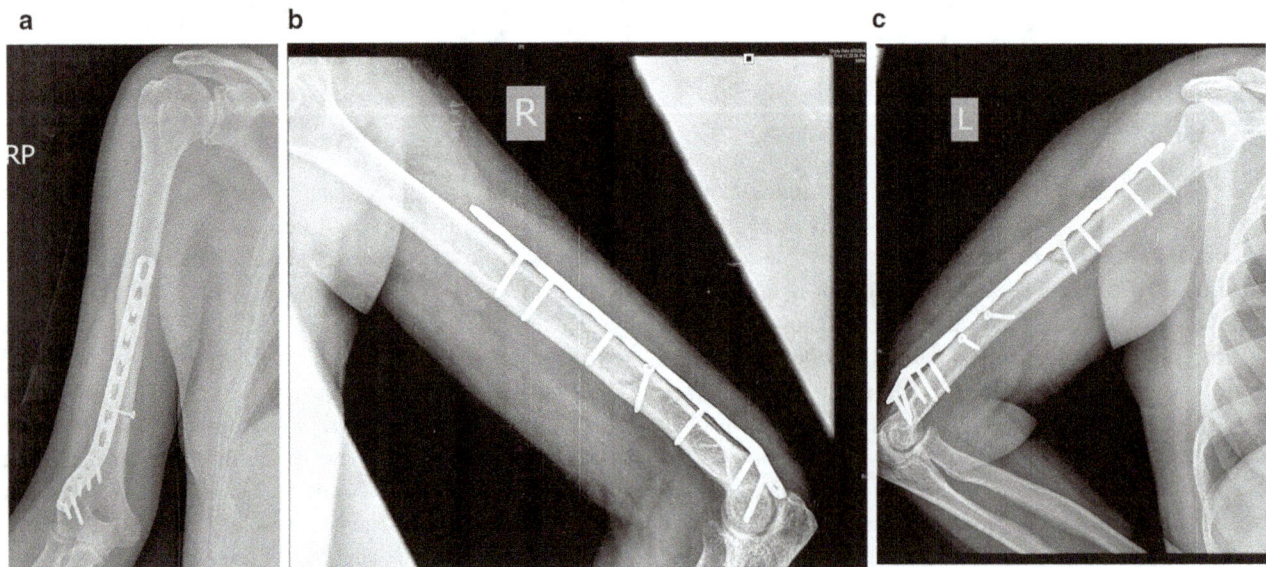

Fig. 9 Post-op X-ray images

be extended proximally and distally; proximal extension is by elevating the triceps off the humerus and mobilizing the radial nerve, and distal extension can be accomplished by converting the approach into an olecranon osteotomy approach, TRAP approach [29] or Bryan and Morrey [30] approach if there is an intra-articular extension of the shaft fracture. Triceps-reflecting anconeus pedicle (TRAP) approach involves complete detachment of triceps from proximal ulna along with anconeus using sharp dissection. The entire flap is then lifted off the posterior aspect of distal humerus. Lewisky, Sheppard and Ruth described how the posterolateral approach can be extended proximally and distally to expose most of the posterior humeral shaft and elbow joint for complex fracture treatment. They described the combined olecranon osteotomy, lateral paratricipital sparing and deltoid insertion splitting (COLD) approach [31]. Approximately 94% of the humeral diaphysis can be exposed with the posterolateral approach (Fig. 6c) as compared to the triceps splitting approach which provides exposure to only 76% of the shaft [9]. This enhanced exposure also provides complete visualization of the radial nerve on both sides of the intermuscular septum and since it exploits a relatively blood less plane, this approach can be performed without a tourniquet.

DASH score was used to assess the functional outcome. This questionnaire asks the patient about symptoms as well as their ability to perform certain activities. The questions are answered based on the condition in the last week. If patient did not have an opportunity to perform an activity in the last week, the best estimate is made. It does not matter which hand or arm is use to perform the activity. The normal DASH score in the general population has been reported to be around 10 with a standard deviation of 14.68 [10].

Our study has a few limitations, namely a small sample size, and the lack of a biomechanical study to test and compare the strength of a single column vs. double-column locking plate.

As the plate is pre-contoured, it does not seat equally well in all patients and bending the plate can potentially damage the locking hole screw threads and can also change the screw direction to a certain extent. Improperly locked screws can compromise the stability of the construct, and the change in screw direction can pose a problem in the distal screws which are directed into the capitellum and trochlea. To circumvent this problem, plate bending should be done after blocking the screw holes with locking sleeves and bending the plate only in between the screw holes.

Tejwani et al. [16] in their laboratory study demonstrated that a double plating construct is stiffer than one single-locking plate, especially in varus stress when the medial column is absent. We, however, in our series of 20 patients did not encounter any patient with a comminuted medial column; those who had so, also had some intra-articular extension of the fracture and were treated by conventional dual plating system. The increased stress placed on a single (lateral) column fixation in the absence or comminution of the other (medial) column leads to increased strain over the implant at the fracture site, which can lead to implant failure in absence of union. This can to some extent be negated by using a longer plate with widely spaced screws to increase the working length.

Conclusion

The EADHP system using the modified posterior approach to the humerus is a useful treatment option for managing extra-articular distal humerus fractures. The provision of greater screw hole density of the plate distally and using 3.5-mm screws instead of 4.5 mm allows adequate number of screws to be placed in the distal fragment. Bi-columnar fixation of distal humerus provides increased stability, but requires increased soft tissue dissection. EADHP fixation of distal humerus fractures using the modified posterior approach provides stable fracture fixation with adequate exposure of the radial nerve and >90% of posterior humeral shaft surface.

Informed consent A proper written and informed consent was taken from all the patients.

References

1. Horne G (1980) Supracondylar fractures of the humerus in adults. J Trauma 20:71–74
2. Aitken GK, Rorabeck CH (1986) Distal humeral fractures in the adult. Clin Orthop 207:191–197
3. Sarmiento A, Horowitch A, Aboulafia A, Vangsness CT Jr (1990) Functional bracing for comminuted extra-articular fractures of the distal third of the humerus. J Bone Joint Surg Br 72(2):283–287
4. O'Driscoll SW, Spinner RJ, McKee MD, Kibler WB, Hastings H 2nd, Morrey BF et al (2001) Tardy posterolateral rotatory instability of the elbow due to cubitus varus. J Bone Joint Surg Am 83-A(9):1358–1369
5. Jawa A, McCarty P, Doornberg J, Harris M, Ring D (2006) Extra-articular distal-third diaphyseal fractures of the humerus. A comparison of functional bracing and plate fixation. J Bone Joint Surg Am 88(11):2343–2347
6. McKee MD, Larsson S (2010) Humeral shaft fractures. In: Bucholz RW, Court-Brown CM, Heckman JD, Tornetta P III (eds) Rockwood and Green's fractures in adults, 7th edn. Lippincott William & Wilkins, Philadelphia, p 1015
7. Prasarn ML, Ahn J, Paul O, Morris EM, Kalandiak SP, Helfet DL et al (2011) Dual plating for fractures of the distal third of the humeral shaft. J Orthop Trauma 25:57–63
8. Paris H, Tropiano P, ClouetD'orval B, Chaudet H, Poitout DG (2000) Fractures of the shaft of the humerus: systematic plate fixation. Anatomic and functional results in 156 cases and a

review of the literature. Rev Chir Orthop Reparatrice Appar Mot 86(4):346–359

9. Gerwin M, Hotchkiss RN, Weiland AJ (1996) Alternative operative exposures of the posterior aspect of the humeral diaphysis with reference to the radial nerve. J Bone Joint Surg Am 78(11):1690–1695

10. Hunsaker FG, Cioffi DA, Amadio PC, Wright JG, Caughlin B (2002) The American academy of orthopaedic surgeon's outcomes instruments: normative values from the general population. J Bone Joint Surg Am 84-A(2):208–215

11. Scolaro JA, Voleti P, Makani A, Namdari S, Mirza A, Mehta S (2014) Surgical fixation of extra-articular distal humerus fractures with a posterolateral plate through a triceps-reflecting technique. J Shoulder Elbow Surg 23(2):251–257

12. Capo JT, Debkowska MP, Liporace F, Beutel BG, Melamed E (2014) Outcomes of distal humerus diaphyseal injuries fixed with a single-column anatomic plate. Int Orthop 38(5):1037–1043

13. Jawa A (2010) Treatment of distal diaphyseal humerus fractures. J Hand Surg Am. 35(2):301–302

14. Meloy GM, Mormino MA, Siska PA, Tarkin IS (2013) A paradigm shift in the surgical reconstruction of extra-articular distal humeral fractures: single-column plating. Injury 44(11):1620–1624

15. Zimmerman MC, Waite AM, Deehan M, Tovey J, Oppenheim W (1994) A biomechanical analysis of four humeral fracture fixation systems. J Orthop Trauma 8(3):233–239

16. Tejwani NC, Murthy A, Park J, McLaurin TM, Egol KA, Kummer FJ (2009) Fixation of extra-articular distal humerus fractures using one locking plate versus two reconstruction plates: a laboratory study. J Trauma 66(3):795–799

17. Thomas PR, Richard EB, Christopher GM (2007) AO philosophy and evolution. In: Thomas PR, Richard EB, Christopher GM (eds) AO principles of fracture management, 2nd edn. Thieme, Stuttgart, pp 1–9

18. Yang Qing, Wang Fang, Wang Qiugen, Gao Wei, Huang Jianhua, Xiaofeng Wu et al (2012) Surgical treatment of adult extra-articular distal humeral diaphyseal fractures using an oblique metaphyseal locking compression plate via a posterior approach. Med Princ Pract 21:40–45

19. Chen RC, Harris DJ, Leduc S, Borrelli JJ Jr, Tornetta P III, Ricci WM (2010) Is ulnar nerve transposition beneficial during open reduction and internal fixation of distal humerus fractures? J Orthop Trauma 24(7):391–394

20. Levy JC, Kalandiak SP, Hutson JJ, Zych G (2005) An alternative method of osteosynthesis for distal humeral shaft fractures. J Orthop Trauma 19(1):43–47

21. Liporace FA, Gupta S, Jeong GK, Stracher M, Kummer F, Egol KA et al (2005) A biomechanical comparison of a dorsal 3.5-mm T-plate and a volar fixed-angle plate in a model of dorsally unstable distal radius fractures. J Orthop Trauma 19(3):187–191

22. Stoffel K, Booth G, Rohrl SM, Kuster M (2007) A comparison of conventional versus locking plates in intraarticular calcaneus fractures: a biomechanical study in human cadavers. Clin Biomech (Bristol, Avon) 22:100–105

23. Weinstein DM, Bratton DR, Ciccone WJ 2nd, Elias JJ (2006) Locking plates improve torsional resistance in the stabilization of three-part proximal humeral fractures. J Shoulder Elbow Surg 15:239–243

24. Ratcliff JR, Werner FW, Green JK, Harley BJ (2007) Medial buttress versus lateral locked plating in a cadaver medial tibial plateau fracture model. J Orthop Trauma 21:444–448

25. Higgins TF, Pittman G, Hines J, Bachus KN (2007) Biomechanical analysis of distal femur fracture fixation: fixed-angle screw-plate construct versus condylar blade plate. J Orthop Trauma 21:43–46

26. Gösling T, Schandelmaier P, Marti A, Hufner T, Partenheimer A, Krettek C (2004) Less invasive stabilization of complex tibial plateau fractures: a biomechanical evaluation of a unilateral locked screw plate and double plating. J Orthop Trauma 18(8):546–551

27. Mueller KL, Karunakar MA, Frankenburg EP, Scott DS (2003) Bicondylar tibial plateau fractures: a biomechanical study. Clin Orthop Relat Res 412:189–195

28. Egol KA, Su E, Tejwani NC, Sims SH, Kummer FJ, Koval KJ (2004) Treatment of complex tibial plateau fractures using the less invasive stabilization system plate: clinical experience and a laboratory comparison with double plating. J Trauma 57(2):340–346

29. Shawn WO (2000) Driscoll: the tricep reflecting anconeus pedicle (TRAP) approach for distal humerus fractures and nonunions. Orthop Clin North Am 31(1):91–101

30. Bryan RS, Morrey BF (1982) Extensive posterior exposure of the elbow: a triceps-sparing approach. Clin Orthop 166:188–192

31. Lewicky YM, Sheppard JE, Ruth JT (2007) The combined olecranon osteotomy, lateral paratricipital sparing, deltoid insertion splitting approach for concomitant distal intra-articular and humeral shaft fractures. J Orthop Trauma 21(2):133–139

12

Subjective ulnar nerve dysfunction commonly following open reduction, internal fixation (ORIF) of distal humeral fractures and in situ decompression of the ulnar nerve

Birgitta Svernlöv[1,2] · Jens Nestorson[3,4] · Lars Adolfsson[3,4]

Abstract The aim of this retrospective study was to investigate the frequency of persistent ulnar affection in patients who underwent open reduction and internal fixation (ORIF) of distal humeral fractures without ulnar nerve transposition or mobilisation. Eighty-two patients (53 women), mean age 62 years, were, at a mean of 48 months, reviewed through medical records and a subjective evaluation form concerning ulnar nerve problems. Ulnar nerve affliction, in most cases regarded as mild, was experienced by 22 patients (27%; 14 women) and significantly associated with multiple surgeries. Three patients had been operated with late neurolysis and one with transposition without reported improvement. The proportion of ulnar nerve dysfunction was equally common regardless of medial or lateral plating. ORIF with plate fixation and without ulnar nerve transposition seems to be an acceptable option for patients with distal humeral fractures. The frequency of ulnar nerve affection in our series does not appear higher than previously reported. Subjective ulnar nerve symptoms were, however, relatively common and appear related to the trauma itself, the surgery, or the post-operative management which highlights the need for further analysis of these factors.

✉ Birgitta Svernlöv
birgitta.svernlov@comhem.se

[1] Department of Plastic Surgery, Hand Surgery and Burns, Linköping University Hospital, 581 85 Linköping, Sweden

[2] Faculty of Experimental and Clinical Medicine, Linköping University, Linköping, Sweden

[3] Department of Orthopedic Surgery, Linköping University Hospital, 581 85 Linköping, Sweden

[4] Faculty of Health Science, Linköping University, Linköping, Sweden

Keywords Fracture · ORIF · Transposition · Humeral · Dellon · McGowan

Introduction

Fractures of the distal humerus in adults are estimated to represent 2% of all fractures and are thus relatively infrequent [1]. Usually operative treatment with accurate anatomic reduction and stable internal fixation is indicated [2–6]. Dual-plate fixation has become the treatment of choice for most surgeons during which procedure the ulnar nerve has to be mobilised to some extent and ulnar nerve dysfunction is a common complication following surgical treatment of distal humeral fractures [7]. The ulnar nerve is at high risk of being injured at the initial trauma during surgery and may also be affected by post-operative scar formation [8–12]. The reported incidence of post-operative ulnar neuropathy varies between 0 and 51% with an average of 13% [3, 7, 13–19]. Many authors advocate routine anterior transposition of the nerve [7, 13, 16, 18, 20–24], but some support the idea of placing the nerve back into its epicondylar groove after the internal fixation is completed [3, 14, 19].

The aim of this study was to investigate the frequency of persistent ulnar affection in patients who underwent open reduction and internal fixation (ORIF) of distal humeral fractures without ulnar nerve transposition or mobilisation.

Materials and methods

Between January 2003 and June 2013, 161 patients with distal humeral fractures were operated at our centre. Out of these, 116 adults were treated with internal plate fixation

Table 1 Fracture types according to the *Arbeitsgemeinschaft für Osteosynthesefragen (AO) classification* [25] and demographics

AO classification	Gender M/F	Mean age	Ulnar nerve affection (n = 22) M/F	M/F (%)
A (n = 11)				
A2:1 1	0/1	32	0/0	0
A2:3 2	0/2	83	0/0	0
A3:1 1	0/1	69	0/0	0
A3:2 4	2/2	56	1/1	4.5/4.5
A3:3 3	0/3	62	0/1	0/4.5
B (n = 13)				
B1:3 5	1/4	63	0/1	0/4.5
B2:1 1	1/0	60	0/0	0
B2:3 3	1/2	68	0/0	0
B3:1 1	0/1	66	0/0	0
B3:3 3	2/1	67	2/1	9.0/4.5
C (n = 58)				
C1:2 7	2/5	65	0/2	0/9.0
C1:3 1	0/1	85	0/0	0
C2:1 4	2/2	67	0/1	0/4.5
C2:2 16	5/11	64	1/4	4.5/18.2
C2:3 14	6/8	61	2/1	9.0/4.5
C3:1 1	0/1	54	0/0	0
C3:2 11	4/7	61	1/2	4.5/9.0
C3:3 4	2/2	59	0/1	0/4.5

N = 82

using bilateral or unilateral plates and screws. There were 35 men and 81 women with an average age of 63 years (SD 18.31, range 21–93 years).

The patients' medical records, comprising information about demographics, operative and hospital information, and any complication that occurred in the immediate or later post-operative period, were reviewed. Twenty-four patients, four males and twenty females, were deceased, and two patients, one man and one woman, could not be reached due to foreign citizenships. The rest of the patients were contacted by phone and offered a follow-up; four women and one man were unable to cooperate due to vascular dementia or mental handicap of other origin. Another three women could not participate due to language difficulties. This left 82 eligible patients (71%), 29 males and 53 females, available for follow-up. The average age was 63 years (SD 16.40, range 21–89 years). The mean age of the men was 62 years (SD 18.31, range 18–89 years), and that of the women was 63 years (SD 16.48, range 21–89 years). The average follow-up was 49 months (SD 27.85, range 14–118 months), 48 months (SD 31.41, range 14–118 months) for the male patients, and 49 months (SD 26.21, range 17–115 months) for the female patients.

The mechanism of injury included 49 simple falls, 11 bicycle accidents, ten falls from a height, six motor vehicle accidents, four rotation accidents (e.g. arm wrestling), one skiing accident, and one with a direct blow from a girder. Four were open fractures, and one patient had ipsilateral forearm fractures. The ulnar nerve function was, according to the medical records, preoperatively intact in all cases.

The preoperative images, including CT scans, were examined, and the fractures classified in accordance with the Arbeitsgemeinschaft für Osteosynthesefragen (AO) system (Table 1) [25].

Seventy patients had been operated with bilateral plating using the parallel concept with plates on each column at an angle of approximately 160° between the plates. In two patients the fracture was stabilised with a solitary medial plate, and in ten patients a lateral plate was the only implant used. The exposure included a mid-line triceps split in 45 patients, an olecranon osteotomy in 19, and a lateral or antero-lateral approach in 15 patients. Three patients had a concomitant fracture of the olecranon that was used for approach to the fracture.

The ulnar nerve was identified and decompressed (in situ) from the arcade of Struthers to the medial ulno-humeral joint line. When a medial plate was used, the ulnar nerve was carefully elevated from the humeral metaphysis and the medial intermuscular septum allowing for the plate to be slid underneath. The nerve was elevated together with a sleeve of perineural soft tissues. In all cases operated

Fig. 1 The subjective patient rated questionnaire concerning possible ulnar nerve affliction based on the systems by McGowan and Dellon [30, 31]

THE QUESTIONNAIRE
Please encircle the most appropriate alternative

Male   Female

1) Are you	Right		Left-handed
2) Which arm is operated	Right		Left
3) Do you experience paraesthesia in your right 4th–and 5th fingers	Never	Occasionally	Constantly
4) Do you experience paraesthesia in your left 4th–and 5th fingers	Never	Occasionally	Constantly
5) Do you experience numbness in your right 4th–and 5th fingers	Never	Occasionally	Constantly
6) Do you experience numbness in your left 4th–and 5th fingers	Never	Occasionally	Constantly
7) Do you experience clumsiness in your right hand	Yes		No
8) Do you experience clumsiness in your left hand	Yes		No
9) Do you experience weakness in your right hand	Yes		No
10) Do you experience weakness in your left hand	Yes		No
11) Do your right 4th–and 5th fingers go numb when flexing your elbow	Yes		No
12) Do your left 4th–and 5th fingers go numb when flexing your elbow	Yes		No

How old are you? ....

through a lateral or antero-lateral approach, the triceps and the ulnar nerve had been left undisturbed.

The patients were immobilised in a posterior plaster splint during two to three days. Active exercises monitored by a physiotherapist were initiated immediately after removal of the plaster. Light activities of daily living were allowed at all times, while load bearing and strengthening exercises begun after 6 weeks.

The follow-up consisted of a questionnaire (Fig. 1) addressing subjective symptoms from the ulnar nerve, such as occasional or constant numbness or paraesthesias in the 4th and 5th finger of the hand of the operated elbow; furthermore, experience of subjective weakness and clumsiness in the actual hand; and whether or not the fingers in question went numb in connection with elbow flexion. For each item the alternatives present or absent could be chosen. A diagnosis of ulnar nerve dysfunction was decided when intermittent paraesthesia and numbness in the 4th and 5th fingers, aggravated by elbow flexion, were reported and classified as a mild affection. Intermittent numbness and paraesthesia with additional weakness and clumsiness were graded as

moderate and constant problems, including all these symptoms, as severe nerve affection.

The questionnaire was sent out by mail to the patients with a prepaid return envelope together with a cover letter and an informed consent form for signature to participate in the study. The participants were reassured of the confidential nature of the study.

An independent researcher (BS) carried out the study, which was approved by the regional committee for medical ethics (Dnr 2010/171-31).

Statistical analyses were made using STATISTICA v.12.0 StatSoft, Inc. The Chi square test was used to test the difference in proportions of ulnar nerve affliction between all patients and between those who had been subjected to re-operations; between the different fracture types; between men and women; between patients operated with or without the use of a medial plate; and between patients operated with or without an olecranon osteotomy. T tests for independent groups were used to test whether there was an age difference between patients presented with ulnar nerve affliction or not. p values <0.05 were considered statistically significant.

Results

In reference to the AO classification, 11 fractures were type A, 13 type B, and the remaining 58 type C fractures (Table 1) [25].

In accordance with the medical histories, there were 16 patients with ulnar nerve affection diagnosed during the post-operative follow-up period. At the last follow-up, on average 4 years, 22 patients (27%; 3 AO type A, 4 type B, 15 type C), 14 women and eight men, reported symptoms based on the criteria for ulnar nerve dysfunction, according to the questionnaire. Thirteen patients suffered from mild affections with only occasional paraesthesia and numbness in the 4th and 5th fingers, particularly during elbow flexion; four presented with intermittent numbness or paraesthesias in the 4th and 5th fingers and additionally subjective weakness and/or clumsiness in the hand and were considered as moderately affected. Five patients reported constant problems with all these symptoms and were regarded as severely affected (Table 2).

Four of these 22 patients had undergone a second procedure with a neurolysis, in one patient combined with subcutaneous transposition, in connection with hardware removal. No improvement was reported following these procedures. Ulnar nerve affliction was significantly associated with multiple surgeries ($p < 0.01$). No significant difference was found between gender ($p > 0.93$) or age ($p > 0.54$) and ulnar nerve problems (Table 2).

Post-operative ulnar nerve dysfunction was not related to fracture type ($p = 0.50$). Ten patients had been operated without the use of a medial plate in which cases the fracture had been stabilised using lateral implants only. There was no significant difference in ulnar nerve symptoms between patients operated with bilateral plates or a single ulnar plate on the medial column ($p < 0.81$) and those who were treated with only a lateral plate nor was there any significant difference in ulnar nerve problems between those operated with an olecranon osteotomy or not ($p < 0.54$; Table 2).

Eight patients presented with radial palsy in connection with the injury. None of these were surgically

explored or repaired, and all subsequently resolved without residual symptoms. Twenty-five patients (30%) had undergone reoperation; 15 with hardware removal, four of which with concomitant ulnar neurolysis due to nerve symptoms. Three patients had been operated with bone graft and new osteosynthesis, two due to non-union of the distal humeral fracture, and one because of non-union of an olecranon osteotomy. All of them subsequently went on to union. Two patients were operated with wound revision due to deep infection. Two patients developed avascular bone necrosis of the distal humerus, one was treated with resection of capitellar fragments, and one, with affection of the entire joint surface, was treated with a hemiprosthesis. Three patients were operated with resection of heterotopic bone formation interfering with mobility.

Discussion

Ulnar neuropathy at the elbow is the second most frequent focal peripheral neuropathy of the upper limb, usually presenting with tingling and paraesthesia in the little and ring fingers and weakened hand grip. In the present study, 27% of the patients operated with internal fixation of a distal humeral fracture reported symptoms from the ulnar nerve at a 4-year follow-up.

The issue of ulnar nerve affection associated with internal fixation of distal humeral fractures has been addressed in several studies resulting in varying conclusions; Shin and Ring [18] found a 22% rate of post-operative ulnar nerve palsies after nerve transposition, and according to them, despite adequate release and transposition, irritation and transient sensory changes have occurred in up to 50% of patients in some series. In fact, after ulnar nerve transposition had been performed, 51% of transient ulnar neuropraxia was reported by Holdsworth and Mossad [14]. Furthermore, McKee et al. [5] calculated a 20% rate of ulnar neuropathy after the same procedure. Athwal et al. [26] concluded that 13% of post-operatively developed ulnar neuropathy might have been the result of

Table 2 Ulnar nerve affection related to fracture type, gender (male/female), mean age, re-operation, bilateral or lateral plates, and olecranon osteotomy

Nerve affection ($n = 22$)	Fracture type			Mean age	Re-operation	Bilateral plates	Lateral plates	Olecranon osteotomy
	A ($n = 3$)	B ($n = 4$)	C ($n = 15$)	M/F (56/63)	M/F ($n = 13$)	M/F ($n = 19$)	M/F ($n = 3$)	M/F ($n = 7$)
Mild ($n = 13$)	2	2	9	54/63	4/4	4/7	1/1	1/3
Moderate ($n = 4$)	0	2	2	70/54	1/2	1/2	1/0	0/1
Severe ($n = 5$)	1	0	4	46/70	1/1	1/4	0/0	0/2

Numbers presented are patients

the routine transposition of the ulnar nerve that they performed in connection with ORIF.

Chen et al. [27], comparing the incidence of ulnar neuritis with and without nerve transposition, recognised almost four times (33%) the incidence in those who underwent transposition. The authors concluded that transposition of the ulnar nerve may not be helpful in preventing the development of ulnar neuritis after distal humeral fractures, instead may place the patient at greater risk for neuritis. Kundel et al. [3], on the other side, after performing in situ release of the nerve in question described a 27% prevalence of ulnar neuropathy.

Worden and Ilyas [28], in a review study, identified a 38% incidence of late ulnar neuropathy in connection with ORIF and found no difference between in situ release and anterior transposition. In an attempt to detect factors associated with ulnar neuropathy, Wiggers et al. [19] diagnosed a 16% ulnar neuropathy, regardless of whether the nerve was transposed or not. Furthermore, Vazquez et al. [12] retrospectively evaluated distal humeral fractures treated with or without ulnar nerve transposition. They discovered, irrespective of procedure, the incidence of post-operative neuropathy to be 16% and concluded that transposition of the nerve did not significantly decrease the development of iatrogenic ulnar neuropathy. Additionally, Ruan et al. [11] randomly allocated patients to either anterior subfascial transposition or in situ decompression, of the ulnar nerve in conjunction with ORIF. They found that there was no significant difference between the groups.

The optimal handling of the ulnar nerve is unclear, but anterior transposition may not be necessary as part of the acute surgical treatment of displaced distal humeral fractures [12].

However, the true prevalence of ulnar nerve dysfunction after elbow injury is unknown, since authors of published studies have not successfully distinguished acute injury-related, acute surgery-related, and delayed (subacute or chronic) ulnar neuropathies, and furthermore, in most of these retrospective case series, careful evaluation of ulnar nerve function has not been included [18].

Wiggers et al. [19] looked for risk factors for post-operative ulnar neuropathy, including age, sex, implant over or below the medial epicondyle, and the total number of surgeries. They learned that columnar fracture and application of a medial plate were the only potential risk factor for iatrogenic post-operative ulnar neuropathy, but Vazquez et al. [12] were not able to identify any single factor that significantly contributed to ulnar neuropathy. They investigated transposition of the ulnar nerve or not, age, gender, presence of multiple procedures, use of olecranon osteotomy, poly-trauma, and open versus closed injury. We found no significant difference in ulnar nerve symptoms between patients in whom an ulnar plate was used and those treated with lateral implants only. This might indicate that the main cause is the trauma itself or that ulnar nerve symptoms could occur secondarily to post-operative immobilization, swelling, scarring, and thickening in the fibro-osseous tunnel. The only variable we detected associated with ulnar nerve affection was re-operation, but this association is hampered by the fact that the reason for reoperation in four cases was because of ulnar nerve symptoms.

The reoperation rate of 30% in our series corresponds with the literature, the results of which fall between 21 and 73% with the majorities in or around 40% [4, 7, 16, 17, 23, 27–29].

This study is impaired by some limitations that are related primarily to the inherent weakness of a retrospective report. There is no direct comparison with a group of patients randomly allocated to another treatment of the ulnar nerve in connection with the surgery. Differences in fracture types and trauma mechanisms may have had an impact on the susceptibility of ulnar nerve affection, but the material is of insufficient size for subgroup analysis. Another potential weakness is the subjective patient-rated questionnaire concerning possible ulnar nerve affliction, since this precludes any objective measures of dysfunction. On the other hand, the majority of complaints include minor sensory disturbance and discomfort that may not have been possible to appreciate by a clinical or neurophysiologic examination.

We decided to construct the questionnaire including all subjectively experienced factors previously described associated with an ulnar neuropathy at the level of the elbow, in reference to the examination systems proposed by McGowan [30] and Dellon [31]. A report of tingling, paraesthesia, numbness, clumsiness, weakness as well as increased symptoms associated with elbow flexion was regarded as definitive attributes of a nerve dysfunction. We are aware that comparison with other studies is difficult since many different methods for assessing ulnar nerve dysfunction have been used but since the main complaint of our patients was subjective sensation of intermittent sensory disturbance which is not objectively measurable, we believe that the method used is appropriate. The questionnaire is not validated in relation to other methods, and the results should therefore be cautiously interpreted.

The strengths of our study are the sample size of 82 patients, that all eligible patients participated, the surgeries were performed by experienced orthopaedists in a single centre, the follow-up period of 4 years appears reasonable, and that an independent reviewer, not involved in the surgeries, conducted the survey.

Future studies that objectively and reliably diagnose injury-related, surgery-related, and delayed (sub-acute or chronic) ulnar neuropathies or prospective randomized trials, using transposition or in situ release of the ulnar nerve with strict definitions and objective measures, would be valuable.

Conclusion

ORIF without ulnar nerve transposition seems to be an acceptable option for patients with distal humeral fractures. Late ulnar nerve dysfunction was found to be a relatively common problem following surgically treated distal humeral fractures. The frequency of the discomfort in our study was somewhat disappointing but, according to what can be learnt from the literature, we do not believe that an anterior transposition of the nerve is preferable to in situ decompression.

Acknowledgements The authors wish to thank Rn Terez Zara Hanqvist for planning and booking radiology examinations of the patients in this study.

Funding This research received no specific grant from any funding agency in the public, commercial, or not-for-profit sectors.

Informed consent A proper written and informed consent was taken from all the participants.

References

1. Robinson CM (2006) Fractures of the distal humerus. In: Bucholz RW, Heckman JD, Court-Brown CM (eds) Rockwood's and Green's fractures in adults, vol 6th. Lippincott, Williams & Wilkins, Philadelphia, pp 1051–1116
2. Jupiter JB, Neff U, Holzach P et al (1985) Intercondylar fractures of the humerus: an operative approach. J Bone Joint Surg Am 67:226–239
3. Kundel K, Braun W, Wieberneit J et al (1996) Intraarticular distal humerus fractures: factors affecting functional outcome. Clin Orthop Relat Res 332:200–208
4. Korner J, Lill H, Muller LP et al (2005) Distal humerus fractures in elderly patients: results after open reduction and internal fixation. Osteoporos Int 16:S73–S79
5. McKee MD, Veillette CJ, Hall JA et al (2009) A multicenter, prospective, randomized, controlled trial of open reduction -internal fixation versus total elbow arthroplasty for displaced intraarticular distal humeral fractures in elderly patients. J Shoulder Elbow Surg 18:3–12
6. Adolfsson L, Nestorson J (2012) The Kudo humeral component as primary hemiarthroplasty in distal humeral fractures. J Shoulder Elbow Surg 21:451–455
7. Gofton WT, MacDermid JC, Patterson SD et al (2003) Functional outcome of AO type C distal humeral fractures. J Hand Surg Am 28:294–308
8. Webb LX (2001) Fractures of the distal humerus. In: Bucholz RW, Heckman JD, Court-Brown CM (eds) Rockwood's and Green's fractures in adults, vol 5th. Lippincott, Williams & Wilkins, Philadelphia, pp 953–972
9. Huang TL, Chiu FY, Chuang TY et al (2005) The results of open reduction and internal fixation in elderly patients with severe fractures of the distal humerus: a critical analysis of the results. J Trauma 58:62–69
10. McCarty LP, Ring D, Jupiter JB (2005) Management of distal humerus fractures. Am J Orthop 34:430–438
11. Ruan HJ, Liu JJ, Fan CY et al (2009) Incidence, management, and prognosis of early ulnar nerve dysfunction in type C fractures of distal humerus. J Trauma 67:1397–1401
12. Vazquez O, Rutgers M, Ring DC et al (2010) Fate of the ulnar nerve after operative fixation of distal humerus fractures. J Orthop Trauma 24:395–399
13. Wang KC, Shih HN, Hsu KY et al (1994) Intercondylar fractures of the distal humerus: routine anterior subcutaneous transposition of the ulnar nerve in a posterior operative approach. J Trauma 36:770–773
14. Holdsworth BJ, Mossad MM (1990) Fractures of the adult distal humerus. Elbow function after internal fixation. J Bone Joint Surg Br 72:362–365
15. Södergard J, Sandelin J, Böstman O (1992) Postoperative complications of distal humeral fractures. 27/96 adults followed up for 6 (2–10) years. Acta Orthop Scand 63:85–89
16. Gupta R, Khanchandani P (2002) Intercondylar fractures if the distal humerus in adults: a critical analysis of 55 cases. Injury 33:511–515
17. Soon JL, Chan BK, Low CO (2004) Surgical fixation of intraarticular fractures of the distal humerus in adults. Injury 35:44–54
18. Shin R, Ring D (2007) The ulnar nerve in elbow trauma. J Bone Joint Surg Am 89:1108–1116
19. Wiggers JK, Brouwer KM, Helmerhorst GT et al (2012) Predictors of diagnosis of ulnar neuropathy after surgically treated distal humerus fractures. J Hand Surg Am 37:1168–1172
20. Jupiter JB, Barnes KA, Goodman LJ et al (1993) Multiplane fracture of the distal humerus. J Orthop Trauma 7:216–220
21. Jupiter JB (1995) Complex fractures of the distal part of the humerus and associated complications. Instr Course Lect 44:187–198
22. Ring D, Jupiter JB (1999) Complex fractures of the distal humerus and their complications. J Shoulder Elbow Surg 8:85–97
23. Ring D, Gulotta L, Jupiter JB (2003) Unstable non-union's of the distal part of the humerus. J Bone Joint Surg Am 85-A:1040–1046
24. Ilyas AM, Jupiter JB (2008) Treatment of distal humerus fractures. Acta Chir Orthop Traumatol Cechoslov 75:6–15
25. Müller ME, Nazarian S, Koch P et al (1990) Humerus = 1. The comprehensive classification of fractures of long bones, 1st edn. Springer, Berlin, pp 54–85
26. Athwal GS, Hoxie SC, Rispoli DM et al (2009) Precontoured parallel plate fixation of AO/OTA type C distal humerus fractures. J Orthop Trauma 23:575–580
27. Chen G, Liao Q, Luo W et al (2011) Triceps-sparing versus olecranon osteotomy for ORIF: analysis of 67 cases of intercondylar fractures of the distal humerus. Injury 42:366–370
28. Worden A, Ilyas AM (2012) Ulnar neuropathy following distal humerus fracture fixation. Orthop Clin North Am 43:509–514
29. Huang JI, Paczas M, Hoyen HA, Huang JI, Vallier HA (2011) Functional outcome after open reduction internal fixation of intraarticular fractures of the distal humerus in the elderly. J Orthop Trauma 25:259–265
30. McGowan AJ (1950) The results of transposition of the ulnar nerve for traumatic ulnar neuritis. J Bone Joint Surg Br 32-B:293–301
31. Dellon AL (1989) Review of treatment results for ulnar nerve entrapment at the elbow. Hand Surg Am 14:688–700

13

Management of mid-shaft clavicular fractures: comparison between non-operative treatment and plate fixation in 60 patients

B. M. Naveen[1] · **G. R. Joshi**[1] · **B. Harikrishnan**[1]

Abstract Clavicle fracture is a common injury due to its subcutaneous and relatively anterior position. Fractures affecting the middle third account for majority of all clavicular fractures. Both non-operative and surgical methods have been described for the management of this injury. However, there is no uniform consensus on the definite choice of treatment. Hence, this study was undertaken to compare conservative approach with primary internal plate fixation in mid-shaft clavicular fractures in terms of subjective outcome, functional outcome, the rates of nonunion and malunion and other local complications. Patients were allocated into two groups, each including 30 patients on alternate basis. Group 1 patients were managed conservatively, consisting of a figure-of-eight bandage and a sling, whereas patients of group 2 were treated surgically by plate fixation. Follow-up examination was done at 06 weeks, 03 and 06 months using patient's subjective evaluation, functional outcome, radiographic assessment and other complications. The study showed that time to union was significantly shorter in patients treated surgically and this group also showed a favorable Constant shoulder score at all follow-ups. Though there was no statistically significant difference between the groups with regard to complication rate, subjective outcome or functional outcome, the surgical intervention group fared better especially when considering overall outcome results. The present study showed that the time to union was lesser, rate of malunion and nonunion was lower, and Constant shoulder scores were higher in the surgical group. This affirms that while conservative treatment remains the treatment of choice for simple undisplaced mid-shaft clavicle fractures, for displaced and comminuted fractures the surgical intervention gives better outcomes and early functional recovery in young active adults.

Keywords Clavicle · Fracture · Mid-shaft · Plating

Introduction

Clavicle fracture is one of the most common injuries around the shoulder girdle [1]. It has been reported that fractures of the clavicle account for approximately 2.6% of all fractures [2]. Incidence in males is usually highest in second and third decade which decreases thereafter as per age [3]. In females, it is usually bimodal, with peak incidence in young and elderly [4]. Allman [5] classified clavicle fractures into three groups based on their location along the bone. The middle-third fractures are most common and account for approximately 80–85% all clavicular fractures [6]. The narrow cross section of the bone in the middle shaft combined with typical muscle forces acting over it predispose to fracture the bone in this locality. Further, Robinson modified Allman classification based on the degree of displacement and comminution [3].

Most mid-shaft clavicle fractures generally unite with any method of immobilization. Hence, non-operative treatment was the established and accepted modality of these fractures. This was evident by extremely low nonunion rates shown by various studies done earlier [7, 8]. However, certain recent studies have shown suboptimal outcomes and a very high nonunion rates when displaced fractures are managed conservatively [9, 10]. Other shortcomings of non-operative treatment brought out were

✉ B. M. Naveen
drnaveenbm@yahoo.co.in

[1] Department of Orthopaedics, Armed Forces Medical College (AFMC), Pune 411040, India

functional impairment of the shoulder and a non-cosmetic bump at the base of the neck possibly due to shortening of the clavicle and exuberant callus formation [9]. Restoration of normal length and alignment by surgical methods can prevent these drawbacks of conservative treatment. Good outcome with high union rates and low complication rates has been reported with various surgical modalities of primary fixation of the displaced fractures [11–14]. However, operative treatment has also got its own disadvantages such as surgical site infection, hypertrophic scar, hardware prominence and a repeat surgery for implant removal at times. Since mid-shaft clavicular fractures generally unite with most of the treatment modalities, clinical trials performed to compare these therapeutic options are rare. In addition, there is no uniform consensus yet on the definite choice of treatment for displaced mid-shaft clavicular fractures.

In the younger age group, apart from isolated clavicle fractures poly-traumatic injuries are also very common, and clavicular mid-shaft fracture remains a frequent entity. In such situations, the choice of treatment remains a constant dilemma for achieving maximum pre-fracture functional status. Hence, in this study we endeavored to find an evidence-based answer to select the better approach for the management of acute displaced mid-shaft clavicular fractures. The aim of this study was to compare sixty patients with mid-shaft clavicular fractures treated either by conservative approach or primary internal plate fixation in terms of functional outcome, the rate of nonunion, malunion and overall local complications up to 6 months after treatment. In addition, it was also intended to study the clinical response in terms of subjective outcome and the advantages and disadvantages of both the treatment modalities.

Materials and methods

A comparative study of management of mid-shaft clavicle fractures (Robinson type 2b) was carried out at a tertiary care teaching hospital between Jun 2011 and Jun 2013. Study population included patients in age group of 20 and 50 years with completely displaced fracture of the mid-shaft clavicle. Patients with severe brain injury, intubated patients, those with open fractures or ipsilateral limb fracture and those with injury precluding operative fixation within 7 days of admission were excluded from the study.

It is a non-randomized comparative trial with equal allocation, consisting of 60 patients with freshly diagnosed mid-shaft clavicular fractures. Group 1 consisted 30 patients who were managed conservatively and group 2 had 30 patients who were treated surgically. Patients were

allocated into both the treatment groups on alternate basis, i.e., group 1 followed by group 2 (Table 1).

In the outpatient department of the hospital, the surgeon or orthopedic resident identified the patients eligible for the study and the study protocol was instituted. Patients were informed in detail by the treating surgeon regarding the advantages and disadvantages of both operative and non-operative care. The nature of the study was explained to all the patients in their own language that they understand and necessary consent was obtained after the patients gave their willingness to participate in the study.

Group 1 patients were managed conservatively, consisting of a figure-of-eight bandage (Fig. 1a–d) and a sling, whereas patients of group 2 were treated surgically by plate osteosynthesis (Fig. 2a–d). Patients allocated to plate fixation group underwent the operation within seven days after the injury. An 8–10 cm skin incision was placed on the line joining sternal notch to anterior edge of acromion centered over fracture site on the affected side. Platysma was released from lateral side and supraclavicular nerves protected wherever possible. Subsequently the clavipectoral fascia was incised and elevated. Fractures fragments identified and reduced under vision. The plate (3.5 mm DCP) was contoured and applied over the superior aspect of the clavicle taking care not to injure the underlying neurovascular structures. Comminuted fragments secured with lag screws wherever possible.

A rehabilitation protocol was started after removal of the bandage in group 1 and immediately after plate fixation in group 2. Gentle pendulum exercises of the shoulder in the sling/arm pouch were allowed as per pain tolerance

Table 1 Flowchart representation of patient recruitment and the follow-up rates

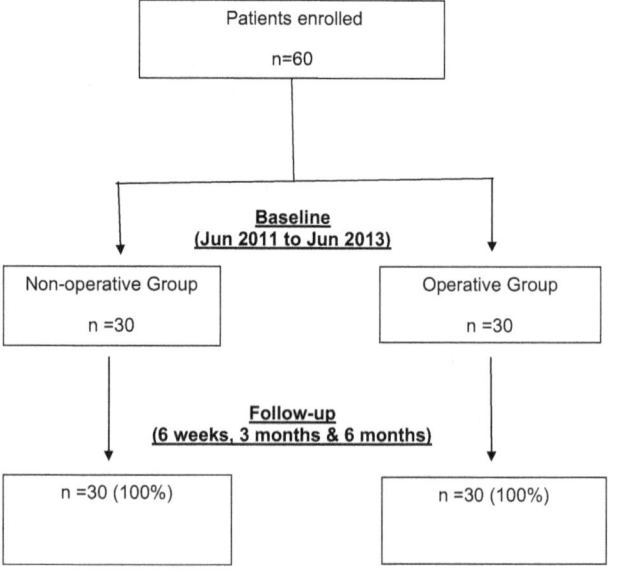

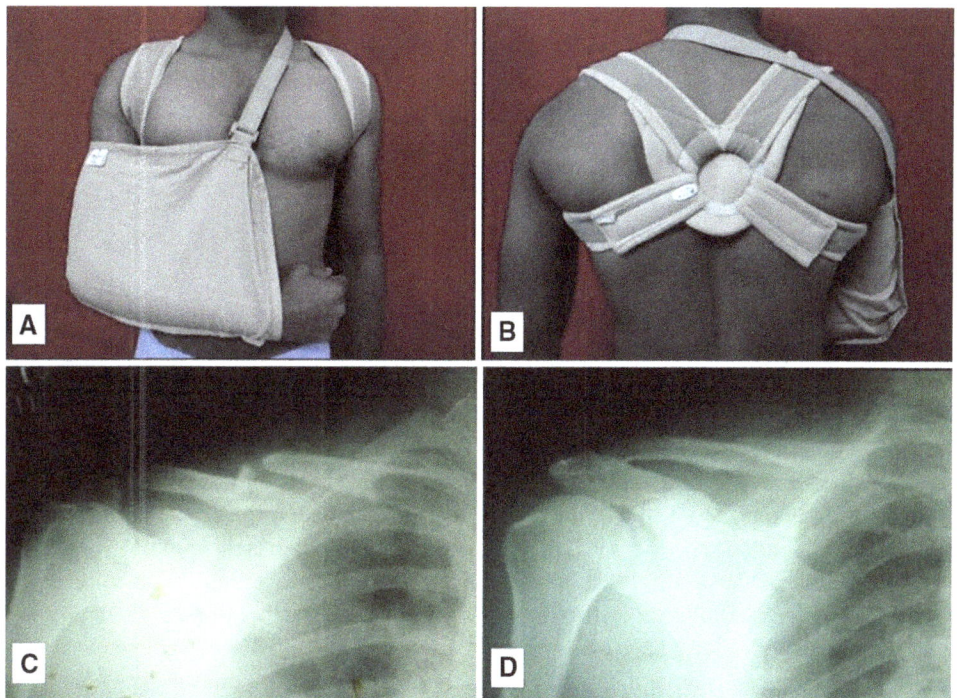

Fig. 1 a Figure-of-eight bandage with shoulder arm pouch-anterior view. **b** Figure-of-eight bandage with shoulder arm pouch-posterior view. **c** Initial radiograph of the fracture at presentation. **d** Fracture union after 6 months of conservative treatment

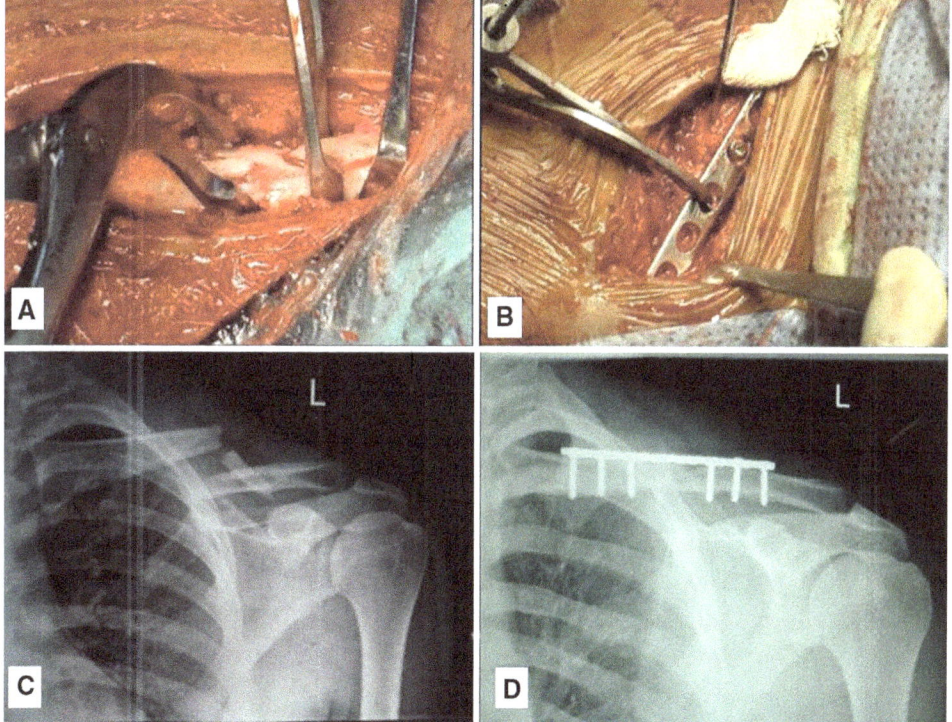

Fig. 2 a Intra-operative fracture reduction. **b** Fracture fixation with 3.5 mm DCP. **c** Radiograph before fracture fixation. **d** Fracture union after 6 months of surgical treatment

immediately after surgery in surgical treated group and after 3 weeks in conservative group. At 3 weeks, gentle active range of motion of the shoulder was allowed with abduction limiting to 90°. Subsequently, active range of motion exercises that are to be performed at home is advised. At four to 6 weeks, active to active assisted range of motion in all planes was allowed. When fracture union (defined as radiographic union with no pain or motion with manual stressing of the fracture) was evident, muscle strengthening exercises were also allowed. At eight to 12 weeks, isometric and isotonic exercises were prescribed to the shoulder girdle muscles with a return to full activities (including sports) at 3 months.

Regular follow-up was done every fortnight for initial 6 weeks, then at 06 weeks, 03 and 06 months using patient's subjective evaluation, functional outcome and radiographic assessment. Patients' subjective evaluation was investigated by direct interview at the follow-up visits. Functional outcome was graded on the standardized clinical evaluation and completion of the Constant and Murley score [15]. Fracture healing was monitored by periodic radiographic examinations on two planes. The fracture was considered to be united when there was no tenderness at the fracture site with full function of the limb clinically and when the bridging callus was seen radiologically. Both the clinical and radiologic unions were assessed by an independent surgeon. An adverse event or complication was defined as any event that necessitated another operative procedure or additional medical treatment.

Statistics

The data analysis was done using SPSS software version 17. We have used Fisher's exact test, Chi-square test and 2 independent sample t-tests to find the association/ significance between group 1 and group 2. The observed results were determined to be significant if the P value was <0.05 and not significant if it was >0.05.

The institute's ethics committee approval was taken before the commencement of study.

Results

There was no statistically significant difference between the group 1 and group 2 with regard to demographic parameters such as mode of injury, age and sex of patients, side affected, presence of associated injuries and type of fracture as per Robinson's classification (Table 2).

The time to union was significantly shorter ($P < 0.05$) in patients treated surgically (Fig. 3). The fracture united in 93% of the patients in group 1, whereas all patients had fracture union in group 2. Fracture union was early and seen in more number of patients in group 2 as compared to group 1. Around 73% of patients were fully satisfied, with the treatment at the end of 6 months in group 1, as compared to 83% in group 2 with the treatment (Fig. 4).

The mean Constant score was higher in the surgically treated group in comparison with conservatively managed group at the end of 6 weeks, 3 and 6 months, and it was statistically significant (Table 3).

Nine patients (30%) in group 1 had various complications such as malunion with cosmetic deformity, nonunion and restriction of shoulder movements, as compared to 6 patients (20%) in group 2 who had scar-related problems and hardware prominence along with the one malunion (Table 4). Malunion and nonunion rates were higher in conservative group in comparison with the surgical group. However, complications of surgical group were generally related to surgical technique and the implant. Overall, the complication rate in the conservative group was relatively higher.

Discussion

In the past, conservative management was the mainstay of treatment for all clavicle fractures in middle third irrespective of displacement and comminution as clavicle has excellent power of remodeling. Conservative treatment with figure-of-8 bandage aligns the displaced fragments in an acceptable manner and results in a good functional outcome. However, a recent meta-analysis revealed higher nonunion rates for displaced fractures treated non-operatively (15%) than operatively (2.2%) with modern internal fixation techniques [10]. Multiple recent trials have also revealed higher incidence of residual pain, nonunion, malunion, shoulder weakness, decreased shoulder

Table 2 Patient demographics and P value between the two groups

Demographic parameters	Group 1	Group 2	P value (<0.05 taken as significant)
Age (mean)	35.20	32.43	0.219
Sex			
Male	27	26	0.999
Female	3	4	
Mode of injury			
RTA	20	19	0.999
Fall	7	7	
Sports injury	3	4	
Side affected			
Dominant	13	12	0.999
Non-dominant	17	18	
Presence of associated injuries			
Present	6	8	0.542
Absent	24	22	
Robinsons classification			
2B1	10	15	0.295
2B2	20	15	

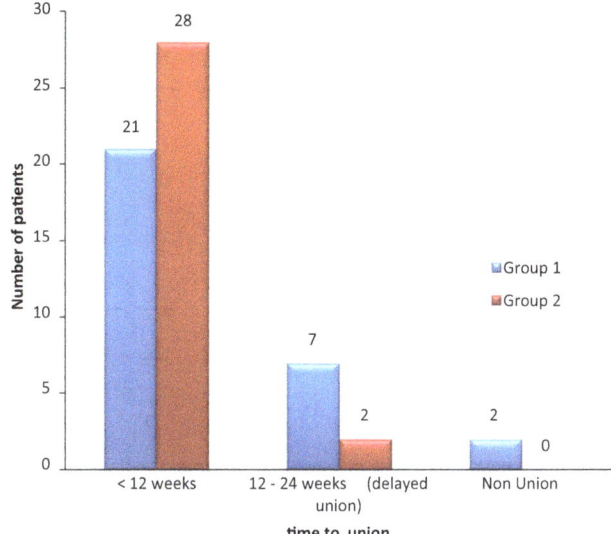

Fig. 3 Time to union with respect to treatment group

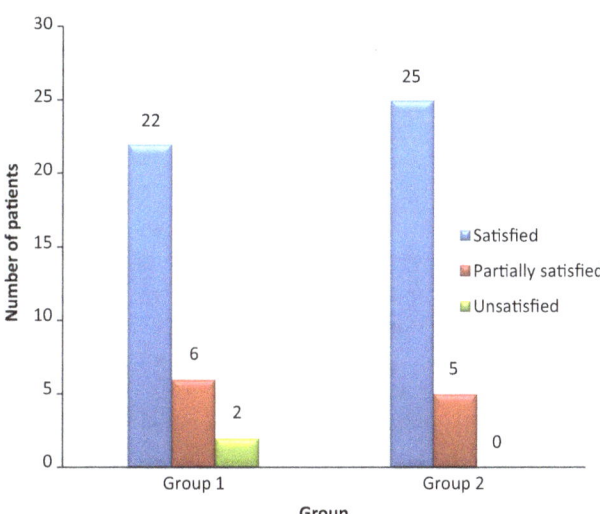

Fig. 4 Subjective evaluation at six months follow-up

Table 3 Comparison of Constant shoulder score between the groups at 6 weeks, 3 and 6 months

Constant score at	Group 1		Group 2		P value
	Mean	SD	Mean	SD	
Sixth week	63.87	5.75	71.80	4.87	<0.001
Third month	75.77	5.96	83.63	4.82	<0.001
Sixth month	89.60	6.64	94.00	2.99	0.001

endurance, inferior patient and surgeon-oriented outcome scores, and lower overall satisfaction after non-operative management of mid-shaft clavicle fractures [12, 16]. The operative management of these fractures with plating or nailing was reserved only for a subset of population with open fractures or highly displaced fractures.

The existing literature reports two sets of incidence of these fractures: The first is the largest and is associated with young active population (sports, motor vehicle accidents), whereas the second is associated with elderly individuals (osteoporotic fractures with simple falls) [4]. A direct blow to the shoulder is the most common mechanism of injury that produces a mid-shaft fracture of the clavicle. As the shoulder is subjected to a high compression force from lateral side, the clavicle and its articulations are the main areas to get affected as they resist these forces. Most (85%) clavicle fractures occur in the mid-shaft as the bone is narrowest and enveloping soft tissue structures (which may help dissipate injury force) are most scarce [17]. In our study, the age group was 20–50 years. The mean age was 35.2 years in group 1 and 32.4 years in group 2. The dominant side was affected in 25 cases (41.66%) out of 60 subjects, whereas remaining 35 cases (58.34%) had fracture on the non-dominant side which similar to the incidence reported in the literature [18, 19]. Functional impairment of the shoulder and the upper limb can be extremely variable. A careful clinico-radiologic assessment is absolutely necessary to exclude associated chest injuries, such as pneumothorax or haemothorax, which are reported in the literature to occur at rates of up to 3% [8]. In the present study, 14 patients (23.3%) had associated injuries. However, none of these patients had pneumothorax or haemothorax or neurovascular injury.

Generally, the clavicle fractures undergo operative fixation within first 10–14 days from the time of injury. However, various studies report increased number of complications, if the primary fixation is delayed for more than 2 weeks [20]. All patients underwent surgery within first 7 days in our study which might have contributed to higher rates of bony union. The advantages of plate fixation include immediate rigid stabilization and pain relief and it also facilitates early mobilization. The rehab protocol instituted in both the treatment groups has been discussed in the previous section. The early mobilization in the surgical group helped the patients to maintain their shoulder strength and early shoulder function, whereas conservatively treated patients had their shoulder immobilized for 3 weeks, which might have resulted in shoulder weakness and delayed shoulder function. Hence, the functional outcome as measured by Constant shoulder score was higher in surgically treated patients at all follow-ups in comparison with non-surgical group. Moreover, the earlier rehabilitation might have contributed to higher rates of bony union and early functional recovery as evident from our results.

The average duration required for union in conservative group was 11.29 weeks, as compared to 9.27 weeks in operative group. There is a statistically significant difference in the mean duration to union in both the groups

Table 4 Various complications in both the groups and their *P* value

	Treatment group		Total	*P* value
	Group 1	Group 2		
Malunion with cosmetic deformity	6	1	7	0.103
Nonunion	2	0	2	0.492
Scar problems	0	3	3	0.237
Hardware prominence	0	2	2	0.492
Restriction of ROM	1	0	1	0.999
Total	9 (30%)	6 (20%)	15 (25%)	0.371

similar to other studies [20, 21]. Majority of the patients in conservative group returned to their pre-injury activity levels by around 16 weeks, whereas in the surgical group it was around 12 weeks.

Previous studies in adults have shown a higher rate of patient satisfaction after non-operative treatment of clavicle fractures [16, 22]. But, patient-reported satisfaction scores may be superior with an early surgical stabilization in some circumstances. A multicenter trial reported better functional outcomes, lower malunion and nonunion rates, and a shorter overall time to union in operatively treated clavicle fractures after plate fixation [12]. In our study, the mean Constant shoulder score for group 1 was 63.87, 75.77 and 89.60 at 6 weeks, 3 and 6 months, respectively. However, for group 2, it was 71.80, 83.63 and 94.00 at 6 weeks, 3 and 6 months, respectively. There was a difference of 7.93 points in favor of surgical group at 6 weeks, 7.86 points at 3 months and 4.40 points at 6 months. At the end of 6 months, 93.33% patients achieved an excellent result (Constant score >90) in the surgically treated group as compared to 80% in the conservative group. 6.66% of the patients had a good score in surgical group (Constant score between 70 and 90) as compared to 13.33% in the conservative group. 6.66% patients had poor score in the conservative group (Constant score <70) as compared to none in the surgical group.

Earlier trials have analyzed the risk of shoulder dysfunction after conservative treatment, which generally was attributed to shortening of the bone segment, residual bone deformity, loss of force and persistent pain [23]. Some studies have observed lesser number of consolidation defects after surgical fixation as compared to conservative treatment, whereas others have demonstrated a 37% risk of adverse events after a surgical procedure possibly due to invasion of the periosteal structures that can lead to nerve damage, blood loss and post-traumatic hematoma, which can delay fracture healing [19].

In our study, we had a total of 15 patients (25%) out of 60 with complications across both groups. Out of 15 patients with complications, 9 patients (30%) belonged to non-surgical group and 6 patients (20%) belonged to surgical group. Though the difference was not significant when total number

of complications was taken into account in both the groups, symptomatic malunion and nonunion was more common in conservative group than the surgical group. There were no surgical site infection, complex regional pain syndrome or neurovascular problems in any of our subjects. The study results are in line with more dated reports of outcomes of operative treatment of displaced mid-shaft clavicular fractures that show a complication rate of 23% and more. Some trials indicate that although clavicular deformities are complex and hard to analyze, shortening by 1.5–2 cm may result in an increased incidence of clinical symptoms. Shortening is one parameter which can be measured [23]. In the present study, there were six patients (20%) with symptomatic malunion with a cosmetic deformity in conservative group as compared to one patient (3.33%) in the surgical group. This patient in the surgical group had premature loading of the injured extremity because of which the plate got bent and resulted in malunion.

Several recent studies have shown high union rates with surgical management using a variety of internal fixation devices, including plating and IM pin or rod fixation [11]. In addition, there is also strong evidence that the nonunion rate after conservative treatment may be higher than previously reported, particularly in certain patients and fracture types. In this study, we had 2 nonunions (6.66%) out of 30 patients in conservative group as compared to none in surgical group. These two patients with nonunion underwent operative treatment at a later date. Our results with regard to various complications compare well with the existing literature and the published studies on the subject.

Our study has few strengths and limitations. Though the sample size is small and was not calculated prior to the study, the study has the sufficient power (>90%) to identify a standardized effect size in the Constant score of 0.5 at the final follow-up. It is a prospective non-randomized comparative trial, wherein there was no selection bias and the baseline demographic characteristics of the subjects in both the groups were almost similar, which reduced the chance of any other bias in the outcome. However, certain residual confounding factors in the results cannot be excluded as only a few were considered. The major strength of the study was the 100% follow-up in both the groups, though it was only 6 months.

From our study, we have noticed that in the surgical group, time to union was shorter with almost 100% union rates. More patients were satisfied and subjective outcome was better. The Constant shoulder scores were also significantly higher at all follow-ups. The numbers of complications were lesser and many of them were implant related and surgical technique related. On the other side, patients treated conservatively took longer time to unite and had more number of malunions and nonunions. Subjective outcome was inferior as compared to surgical group, and Constant shoulder scores were also lower at all follow-ups. Hence, in a young, active patient, surgical fixation of an acute displaced mid-shaft clavicle fracture in the form of plating appears to result in improved outcome. Plate fixation in these individuals is a reasonable option to maintain anatomic reduction and achieve union with restoration of maximal shoulder function.

The limited complications of surgical group seen in the present study were implant and surgical technique related and can be minimized with better availability of modern implants and good surgical technique. Recently, with the advent of pre-contoured locking plates, the incidence of hardware prominence has decreased. These plates are particularly beneficial in osteoporotic and severely comminuted fractures. The usage of pre-contoured anatomic clavicle plates and an anteroinferior approach for the fixation may minimize many of these complications. The conservative treatment remains the gold standard in treatment of simple undisplaced mid-shaft clavicle fractures, but for displaced and comminuted fractures surgical intervention is appropriate especially in young active adults. If implants and expertise is available, with a good surgical technique operative treatment might give satisfactory and superior results over nonoperative treatment. Although certain multicenter trials support the use of primary operative fixation for diaphyseal fractures [12], the quantum of this treatment effect on the outcome may not be sufficient enough to justify a surgical treatment to all patients.

In conclusion, anatomic reduction with plate fixation and early mobilization of displaced clavicle fractures is a viable treatment option, especially in young active adults with good outcomes and no major complications. There is also a need for further large multicenter prospective randomized controlled trials in order to generalize this preference of operative fixation over non-operative management in acute displaced mid-shaft clavicular fractures for all patients.

Informed consent Informed consent was obtained from all individual participants included in the study.

References

1. Curtis RJ, Dameron TB, Rockwood CA (1991) Fractures and dislocations of the shoulder in children. In: Rockwood CA, Wilkins KE, King RE (eds) Fractures in children, 3rd edn. JB Lippincott, Philadelphia, pp 829–919
2. Craig EV (1998) Fractures of the clavicle. In: Rockwood CA, Matsen FA (eds) The shoulder, 3rd edn. WB Saunders, Philadelphia, pp 428–482
3. Robinson CM (1998) Fractures of the clavicle in the adult. J Bone Joint Surg Br 80B:476–484
4. Nordqvist A, Petersson C (1994) The incidence of fractures of the clavicle. Clin Orthop Relat Res 300:127–132
5. Allman FL Jr (1967) Fractures and ligamentous injuries of the clavicle and its articulation. J Bone Joint Surg Am 49(4):774–784
6. Stanley D, Trowbridge EA, Norris SH (1988) The mechanism of clavicular fracture. A clinical and biochemical analysis. J Bone Joint Surg Br 70B:461–464
7. Neer CS (1960) Nonunion of the clavicle. JAMA 172:1006–1011
8. Rowe CR (1968) An atlas of anatomy and treatment of mid-clavicular fractures. Clin Orthop 58:29–42
9. Hill JM, McGuire MH, Crosby LA (1997) Closed treatment of displaced middle-third fractures of the clavicle gives poor results. J Bone Joint Surg Br 79B:537–539
10. Zlowodzki M, Zelle BA, Cole PA et al (2005) Treatment of midshaft clavicle fractures: systemic review of 2144 fractures. J Orthop Trauma 19:504–507
11. Ali Khan MA, Lucas HK (1978) Plating of fractures of the middle third of the clavicle. Injury 9:263–267
12. Canadian Orthopaedic Trauma Society (2007) (MD McKee, principal investigator). Plate fixation versus nonoperative care for acute, displaced midshaft fractures of the clavicle. J Bone Joint Surg 89A:1–11
13. Chen CH, Ch WJ, Shih CH (2002) Surgical treatment for distal clavicle fractures with coracoclavicular ligament disruption. J Trauma 52:7–8
14. Flinkkila T, Ristiniemi J, Hyvonen P et al (2002) Surgical treatment of unstable fractures of the distal clavicle: a comparative study of Kirschner wire and clavicular hook plate fixation. Acta Orthop Scand 73:50–53
15. Constant CR, Murley AH (1987) A clinical method of functional assessment of the shoulder. Clin Orthop Relat Res 214:160–164
16. Eskola A, Vainionpaa S, Myllynen P, Patiala H, Rokkanen P (1986) Outcome of clavicular fracture in 89 patients. Arch Orthop Trauma Surg 105(6):337–338
17. Robinson CM, Cairns DA (2004) Primary nonoperative treatment of displaced lateral fractures of the clavicle. J Bone Joint Surge Am 86A:778–782
18. De Giorgi S, Notarnicola A, Tafuri S, Solarino G, Moretti L, Moretti B (2011) Conservative treatment of fractures of the clavicle. BMC Res Notes 8(4):333
19. Vander Have KL, Perdue AM, Caird MS, Farley FA (2010) Operative versus nonoperative treatment of midshaft clavicle fractures in adolescents. J Pediatr Orthop 30(4):307–312
20. van der Woude P, van der Vlies CH, Jean MFH (2012) Operative treatment of displaced midshaft clavicular fracture: is it the best management? Curr Orthop Pract 23(2)
21. Altamimi SA, McKee MD (2008) Canadian Orthopaedic Society. Nonoperative treatment compared with plate fixation of displaced midshaft clavicle fractures. Surgical technique. J Bone Joint Surg Am. 90(90 Suppl 2 Pt 1):1–8
22. Nordqvist A, Petersson CJ, Redlund-Johnell I (1998) Mid-clavicle fractures in adults: end result study after conservative treatment. J Orthop Trauma 12(8):572–576

14

Femoral shaft osteotomy for obligate outward rotation due to SCFE

Peter M. Stevens[1] · Lucas Anderson[1] · Bruce A. MacWilliams[1]

Abstract Slipped capital femoral epiphysis (SCFE) is an adolescent disease that leads to retroversion of the femoral neck and shaft, relative to the head. Observing that patients with SCFE must walk with an outward foot progression angle and externally rotate the leg in order to flex the hip, we have been performing a femoral shaft rotational osteotomy wherein we rotate the lower femur 45° inward, relative to the upper femur. By correcting retroversion, our goal is to improve functional hip and knee motion, thereby mitigating the effects of SCFE impingement. This is a retrospective review of five hips in four patients (two boys and two girls), average age 14.7 years (range 11 + 7–18 years) who underwent femoral midshaft rotational osteotomy for correction of acquired retroversion of the femur secondary to severe SCFE. We compared clinical findings at the outset to those at an average follow-up of 46 months (range 24–74 months). Pre- and post-gait analysis was performed in three patients. Two of the patients underwent elective arthroscopic osteochondroplasty to alleviate residual FAI: contralateral arthroscopy is pending in one. The first patient in this series received a hip arthroplasty, 62 months after his osteotomy, at age 23. Following midshaft osteotomy, all patients experienced improvement in comfort, gait and activities of daily living. With the patella neutral, they had improved range of hip flexion from an average preoperative flexion of <25° to a postoperative flexion of >90°. Two patients (both male) had delayed union and some loss of correction, secondary to broken interlocking screws; each healed with reamed, exchange nailing. The interlocking screws have since been redesigned and enlarged. Femoral shaft rotational osteotomy restores the functional range of hip motion, while correcting obligate out-toeing and improving knee kinematics. This procedure is technically straightforward, permitting progressive weight bearing, while avoiding the risk of AVN. Osteochondroplasty for residual FAI can be deferred, pending the outcome.
Level of evidence III: retrospective series—no controls.

Keywords Slipped capital femoral epiphysis · SCFE · Femoral retroversion · FAI · Femoroacetabular impingement · Femoral osteotomy

Introduction

Slipped capital femoral epiphysis (SCFE) is an injury to the femoral capital physis. The metaphysis displaces anterosuperiorly relative to the femoral head and produces a varus and retroverted proximal femoral deformity. This deformity can lead to femoroacetabular impingement (FAI) where, in hip flexion, the anterior head–neck junction abuts the anterolateral labrum resulting in pathological compressive and shearing forces to the labral tissues and peripheral cartilage (Fig. 1). The pathomechanics associated with FAI secondary to SCFE has been shown to cause chondrolabral damage in the form of labral degeneration and peripheral acetabular cartilage damage [1–3]. In symptomatic FAI related to SCFE, treatment options range from arthroscopic osteochondroplasty, surgical dislocation and osteochondroplasty (SDO), subcapital realignment, intertrochanteric flexion—valgus osteotomy—as well as hip arthroplasty.

The retroversion associated with severely malunited capital epiphyses not only can result in functional limitations in hip flexion and inward rotation but, additionally,

✉ Peter M. Stevens
  peter.stevens@hsc.utah.edu

[1] Department of Orthopaedics, University of Utah,
  Salt Lake City, UT 84113, USA

Fig. 1 a Normal version of the adolescent or adult femur = 11° and the foot progression angle is neutral. **b** Acquired retroversion (40° depicted) may be under-recognized because this is interpreted as varus or extension on plain radiographs. **c** The clinical manifestations include outward foot progression angles noted during gait. **d** Attempted inward rotation of the hip causes anterolateral impingement, exacerbated by attempted hip flexion. This produces an obligatory outward rotation when walking or sitting. **e** The rationale for an anteverting osteotomy is shown here, mitigating the impingement in flexion while restoring the neutral foot progressing angle and improving knee kinematics

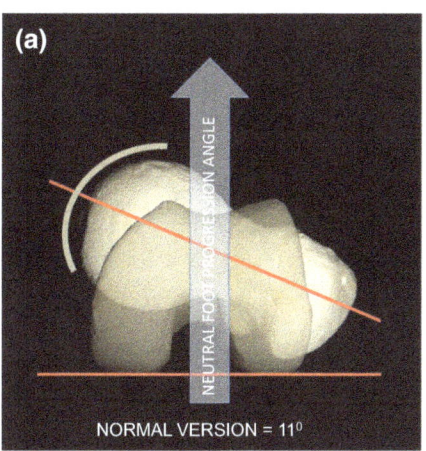
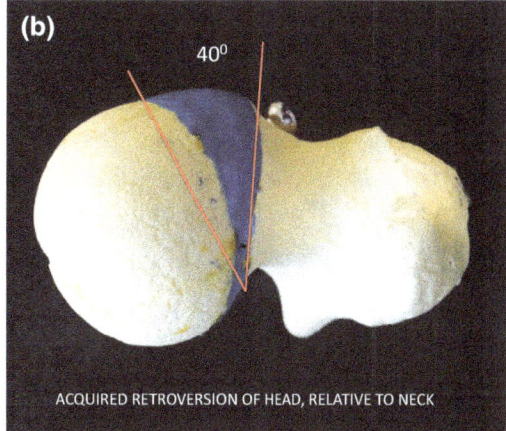
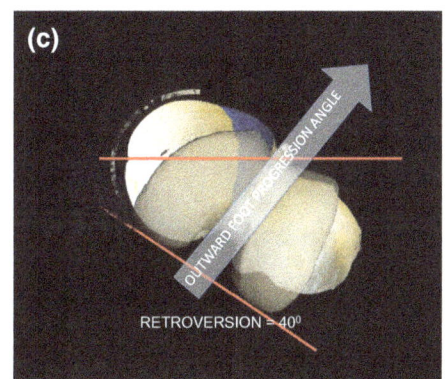
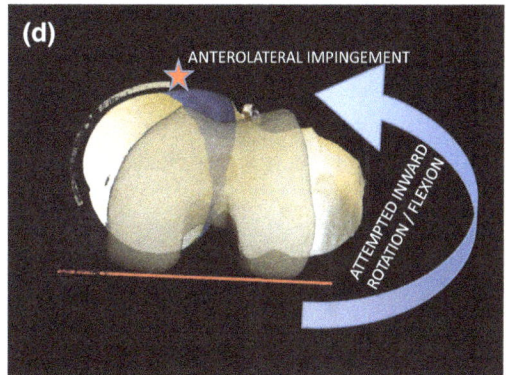
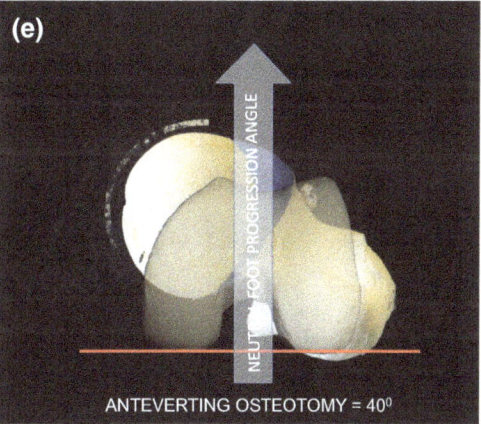

produces an outward foot progression angle during ambulation. This compromises knee kinematics. Patients with bilateral SCFE may have difficulty with daily activities including sitting upright in a chair, tying their shoes, riding a bicycle and driving a car. They complain of knee pain often in addition to hip pain and limited motion.

Consequent to the negative impact of the hip retroversion, we have adopted a strategy for managing symptomatic malunited SCFE by a midshaft and 45° inward rotation femoral shaft osteotomy (FSRO). The goal is to restore a functional range of motion for the involved hip and ipsilateral knee and restore a foot-forward gait. An osteotomy of the proximal femur is avoided and

arthroscopic treatment of FAI can be pursued electively. The purpose of this study was to report on the preliminary outcome of a series of SCFE patients treated with an anteverting midshaft osteotomy of the femur for outward rotation in flexion and gait in lieu of the traditional femoral neck or intertrochanteric osteotomy.

Patients and methods

Between January 2003 and January 2012, four patients (five limbs) with SCFE were treated with femoral shaft rotational osteotomies (FSRO). There were two female and two male patients (one male bilateral FRSO), with an average age of 14.7 years old (range 11 + 7–18 years old) at time of surgery. This retrospective study was approved by the Institutional Board Review.

Three of the hips had prior in situ pinning of their SCFE; the other two had not had any prior intervention for unrecognized SCFE. The indication for surgery in this group of patients included acquired gait disturbance (obligate out-toeing), marked limitation of hip flexion (<25°) and hip or knee pain that interfered with activities of daily living. One patient had mild chondrolysis at presentation (diagnosed from 1 mm of relative narrowing of the articular clear space as compared to the uninvolved hip). This was not exacerbated post-osteotomy.

Clinical

The gait pattern revealed an outward foot progression angle of at least 30° preoperatively. Patients were unable to sit upright in a chair and lean forward to tie their shoe laces. The preoperative examination included a standard torsional profile measured in the prone position. Inward rotation of the involved hip was limited to 0° (or even less) typically as compared to outward rotation >90°. Based on these findings, 45° of rotational correction was undertaken at the time of the midshaft osteotomy. In the supine position, the range of hip flexion (<25°—patella neutral) was compared to flexion past 90° when the hip was rotated 45° outward (Fig. 2). This small retrospective series of patients did not lend itself to patient-reported outcomes or functional hip or knee scores.

Imaging

Plain radiographs included a full-length standing AP legs (to assess the mechanical axis and relative limb lengths) along with a standing AP of the pelvis and frog lateral view. Each hip was judged to be a stable SCFE of

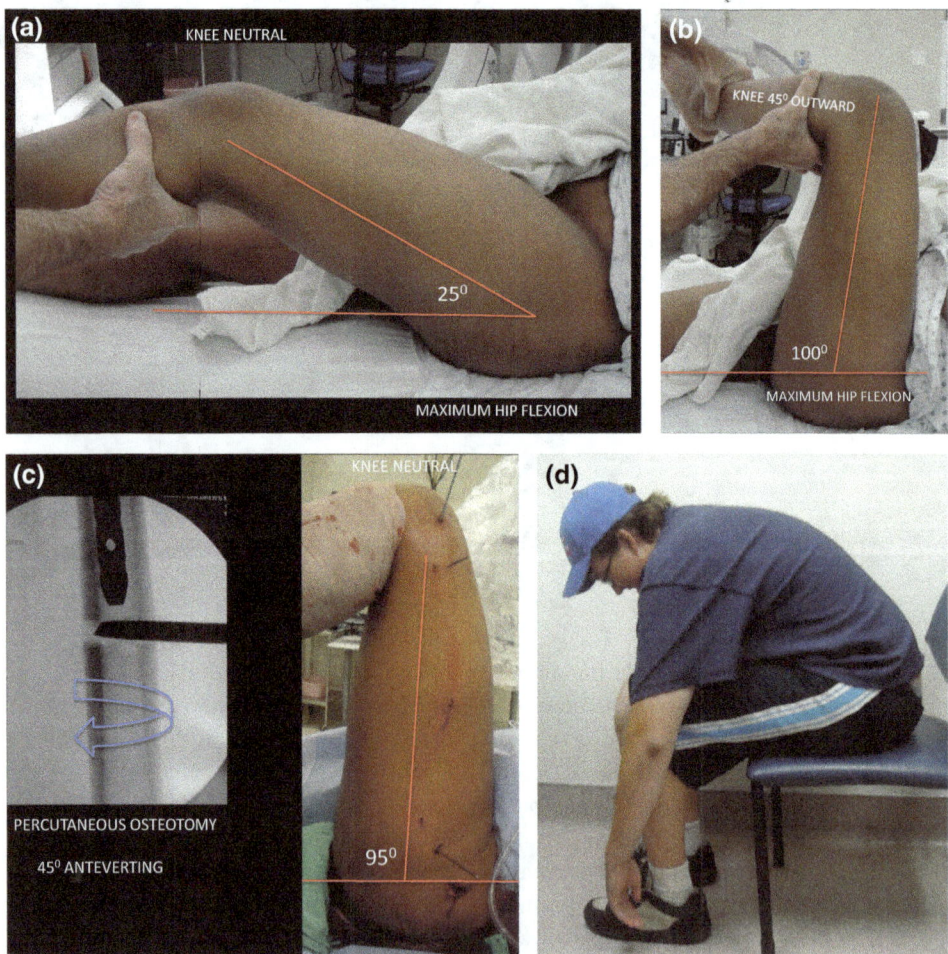

Fig. 2 a Preoperative attempt to flex the hip with the knee held neutral demonstrates the blockage due to FAI. **b** By simply rotating the hip outward 40°, hip flexion is permitted past 90°. **c** The anteverting femoral osteotomy resolves the clinical problems at the knee while improving functional ROM of the hip. **d** Functional range of hip flexion, maintained 4 years post-rotational osteotomy. This was not possible pre-osteotomy

intermediate severity. We did not grade the slip angle specifically because of the likelihood of projectional artifact and inter-observer error. Advanced imaging, such as MRI or CT scan with 3D reconstruction, was not undertaken as the osteotomy was away from the hip joint and should not change angles or coverage. We reasoned the abnormal head–neck offset could be dealt with subsequently, as needed, via hip arthroscopy. This has been undertaken in two of the hips and a third is pending.

Gait analysis

Pre- and post-operative computational gait analysis was performed on three of four subjects. A standard marker model was applied, and data were collected using a ten camera motion capture system (Vicon, Centennial CO, USA) and four force platforms (AMTI, Watertown, MA, USA) as the subjects ambulated at a self-selected velocity along a 10-m walkway [4]. Temporal parameters, kinematics and kinetics of the hip, knee and ankle, and an overall measure of gait kinematics are reported using the gait deviation index (Fig. 3) [4].

Surgical technique for FRSO

The patient was placed supine on a standard radiolucent table with a radiolucent bump under the ipsilateral hip. The degree of hip flexion, with the patella forward, was noted and compared to hip flexion with the knee rotated 45° of outward. In each case, flexion past 90° was obtained (Fig. 2a, b). A trochanteric entry intramedullary rod, avoiding the piriformis fossa penetration, was utilized for stabilization post-osteotomy. Rotational guide pins (7/64 Steinman pins) were inserted into the proximal and distal femur to anticipate inward rotation correction of 45°. The osteotomy was performed percutaneously, at the midshaft level, connecting transverse drill holes with an Ilizarov osteotome and applying torque with a wrench. The distal interlocking screw was inserted first, using the perfect circle method, followed by the proximal screw via a jig [5]. Patients were permitted progressive weight bearing with crutches and physical therapy was utilized when needed to address abductor and quadriceps weakness and range of motion.

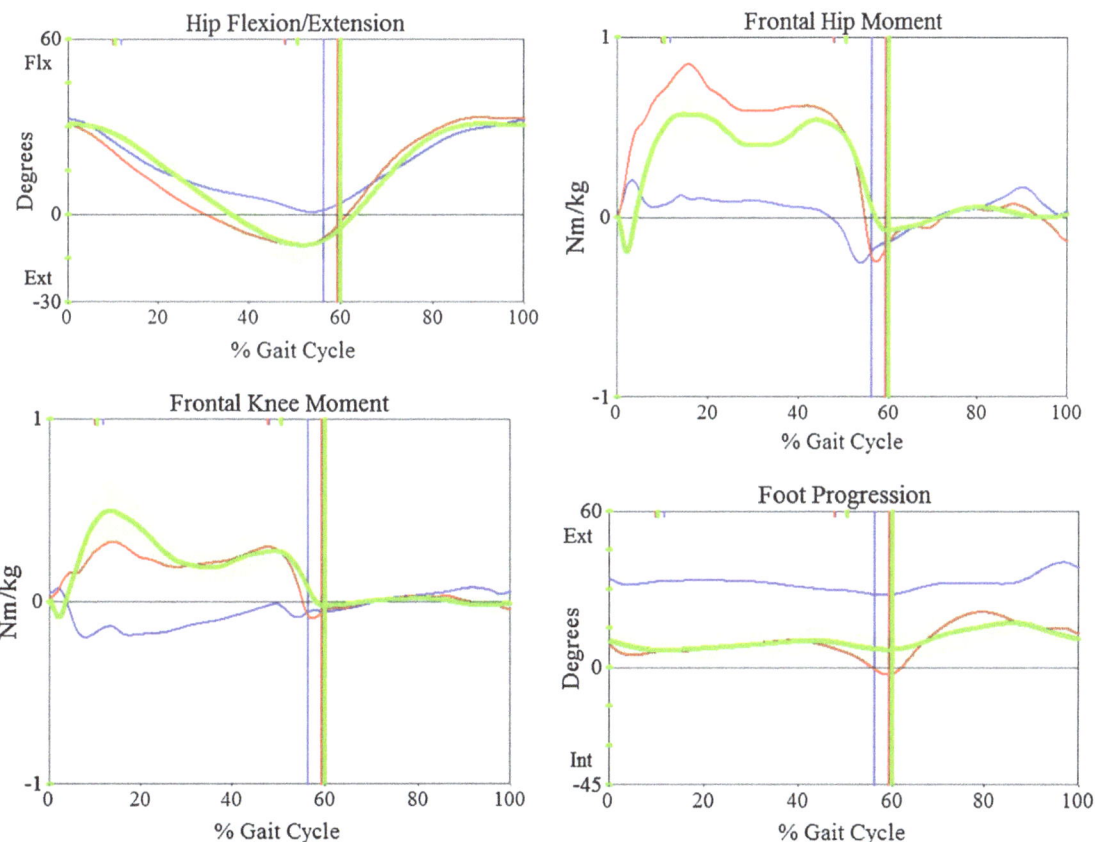

Fig. 3 Movement analysis graphs depicting improvement, not only at the hip, but the ipsilateral knee as shown −/*blue* + preoperative/ *red* = post-anteverting osteotomy/*green* = control (color figure online)

Results

The mean follow-up was 44 months (range 24–74 months). The prone rotational profile was improved uniformly with an average of 40° inward and 60° of outward rotation of the hips (as compared to 0° inward and 90° outward preoperatively). The foot progression angle had improved from 35° outward to within normal range (0°–15°). Hip flexion, limited to 20° preoperatively, was maintained past 90° with the knee(s) in neutral. The patients were able to sit in a chair, with the knee(s) facing forward and bend over to tie their shoe laces (Fig. 2d).

There were no intra-operative or immediate postoperative complications. Osteonecrosis was absent on follow-up. There were two long-term postoperative complications; both male patients experienced interlocking screw fatigue failure and some loss of rotational correction requiring revision intramedullary fixation at 5 and 8 months after the index procedure. In both cases, the desired rotational correction was achieved ultimately. The interlocking screw failure has since been addressed by a redesign of the core diameter of 3.0–3.75 mm.

One patient underwent an arthroscopic osteochondroplasty in conjunction with extraction of screws and rod. Another patient underwent the same for ongoing impingement symptoms 6 months after rotational osteotomy. This patient had hip chondrolysis on presentation. The first (and oldest) patient eventually underwent a total hip arthroplasty at age 23, 5 years after rotational osteotomy. The joint surgeon reported no challenges or extenuating circumstances resulting from the prior diaphyseal osteotomy.

Gait study

This series was too small to establish significant differences from pre- and postoperative gait analysis (Fig. 3). The investigation remains informative on the overall impact of retroversion from chronic SCFE. Knee pain that is commonly associated with SCFE is probably due to the retroversion which has a negative impact upon knee kinematics. As a result, pre- and postoperative torsional profiles and comparative gait analysis are planned for a group of patients undergoing arthroscopic osteochondroplasty.

Discussion

The proximal femoral abnormalities characteristic of SCFE are a well-known cause of femoroacetabular impingement (FAI) [6–8]. The pistol grip deformity from hip varus and retroversion causes a decreased head/neck offset [9]. This deformity causes abutment of the head–neck junction

within the acetabulum which leads to intra-articular chondrolabral damage frequently [10–12]. Typically, the degree of slip is graded according to plain AP and frog lateral radiographic images, but these fail to illustrate the acquired retroversion from SCFE. While CT scans with 3D reconstruction may demonstrate the complex nature of this deformity, these imaging modalities are typically focused upon the hip and do not include the distal femur. Consequently, the contribution of retroversion is not recognized. It is the clinical examination that puts the acquired retroversion and knee malorientation in perspective; this should include noting the foot progression angle, the prone torsional profile and the range of hip flexion with the knee neutral and limb rotated outward. This correlates well with the forced outward orientation of the limb when attempting to flex the knee and hip in the supine position. It explains the obligate out-toeing and altered knee kinematics and pain that should be addressed in corrective surgery.

The treatment approach to the patient with symptomatic FAI secondary to malunited SCFE has focused on the proximal femur and remains controversial. Treatment strategies range from watchful waiting to surgical intervention which has included one or more of the following: arthroscopy, intertrochanteric osteotomy, surgical dislocation and osteochondroplasty, arthrodesis and total hip arthroplasty [13, 14]. Fabricant et al. [15] noted that treatment of FAI may have less benefit in patients with relative femoral retroversion. Several groups have demonstrated clinical improvement with intertrochanteric osteotomy and base of neck extra-capsular osteotomies [16, 17]. Surgical dislocation (or arthroscopy) with osteochondroplasty alone can be used to improve the head–neck offset and address chondrolabral lesions. However, the reported outcomes have focused on pain relief and improvement in femoral head-to-neck offset. Leunig et al. [18] advocated for simultaneous in situ pinning and osteochondroplasty of the head–neck junction to improve offset in mild SCFE deformities. However, this technique lacks the power to resolve the obligate out-toeing that is so often associated with severe slips and may not improve knee kinematics.

Subcapital correction osteotomy has gained attention recently because it permits correction of both the varus and retroversion deformity of the proximal femur without creating other deformities. Numerous studies have discussed the use of subcapital cuneiform osteotomies to correct SCFE deformities in skeletally immature patients with concerning rates of AVN and chondrolysis [19–22]. Ziebarth and Huber each reported on a series of modified Dunn osteotomies and Slongo reported on open reductions in acute SCFE's, each utilizing the surgical dislocation technique described by Ganz with minimal risk of AVN and chondrolysis [10, 23]. However, a recent series on the subcapital correction osteotomy for SCFE deformities in patients with closed physes utilizing the surgical dislocation technique reported a concerning rate of AVN despite good results in the majority of patients [24].

Intertrochanteric osteotomy has been used to address varus and retroversion deformities; however, it has its own set of complications including AVN, nonunion and malunion [25]. For the surgeon who uses this as their "go to" method to address severe SCFE deformities, we would suggest on making a goal of gaining 35°–45° of anteversion through rotation of the fragments in addition to the valgus correction gained. We believe the retroversion is the greater cause of impingement and obligate out-toeing when walking and sitting while the varus deformity is more related to the limb length inequality and trochanteric impingement.

While femoral shaft rotational osteotomy does not address the proximal femoral deformity directly, this technique recovers a functional range of hip motion and allows them to walk with their "hip" externally rotated (but foot neutral), thereby mitigating the effects of FAI. This also allows patients to sit more naturally as demonstrated by the improvement in hip flexion and normalization of their internal–external rotational range from their hips, both prone and at 90° of flexion. This osteotomy is comparatively safe and well tolerated with no associated risks of iatrogenic necrosis or chondrolysis.

Limitations

Our study has several limitations. This is a retrospective series of a small number of patients with short follow-up. Given the lack of a control group and short follow-up, we cannot comment on the influence on hip arthritis. Furthermore, we recognize that a rotational osteotomy alone does not address the head–neck offset abnormalities or chondrolabral pathology of the acetabulum. However, if the patient continues to manifest symptoms (three of five hips in this series), these issues can be addressed either at the time of derotation or subsequently, through a small Smith–Peterson approach or arthroscopically if the patient continues to be symptomatic. Finally, we had two non-unions/delayed unions, with loss of correction, treated with revised reamed nailing. These complications are related to choice of hardware rather than a flawed surgical strategy. Both patients broke single 4.5 mm screws (core diameter of 3.0 mm) and appeared to have lost enough of the rotational correction to warrant revision surgery. While we have had success using single interlock screws both proximal and distal for rotational osteotomies in miserable malalignment patients, we have found that SCFE patients (more often male and larger) are at an increased risk of

fixation failure [26]. We now use a 3.75-mm-core-diameter bolt preferentially.

Due to the acquired retroversion, patients with symptomatic FAI secondary to SCFE deformities have significant functional limitations, including obligate outward rotation when walking and during hip flexion. Femoral shaft rotational osteotomy is a familiar and safe technique that may normalize knee kinematics, while improving gait and hip flexion, hip biomechanics and short-term hip outcomes, without posing the risk of serious complications.

Informed consent Proper informed consent was established with all subjects.

References

1. Abraham E, Gonzalez MH, Pratap S, Amirouche F, Atluri P, Simon P (2007) Clinical implications of anatomical wear characteristics in slipped capital femoral epiphysis and primary osteoarthritis. J Pediatr Orthop 27:788–795. doi:10.1097/BPO.0b013e3181558c94
2. Goodman DA, Feighan JE, Smith AD, Latimer B, Buly RL, Cooperman DR (1997) Subclinical slipped capital femoral epiphysis. Relationship to osteoarthrosis of the hip. J Bone Joint Surg Am 79:1489–1497
3. Leunig M, Slongo T, Kleinschmidt M, Ganz R (2007) Subcapital correction osteotomy in slipped capital femoral epiphysis by means of surgical hip dislocation. Oper Orthop Traumatol 19:389–410. doi:10.1007/s00064-007-1213-7
4. Schwartz MH, Rozumalski A (2008) The Gait Deviation Index: a new comprehensive index of gait pathology. Gait Posture 28:351–357. doi:10.1016/j.gaitpost.2008.05.001
5. Stevens PM, Anderson D (2008) Correction of anteversion in skeletally immature patients. J Pediatr Orthop 28:277–283. doi:10.1097/BPO.0b013e318168d962
6. Beck M, Kalhor M, Leunig M, Ganz R (2005) Hip morphology influences the pattern of damage to the acetabular cartilage: femoroacetabular impingement as a cause of early osteoarthritis of the hip. J Bone Joint Surg Br 87:1012–1018. doi:10.1302/0301-620X.87B7.15203
7. Ganz R, Leunig M, Leunig-Ganz K, Harris WH (2008) The etiology of osteoarthritis of the hip: an integrated mechanical concept. Clin Orthop Relat Res 466:264–272. doi:10.1007/s11999-007-0060-z
8. Harris WH (1986) Etiology of osteoarthritis of the hip. Clin Orthop Relat Res 213:20–33
9. Rab GT (1999) The geometry of slipped capital femoral epiphysis: implications for movement, impingement, and corrective osteotomy. J Pediatr Orthop 19:419–424
10. Slongo T, Kakaty D, Krause F, Ziebarth K (2010) Treatment of slipped capital femoral epiphysis with a modified Dunn procedure. J Bone Joint Surg Am 92:2898–2908. doi:10.2106/JBJS.I.01385
11. Clinical implications of anatomical wear characteristics in slipped capital femoral epiphysis and primary osteoarthritis. J Pediatr Orthop (2007)
12. Leunig M, Casillas MM, Hamlet M, Hersche O, Nötzli H, Slongo T et al (2000) Slipped capital femoral epiphysis: early mechanical damage to the acetabular cartilage by a prominent femoral metaphysis. Acta Orthop Scand 71:370–375. doi:10.1080/000164700317393367

13. Castañeda P, Macías C, Rocha A, Harfush A, Cassis N (2009) Functional outcome of stable grade III slipped capital femoral epiphysis treated with in situ pinning. J Pediatr Orthop 29:454–458. doi:10.1097/BPO.0b013e3181aab7c3

14. Diab M, Daluvoy S, Snyder BD, Kasser JR (2006) Osteotomy does not improve early outcome after slipped capital femoral epiphysis. J Pediatr Orthop B 15(2):87–92

15. Fabricant PD, Fields KG, Taylor SA, Magennis E, Bedi A, Kelly BT (2015) The effect of femoral and acetabular version on clinical outcomes after arthroscopic femoroacetabular impingement surgery. J Bone Joint Surg Am 97:537–543. doi:10.2106/JBJS.N.00266

16. El-Mowafi H, El-Adl G, El-Lakkany MR (2005) Extracapsular base of neck osteotomy versus Southwick osteotomy in treatment of moderate to severe chronic slipped capital femoral epiphysis. J Pediatr Orthop 25:171–177

17. Salvati EA, Robinson JH Jr, O'Down TJ (1980) Southwick osteotomy for severe chronic slipped capital femoral epiphysis: results and complications. J Bone Joint Surg Am 62(4):561–570

18. Leunig M, Horowitz K, Manner H, Ganz R (2010) In situ pinning with arthroscopic osteoplasty for mild SCFE: a preliminary technical report. Clin Orthop Relat Res 468:3160–3167. doi:10.1007/s11999-010-1408-3

19. Fish JB (1984) Cuneiform osteotomy of the femoral neck in the treatment of slipped capital femoral epiphysis. J Bone Joint Surg Am 66:1153–1168

20. Gage JR, Sundberg AB, Nolan DR, Sletten RG, Winter RB (1978) Complications after cuneiform osteotomy for moderately or severely slipped capital femoral epiphysis. J Bone Joint Surg Am 60:157–165

21. Heyman CH, Herndon CH (1950) Legg–Perthes disease; A method for the measurement of the roentgenographic result. J Bone Joint Surg Am 32:767–778

22. Martin PH (1948) Slipped epiphysis in the adolescent hip a reconsideration of open reduction. J Bone Joint Surg Am 30:9–19

23. Ziebarth K, Zilkens C, Spencer S, Leunig M, Ganz R, Kim Y-J (2009) Capital realignment for moderate and severe SCFE using a modified Dunn procedure. Clin Orthop Relat Res 467:704–716. doi:10.1007/s11999-008-0687-4

24. Anderson LA, Gililland JM, Pelt CE, Peters CL (2013) Subcapital correction osteotomy for malunited slipped capital femoral epiphysis. J Pediatr Orthop 33:345–352. doi:10.1097/BPO.0b013e31827d7e06

25. Parsch K, Zehender H, Bühl T, Weller S (1999) Intertrochanteric corrective osteotomy for moderate and severe chronic slipped capital femoral epiphysis. J Pediatr Orthop B 8:223

26. Stevens PM, Gaffney CJ, Fillerup H (2016) Percutaneous rotational osteotomy of the femur utilizing an intramedullary rod. Strategies Trauma Limb Reconstr 11(2):129–134

15

Accuracy in identifying the elbow rotation axis on simulated fluoroscopic images using a new anatomical landmark

J. K. Wiggers[1] · R. M. Snijders[1] · J. G. G. Dobbe[2] · G. J. Streekstra[2] · D. den Hartog[3] · N. W. L. Schep[1,4]

Abstract External fixation of the elbow requires identification of the elbow rotation axis, but the accuracy of traditional landmarks (capitellum and trochlea) on fluoroscopy is limited. The relative distance (RD) of the humerus may be helpful as additional landmark. The first aim of this study was to determine the optimal RD that corresponds to an on-axis lateral image of the elbow. The second aim was to assess whether the use of the optimal RD improves the surgical accuracy to identify the elbow rotation axis on fluoroscopy. CT scans of elbows from five volunteers were used to simulate fluoroscopy; the actual rotation axis was calculated with CT-based flexion–extension analysis. First, three observers measured the optimal RD on simulated fluoroscopy. The RD is defined as the distance between the dorsal part of the humerus and the projection of the posteromedial cortex of the distal humerus, divided by the anteroposterior diameter of the humerus. Second, eight trauma surgeons assessed the elbow rotation axis on simulated fluoroscopy. In a preteaching session, surgeons used traditional landmarks. The surgeons were then instructed how to use the optimal RD as additional landmark in a postteaching session. The deviation from the actual rotation axis was expressed as rotational and translational error ($\pm$SD). Measurement of the RD was robust and easily reproducible; the optimal RD was 45%. The surgeons identified the elbow rotation axis with a mean rotational error decreasing from 7.6° $\pm$ 3.4° to 6.7° $\pm$ 3.3° after teaching how to use the RD. The mean translational error decreased from 4.2 $\pm$ 2.0 to 3.7 $\pm$ 2.0 mm after teaching. The humeral RD as additional landmark yielded small but relevant improvements. Although fluoroscopy-based external fixator alignment to the elbow remains prone to error, it is recommended to use the RD as additional landmark.

Keywords Fluoroscopy · Elbow · Rotation axis · Landmark · Segmentation

Introduction

Hinged external elbow fixation is used to treat persistent instability of the ulnohumeral joint, either following closed reduction of an elbow dislocation or following operative treatment of complex elbow fractures. This treatment theoretically mitigates postoperative stiffness because it allows immediate active and passive motion of the elbow joint, while the joint remains stable [1–6].

Though encouraging outcomes have been reported with external fixators, complications are numerous, including nerve injury, deep infection, increased motion resistance, pin site infection, pin loosening and pin breakage [7]. Some of these complications are explained by incongruence between the rotation axis of the fixator hinge and the anatomical rotation axis of the elbow [7–9]. There are two

J. K. Wiggers and R. M. Snijders have contributed equally to this work.

✉ J. K. Wiggers
    j.k.wiggers@amc.nl

[1] Trauma Unit, Department of Surgery, Academic Medical Center, Meibergdreef 9, 1105 AZ Amsterdam, The Netherlands

[2] Department of Biomedical Engineering and Physics, Academic Medical Center, Amsterdam, The Netherlands

[3] Trauma Research Unit, Department of Surgery, Erasmus Medical Center, Rotterdam, The Netherlands

[4] Department of Surgery, Maasstad Hospital, Rotterdam, The Netherlands

explanations for this incongruence. First, the elbow rotation axis has an 'instant center of rotation,' meaning that the rotation axis is not fixed in three-dimensional space but moves like a twist around a screw. Therefore, it is impossible to place a hinged fixator in perfect alignment with the rotation axis of the elbow, as the latter migrates during flexion and extension. The second reason for incongruence is that surgeons often misidentify the correct elbow rotation axis during surgery, which is potentially preventable.

To position the axis of the fixator hinge, it is essential to identify the elbow rotation axis on fluoroscopy and drill an axis pin (Kirschner wire) through it. However, we showed in a previous fluoroscopic simulation study that the intra-operative accuracy to identify the elbow rotation axis is low and associated with substantial error [10]. Madey et al. [10] showed that applying an external fixator with 5° or 10° incongruence relative to the elbow axis, which was a common error in our previous fluoroscopic simulation study, results in a 3.7- and 7.1-fold increase in motion resistance, respectively [8]. Such incongruence often results in morbidity and secondary procedures. In a recent prospective study of hinged external elbow fixation, 19% of patients had elbow incongruence resulting from fixator malalignment, and these patients all required secondary procedures for fixator realignment or replacement [6].

To identify the elbow rotation axis on fluoroscopy, it is required to obtain an 'optimal lateral image,' which should be orientated perpendicular to the rotation axis (i.e., an on-axis image). Traditionally, surgeons aim to overlap the capitellum and the trochlear sulcus until these structures form concentric circles with the centers of these circles representing the axis of rotation [9]. However, orientation with this method alone is limited to the coronal plane (abduction/adduction) and arguably causes rotational errors in the transverse plane (internal/external rotation). In other words, the circles of the capitellum and trochlea can overlap, while there is still unwitnessed rotational error of the lateral image in the transverse plane, as previously demonstrated in a study by Bottlang et al. [11].

Additional radiographic landmarks may improve identification of the optimal lateral image and elbow rotation axis and may eventually improve external fixator alignment. A landmark that could help orientation in the transverse plane is the relative distance (RD) of the humerus [11]. This landmark, developed by Bottlang et al., is based on the relative position of the dense projection of the posteromedial cortex within the boundaries of the distal humerus. The RD is obtained by measuring the distance between the dorsal side of the humerus and the projection of the posteromedial cortex, subsequently dividing this distance by the diameter of the humerus (Fig. 1). Bottlang et al. [11] designed this measure in a study with cadaveric

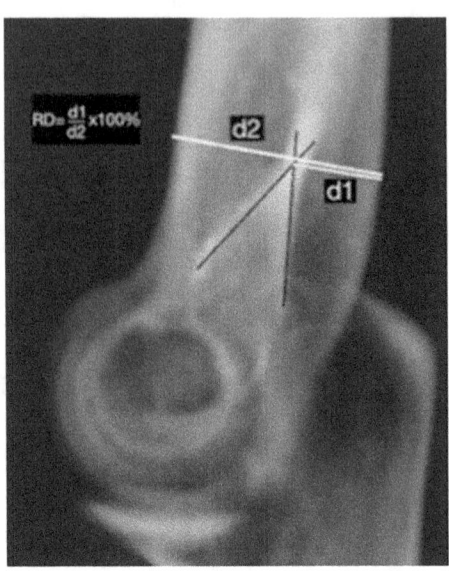

Fig. 1 Digitally reconstructed radiograph (DRR) of the humerus in lateral view, depicting how the relative distance (RD) of the humerus is measured. The RD is defined as RD = $(d1/d2) \times 100\%$, with $d1$ the distance from the dorsal side of the humerus to the projection of the posteromedial cortex (measured at the intersection point of the cortical lines, as represented by the intersection of the drawn black lines in the figure) (mm), and with $d2$, anteroposterior diameter of the humerus (mm). The *lines d1* and *d2* are measured perpendicular to the bone axis. Finally, the RD is calculated as the length ratio of $d1$ and $d2$ and expressed as a percentage

bones and electromagnetic motion tracking data, but these measures have not been validated in healthy volunteers.

In the first part of this study, we determined the elbow rotation axis using 3D image analysis in five healthy volunteers and subsequently assessed the RD value that corresponds to the optimal lateral fluoroscopic image of the humerus in vivo. The second part of this study was designed to assess potential improvements in surgical accuracy to identify the elbow rotation axis, after surgeons have been instructed how to use the optimal RD value as additional landmark on fluoroscopy.

Methods

Compliance with ethical standards

This study was approved by the local ethical committee, and was conducted in accordance with the Declaration of Helsinki. Informed consent was obtained from all individual participants included in the study.

Data acquisition

The non-dominant left elbow of five healthy male volunteers with normal elbow function and no history of trauma, was CT-scanned in incremental flexion angles (0°, 35°, 65°, 100°, 135°) [12]. Scans were made using a Brilliance 64-channel CT scanner (Philips Healthcare, Best, the Netherlands) (120 kV, slice thickness 0.9 mm, increment 0.33 mm, isotropic voxel spacing of 0.33 mm). In the neutral position (0°), the elbow was scanned at a high dose (150 mAs) for adequate virtual modeling of the bone by image segmentation, and at a low dose (50 mAs) for the remaining states of elbow flexion, to limit the radiation expose.

Calculation of the actual elbow rotation axis

The actual elbow rotation axis is calculated from the CT scans with the elbow in different states of flexion, as described previously [10]. In short, the humerus and ulna were manually segmented from a high-dose scan at 0° flexion, and subsequently aligned, by 3D image registration, with low-dose CT images containing the elbow in subsequent states of flexion. Taking the humerus as fixed reference bone, the ulna will now show a rotation between the segmented state, at 0° flexion, and its position after registration to each of the subsequent flexion images. These rotations evolve about their respective so-called helical axes. Since the helical axes found for elbow rotation between 0° and incremental flexion do not completely overlap due to the previously mentioned 'instant center of rotation' of the elbow, we used the average of the four helical axes as the elbow rotation axis, referred to as the 'calculated rotation axis' in this study.

Measuring the in vivo relative distance

In the first part of this study, we measured the RD that corresponds to an optimal lateral fluoroscopic image of the humerus in vivo. Digitally reconstructed radiographs (DRRs) of the CT scans were used to simulate fluoroscopic images (Fig. 2). Each DRR could be projected into the plane perpendicular to the calculated rotation axis, hence providing an optimal lateral image of the elbow. Because the actual elbow rotation axis may slightly vary over the flexion–extension trajectory, we constructed two evaluation sets of optimal lateral elbow images, both based on the same average elbow rotation axis: one set including images of the five elbows in extension (0° flexion) and one set including images of the five elbows in 100° flexion. Subsequently, three observers (RS, JD and GJ) measured the RD in the two sets of elbow images. Figure 1 shows how the RD was measured.

Accuracy of assessing the rotation axis using the relative distance

In the second part of this study, we assessed potential improvements of surgeons in finding the elbow rotation axis on fluoroscopic images after the surgeons have been instructed to use the RD of the humerus in addition to traditional landmarks. A custom-made software application was used to simulate fluoroscopy of the elbow. The application produces real-time DRR images and enables the operator to freely rotate and translate the CT volume

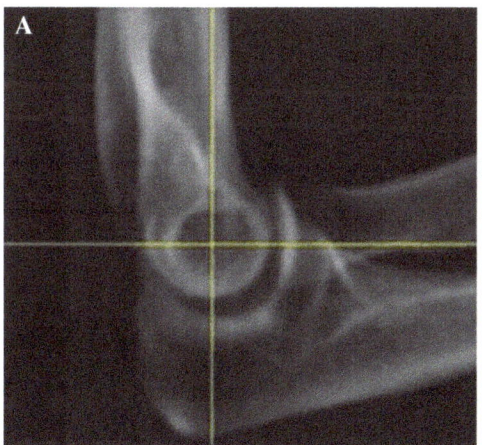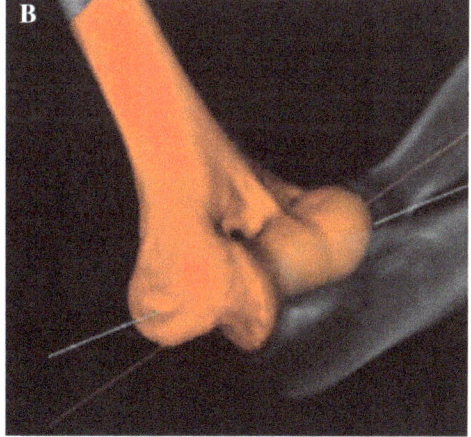

Fig. 2 a Digitally reconstructed radiograph (DRR) that simulates fluoroscopic images. The figure shows an optimal lateral image of the elbow that is orientated perpendicular to the rotation axis. Surgeons were able to freely rotate the elbow CT to generate DRRs from different projection angles in search of this optimal lateral image and used the crosshair cursor to indicate the position of the rotation axis, **b** example of an axis estimated by one of the surgeons (*red line*) and the calculated rotation axis (*white line*) in a 3D reconstructed image, showing the surgeons' error

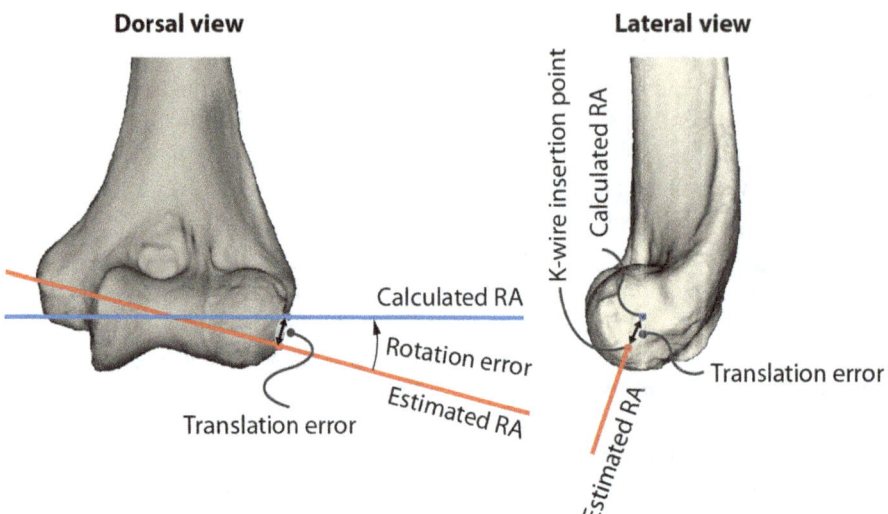

Fig. 3 Dorsal and lateral view of the humerus showing the calculated elbow rotation axis (*blue*) and the rotation axis estimated by the surgeon (*red*) by inserting a K-wire. The deviation from the calculated axis is expressed in terms of a rotation error and a translation error.

The rotation error describes the projection angle between both axes, while the translation error is defined by the Euler (shortest) distance between the K-wire insertion point and the entry point that corresponds to the calculated rotation axis on the lateral epicondyle

containing the elbow [13]. Operators are enabled to position the CT volume until the resulting elbow DRR is felt to represent the optimal lateral image perpendicular to the elbow rotation axis. Operators then center the image at the expected position of the rotation axis, and an 'axis definition' is subsequently ejected at the crosshair cursor position (Fig. 2).

Eight surgeons were invited to determine the elbow rotation axis on simulated fluoroscopy images in two sessions. During each session, the five available scanned elbows were presented three times in random order and each time with a different starting image, resulting in 15 axis definitions per surgeon for each session. In the first session, surgeons were instructed to use traditional landmarks that they normally use in clinical practice, including the overlapping centers of the capitellum, trochlear sulcus and trochlea. After completion of the first session, the surgeons were instructed how to use the humeral RD as anatomical landmark, including the RD corresponding to an optimal lateral image as defined in the first part of the study. Teaching consisted of a 10-min lecture with explanatory figures how to use the humeral RD as landmark. The figures used during teaching were similar to Figs. 1 and 2. After teaching and a break of approximately 30 min, the surgeons conducted the second session of the experiment. They again determined the elbow rotation axis on fluoroscopy, now using the humeral RD as a landmark in addition to the traditional landmarks. All axis definitions provided by the surgeons (i.e., from both the first and second session) were compared with the calculated rotation axis, which provided measures for off-axis alignment by the surgeons before and after teaching of the humeral RD. Off-axis alignment was expressed as rotation error, which is a measure of orientation and expressed as an angle, and as surface translation error, which is measured on the surface of the lateral epicondyle and expressed in millimeters (Fig. 3) [10, 11]. The surface translation error is defined by the Euler (shortest) distance between the entry point of the elbow rotation axis on the lateral epicondyle and the location where the surgeon's axis definition enters the lateral epicondyle, and thus represents the 'K-wire insertion error' if a surgeon would normally start drilling the fixator axis at this location. Finally, the mean rotation and translation error values were compared between the first (preteaching) and second (postteaching) experiment session.

Statistical analysis

The RD corresponding to an on-axis lateral image of the elbow (i.e., 'the optimal RD'), as measured by three observers, is expressed as an average with corresponding standard deviation (SD). Correlation between the optimal RD for elbows in flexion and extension was analyzed with a Pearson correlation coefficient; interobserver agreement was assessed with an intraclass correlation coefficient.

Paired-sample t tests were used to compare the mean error parameters between elbow axis determination with and without the RD as additional assessment parameter (i.e., preteaching and postteaching).

Results

Optimal in vivo relative distance

The mean optimal RD measured 45.9% (SD 5.0) for elbows in extension and 45.6% (SD 5.6) for elbows in flexion. A difference of the optimal RD for elbows in extension and flexion could not be detected ($P = 0.94$); measurements of the optimal RD for elbows in extension and flexion had strong correlation (correlation coefficient 0.80) [14]. The intraclass correlation coefficients for measuring the optimal RD of elbows in extension and flexion were 0.82 and 0.90, respectively, which showed strong interobserver agreement [15].

Improvements in Surgical Accuracy

The first and second experiment sessions both resulted in 120 axis definitions (8 surgeons × 5 specimens × 3 axis definitions). All surgeons' axis definitions were compared with the CT-based calculated rotation axis, as illustrated in Fig. 2b. The mean rotational error in identifying the elbow rotation axis decreased from 7.6° (SD 3.4; range 0.61–17.66) before teaching to 6.7° (SD 3.3; range 0.37–16.50) after teaching (i.e., after surgeons had been instructed how to use the optimal RD as additional landmark) ($P = 0.03$). The mean translational error decreased from 4.2 mm (SD 2.0; range 0.78–11.46 mm) before teaching to 3.7 mm (SD 2.0; range 0.23–9.33) after teaching ($P = 0.01$).

Discussion

Hinged external elbow fixation enables early mobilization after complex elbow dislocation and residual instability, but alignment of the fixator may cause complications and require revision procedures [6]. In this study, we assessed the RD of the humerus as an additional landmark to identify the elbow rotation axis on fluoroscopy images. The technique is easy to use intraoperatively and does not require extra equipment. First, we showed that the in vivo RD corresponding to an optimal on-axis lateral fluoroscopic image averaged 45%. We also showed that measurement of the optimal RD was robust, as evidenced by good interobserver agreement and high correlation between measurements for elbows in extension and flexion. Secondly, we showed that a 10-min teaching program with explanatory figures about the use of the optimal RD (Figs. 1, 2) improved the surgical accuracy in determining the elbow rotation axis, albeit these improvements were small.

Bottlang introduced the RD as an anatomical landmark and suggested the RD should read 27% ± 3.7% to find the optimal lateral image in the transverse plane. The difference in optimal RD between that study and the present study can be explained by the fact that Bottlang used cadaveric bones, whereas the present study was based on simulated in vivo elbow fluoroscopy. Moreover, Bottlang used electromagnetic motion tracking data to determine the elbow rotation axis, but the present study incorporated a CT segmentation technique that has proven to be accurate with rotational errors of (mean ± SD) 0.1° ± 0.1° and translation errors of 0.4 ± 0.1 mm [13]. Our technique of scanning elbows with incremental values of flexion was similar to other recent anatomical studies analyzing elbow rotation axis kinematics [12]. Nonetheless, it seems preferable to validate the determined optimal RD in future studies.

This study showed only a marginal improvement of the surgical accuracy in identifying the elbow rotation axis, but these improvements may still be clinically relevant. This is illustrated in a cadaveric electromagnetic tracking study by Madey et al. [8], who found a linear relation between fixator malalignment and motion resistance. Reducing the rotational error of fixator alignment from 10° to 5° resulted in a 50% decrease in elbow motion resistance. Reducing the rotational error toward a perfect alignment further reduces motion resistance.

Surgical errors in elbow axis definitions were expressed as rotation and translation errors. The rotation error measures the angle between the axis chosen by the surgeon and the calculated rotation axis. The surface translational error represents the shortest distance between the entry points of the axis chosen by the surgeon and the calculated rotation axis on the lateral epicondyle. Both measures are informative of surgical achievements, the latter especially because it provides the distance of the 'K-wire insertion error' if a surgeon would normally start drilling a K-wire to position the fixator axis at the chosen point at the lateral epicondyle. Our previous study measured translational error at the shortest distance anywhere between the calculated elbow rotation axis and the surgeons' axis definition [10]. However, that method is less informative and provides an underestimation of the true translation error.

In this study, the surgeons identified the rotation axis in virtual space but did not actually insert a K-wire. In that respect, the reported surgical errors reflect the X-ray projection that they chose and not their K-wire orientation. This may have underestimated the real intraoperative error, since the actual placement of the K-wires while using fluoroscopy intermittently may add to even larger surgical errors. The study is also limited by its simulation design: we used DRR images to simulate fluoroscopy instead of using real intraoperative fluoroscopy. Nonetheless, the DRR images were designed to resemble the quality of intraoperative fluoroscopy, and the study setting allowed surgeons to freely rotate and translate the elbow similar to the intraoperative setting. One other limitation is that surgeons may get better at determining the axis of rotation with each iteration, which may have biased the improvement in accuracy after teaching surgeons how to use the RD. Furthermore, the study was limited by a low sample size of elbow specimens that were tested, so results regarding significance of the data should be interpreted with caution. It was not possible to increase the number of elbow specimens because it was regarded unethical to subject additional volunteers to the radiation of CT scans. Instead, we tried to circumvent the limitation of low sample size by having the surgeons repeating the rotation axis assessments on the same elbow specimens. This was done in a blinded fashion, so the surgeons were not aware that they were looking at the same elbow again.

Perfect fixator alignment remains a difficult procedure even for highly skilled surgeons due to variation between patients and due to natural variation of the elbow rotation axis during flexion–extension motion [12]. Some surgeons have switched to using a static fixator and no longer use a hinge, but many surgeons adhere to hinged external fixation because it enables early mobilization postoperatively [6]. In choosing the method to intraoperatively align fixator orientation, fluoroscopy is easy to use and requires only standard equipment. However, fluoroscopy seems insufficient to completely eliminate malalignment of external elbow fixators, given the rotation and translation errors described in this study. Preoperative CT may prove useful in the future to tailor intraoperative landmarks, similar to techniques used in knee arthroplasty [16]. For example, Sabo et al. [17] recently explored the value of the posterior humeral cortex on preoperative CT as a landmark to place the humeral component during elbow arthroplasty. As an alternative to fixator axis placement by the surgeon, hinged fixators can also be designed as self-centering devices. This recent development was shown to be effective in a study with seven patients, who all had correct alignment of the external fixator and had no complications [18]. Awaiting the introduction of such developments into common practice, we recommend adding the RD as anatomical landmark when using fluoroscopy for aligning hinged external fixators with the elbow rotation axis.

Acknowledgements The authors are grateful to the surgeons who contributed to the production of this research, including: Dr. T. Schepers, Dr. R. Peters, Dr. P. Kloen, Dr. V. de Jong, Dr. F. Beeres, Prof. Dr. J.C. Goslings, and Prof. Dr. D. Eygendaal.

Informed consent Informed consent was obtained from all individual participants included in the study.

Funding The authors received no financial support for the research, authorship and/or publication of this article.

References

1. Ring D, Hannouche D, Jupiter JB (2004) Surgical treatment of persistent dislocation or subluxation of the ulnohumeral joint after fracture-dislocation of the elbow. J Hand Surg 29(3):470–480
2. Schep NW, De Haan J, Iordens GI et al (2011) A hinged external fixator for complex elbow dislocations: a multicenter prospective cohort study. BMC Musculoskelet Disord 12:130
3. McKee MD, Bowden SH, King GJ et al (1998) Management of recurrent, complex instability of the elbow with a hinged external fixator. J Bone Joint Surg 80(6):1031–1036
4. Sorensen AK, Sojbjerg JO (2011) Treatment of persistent instability after posterior fracture-dislocation of the elbow: restoring stability and mobility by internal fixation and hinged external fixation. J Shoulder Elbow Surg 20(8):1300–1309
5. Ouyang Y, Liao Y, Liu Z, Fan C (2013) Hinged external fixator and open surgery for severe elbow stiffness with distal humeral nonunion. Orthopedics 36(2):e186–e192
6. Iordens GI, Den Hartog D, Van Lieshout EM et al (2015) Good functional recovery of complex elbow dislocations treated with hinged external fixation: a multicenter prospective study. Clin Orthop Relat Res 473(4):1451–1461
7. Cheung EV, O'Driscoll SW, Morrey BF (2008) Complications of hinged external fixators of the elbow. J Shoulder Elbow Surg 17(3):447–453
8. Madey SM, Bottlang M, Steyers CM, Marsh JL, Brown TD (2000) Hinged external fixation of the elbow: optimal axis alignment to minimize motion resistance. J Orthop Trauma 14(1):41–47
9. Chen NC, Julka A (2010) Hinged external fixation of the elbow. Hand Clin 26(3):423–433
10. Wiggers JK, Streekstra GJ, Kloen P, Mader K, Goslings JC, Schep NW (2014) Surgical accuracy in identifying the elbow rotation axis on fluoroscopic images. J Hand Surg 39(6):1141–1145
11. Bottlang M, O'Rourke MR, Madey SM, Steyers CM, Marsh JL, Brown TD (2000) Radiographic determinants of the elbow rotation axis: experimental identification and quantitative validation. J Orthop Res 18(5):821–828
12. Adikrishna A, Kekatpure AL, Tan J, Lee HJ, Deslivia MF, Jeon IH (2014) Vortical flow in human elbow joints: a three-dimensional computed tomography modeling study. J Anat 225(4):390–394
13. Dobbe JG, Strackee SD, Schreurs AW et al (2011) Computer-assisted planning and navigation for corrective distal radius osteotomy, based on pre- and intraoperative imaging. IEEE Trans Bio-Med Eng 58(1):182–190
14. Peacock J, Peacock PJ (2011) Oxford handbook of medical statistics. Oxford University Press, Oxford
15. Everitt BS (2005) Encyclopedia of statistics in behavioral science. Wiley, Hoboken
16. Victor J (2009) Rotational alignment of the distal femur: a literature review. Orthop Traumatol Surg Res 95(5):365–372
17. Sabo MT, Athwal GS, King GJ (2012) Landmarks for rotational alignment of the humeral component during elbow arthroplasty. J Bone Joint Surg 94(19):1794–1800
18. Bigazzi P, Biondi M, Corvi A, Pfanner S, Checcucci G, Ceruso M (2015) A new autocentering hinged external fixator of the elbow: a device that stabilizes the elbow axis without use of the articular pin. J Shoulder Elbow Surg 24(8):1197–1205

16

Percutaneous rotational osteotomy of the femur utilizing an intramedullary rod

Peter M. Stevens[1] · Christian J. Gaffney[1] · Heather Fillerup[1]

Abstract The purpose is to describe the technique and report the results and complications of percutaneous femoral rotational osteotomy, secured with a trochanteric-entry, locked intramedullary rod, in adolescents with femoral anteversion. Our series comprised an IRB approved, retrospective, consecutive series of 85 osteotomies (57 patients), followed to implant removal. The average age at surgery was 13.3 years (range 8.8–18.3) with a female-to-male ratio of 2.8:1. The minimum follow-up was 2 years. Eighty-three osteotomies healed primarily. Two patients, subsequently found to have vitamin D deficiency, broke screws and developed nonunions; both healed after repeat reaming and rod exchange and vitamin supplementation. Preoperative symptoms, including in-toeing gait, tripping and anterior knee pain or patellar instability, were resolved consistently. We did not observe significant growth disturbance or osteonecrosis. We noted a 12.5 % incidence of broken interlocking screws; this did not affect the correction or outcome except for the two patients mentioned above. This prompted a switch from a standard screw (core diameter = 3 mm) to a threaded bolt (core diameter = 3.7 mm). These results have led this technique to replace the use of plates or blade plates for rotational osteotomies.

Keywords Anteversion · Retroversion · Femoral osteotomy · Intramedullary rod · Osseous necrosis

Introduction

Persistent femoral anteversion is a frequent contributing factor to anterior knee pain and patello-femoral instability in adolescents. If left untreated, there may be a suscepti-bility to acute or repetitive injuries that limit sports par-ticipation and lifestyle. Presenting symptoms include anterior knee pain and patellar mal-tracking or frank instability. While retroversion is less common and does not cause knee pain typically, it represents an indication for surgical treatment occasionally. Non-operative measures such as NSAIDs, knee braces and physical therapy are palliative at best. The definitive treatment comprises rota-tional osteotomy of the femur. Once the osteotomy has healed, unrestricted activities are permitted and the rod is removed at an average of 12 months post-osteotomy.

Patients and methods

This is a consecutive series of patients who underwent cor-rection of anteversion between 2010 and 2014. All patients were older than 8 years and had presented with persistent in-toeing, tripping and anterior knee pain with or without patello-femoral instability. The symptoms had been refractory to non-operative management. There are several advantages to deferring osteotomy until after the age of 8 years:

1. there is torsional remodeling potential that may mitigate against the need for surgery before the age of 8 years,
2. after the age of 8 years, recurrence of torsion is rare so an osteotomy need not be repeated,
3. femoral osteotomy (or fracture) in younger children may stimulate overgrowth resulting in iatrogenic limb length inequality,

✉ Peter M. Stevens
peter.stevens@hsc.utah.edu

[1] University of Utah, Salt Lake City, UT, USA

4. there is diminished likelihood of altering trochanteric growth or causing coxa valga,

5. there is appropriate, transtrochanteric instrumentation available that permits stable, antegrade intramedullary nailing of the femur [1, 2].

By employing a quadriceps-sparing, percutaneous osteotomy, the blood loss is minimal and healing rapid with morbidity decreased. The purpose of this review is to report our experience with this less invasive form of osteotomy as compared to the more established or popular plating or blade plate fixation methods, and include complications and outcomes from a single surgeon series.

With IRB approval, a retrospective review was conducted of 57 patients who underwent a percutaneous osteotomy of the femur to correct anteversion (or retroversion) utilizing a trochanteric-entry intramedullary rod for fixation. We evaluated historical complaints and functional limitations as well as clinical findings including anterior knee pain, patellar tracking, gait pattern, comparing the preoperative status to that at the time of rod removal. This cohort comprised 57 patients (15 males and 42 females) ranging in age from 8.8 to 18.3 years (average 13.3 years) at the time of the osteotomy. Bilateral correction was undertaken in 28 and a unilateral osteotomy in the other 29, giving a total of 85 osteotomies. Simultaneous surgical procedures included rotational osteotomy for tibial torsion and guided growth for genu valgum or fixed knee flexion deformity. The etiology of femoral torsion was idiopathic in 53 patients and neurogenic in four. All patients were seen in follow-up until rod removal; this was at an average 10.7 months (range 9–12 months) following osteotomy.

The physical examination included measurement of limb lengths, frontal knee alignment (varus/valgus), observation of the gait pattern and prone torsional profile, noting the degrees of inward and outward hip rotation and the thigh/foot axis. We did not recommend surgery unless the degree of excessive femoral torsion (beyond the normal 11°) measured greater than 20°. The gait pattern was observed with attention to both the foot progression angle and the knee progression angle. The foot progression angle may appear normal in patients with concomitant outward tibial torsion. However, the effects of inward femoral and outward tibial torsion are cumulative, not compensatory, with respect to the patella and knee. For example, a patient with 30° of femoral anteversion and 30° outward thigh–foot axis (tibial torsion) is subject to 60° of torsional stress on the knee. For these patients, simultaneous femoral and tibial osteotomies are justified. We elected not to employ PROMs (patient-reported outcomes) because we did not have an adequate tool to apply for this retrospective series.

The radiographic evaluation included a standing AP view of the legs, with the patellae neutral, upon which we

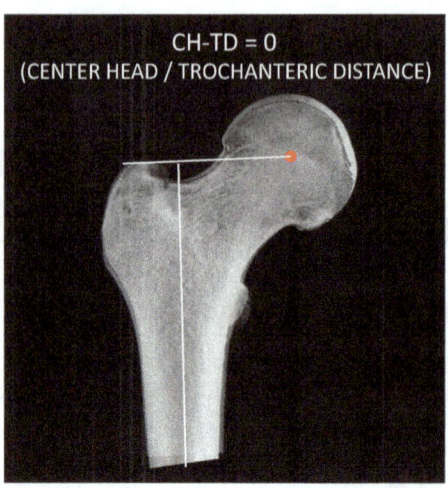

Fig. 1 The center of femoral head to trochanteric tip vertical offset is normally zero. This affords maximum efficiency for the abductors. In preadolescent children, this distance is not measurable on plain radiographs because the tip of the trochanter is not ossified. In our series, transtrochanteric rod insertion did not result in any observed change in the center head/trochanteric distance (CH–TD)

documented limb length discrepancy. This was performed preoperatively and repeated prior to rod removal. We measured the center of femoral head to trochanteric tip vertical offset distance (normally = 0, Fig. 1). Intentionally, we did not record the pre- and postoperative femoral neck-shaft angles because there is projection artifact introduced by patient positioning and parallax distortion, making such measurements unreliable (Fig. 2a, b).

The indications for surgery included tripping, activity related anterior knee (and sometimes hip) pain and patellar mal-tracking or instability. Rotational correction was typically in the 30° range, with a minimum of 20° and maximum of 40°, leaving approximately 10°–15° of normal version of the femur. Patients with bilateral involvement, weighing less than 50 kg, were corrected simultaneously. Sixteen children with outward tibial torsion (pan genu torsion) underwent ipsilateral, simultaneous correction osteotomies. In select cases, concomitant lateral retinacular release (9 knees) or patellar realignment (4 knees) was combined with osteotomy (or undertaken at the time of rod removal). Iatrogenic retroversion was meticulously avoided.

Technique

The entry point for the nail is made, through a 3-cm incision, just lateral to the tip of the trochanter and well away from the piriformis fossa (Fig. 3). Prior to reaming, a 1-cm lateral mid-thigh incision is made and, using a stout 3.5- or 4.2-mm drill bit (Fig. 4a), several transverse drill holes are made for the dual purpose of decompressing the femoral

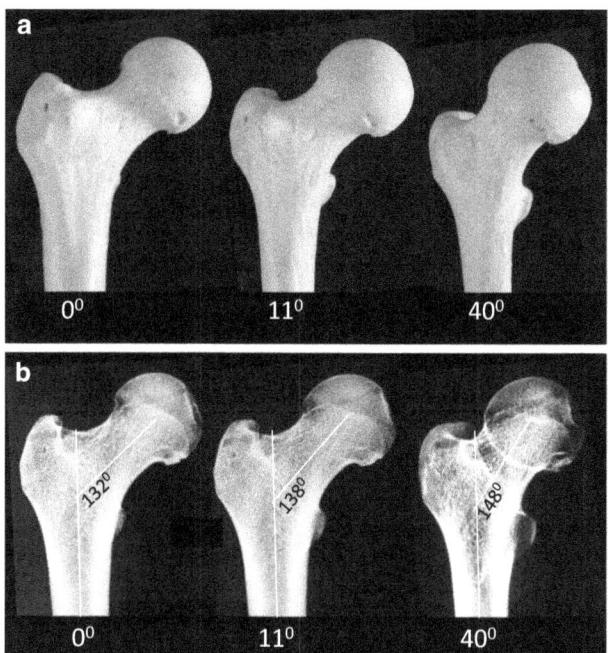

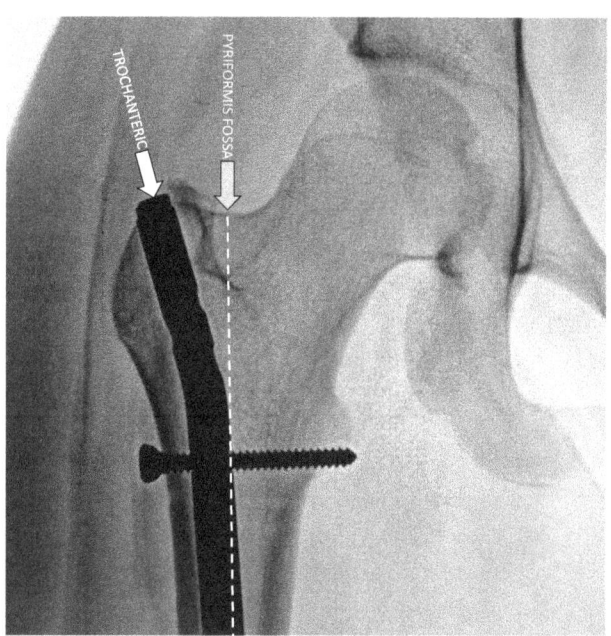

Fig. 2 a As a femur is rotated from orthogonal to 11° of (normal) version, and to simulated 30° of excessive anteversion, the shape of the head and neck, along with the apparent CH–TD appears to change. The projection artifact may lead to spurious conclusions regarding the femoral head–neck offset. **b** The projected femoral neck-shaft is altered as a result of positioning, causing parallax distortion. This is why it is not possible to accurately document the neck-shaft angle on plain AP images. It would also lead the unwary to conclude that, by correcting anteversion with an antegrade intramedullary rod, there is an iatrogenic change in the neck-shaft angle. Therefore, we chose not to measure the neck-shaft angle in this series

Fig. 3 The new generation of trochanteric-entry, antegrade intramedullary femoral rods mitigates against iatrogenic osseous necrosis that had been previously reported with straight, piriformis entry rods. Presumably, the distance from the circumflex vessels protects against physical or thermal trauma during reaming

canal and allowing egress of reaming material to serve as autogenous bone graft. The femur is then reamed sequentially until reaching a diameter that is 2 mm greater than the diameter of the rod to be used (typically 8 or 9 mm).

Rotation is monitored via two smooth 7/64th inch bicortical Steinman pins that are placed at the base of the greater trochanter (anterior or posterior to the rod) and one through the lateral femoral condyle. These are inserted at the angle of desired correction (using triangles to measure) relative to each other such that they will end up parallel once the osteotomy has been completed and the distal fragment rotated. The osteotomy is completed with a ½-inch osteotomy (hexagonal handle) that is torqued with a wrench to complete the cut (Fig. 4b). The distal interlocking screw is placed first under fluoroscopic guidance using the "free hand/perfect circle" technique. The proximal interlocking screw is introduced then using the jig.

Partial weight-bearing with crutches is encouraged; a wheelchair is preferred for school or long distance. With regional nerve block catheters delivering pain relief, patients are discharged the day after surgery typically. Crutch weaning commences 1 month (sooner with the newer locking bolt) following osteotomy and, if radiographs confirm callus formation, permission for progression of activities given.

Results

Clinical

The surgical goals were achieved primarily in all but two cases that required rod exchange for nonunion. In-toeing and tripping were relieved and anterior knee pain abated. Six patients required patellar realignment: four at the time of osteotomy and two subsequent to the rotational correction. There was no recurrence of torsion.

There were two femoral nonunions which required exchange of the rods. The remaining 55 patients had primary, solid radiographic union between 3 and 4 months.

In no instance was the center head to trochanteric distance altered by more than 5 mm, and limb lengths were not changed by more than 8 mm. Importantly, there were no cases of osseous necrosis of the femoral head or neck. This feared complication, reported in the literature, appears to be confined to patients with femoral fractures who are treated with an antegrade rod placed through the piriformis fossa. Some of the cases reported were diagnosed on follow-up radiographs without apparent clinical sequelae.

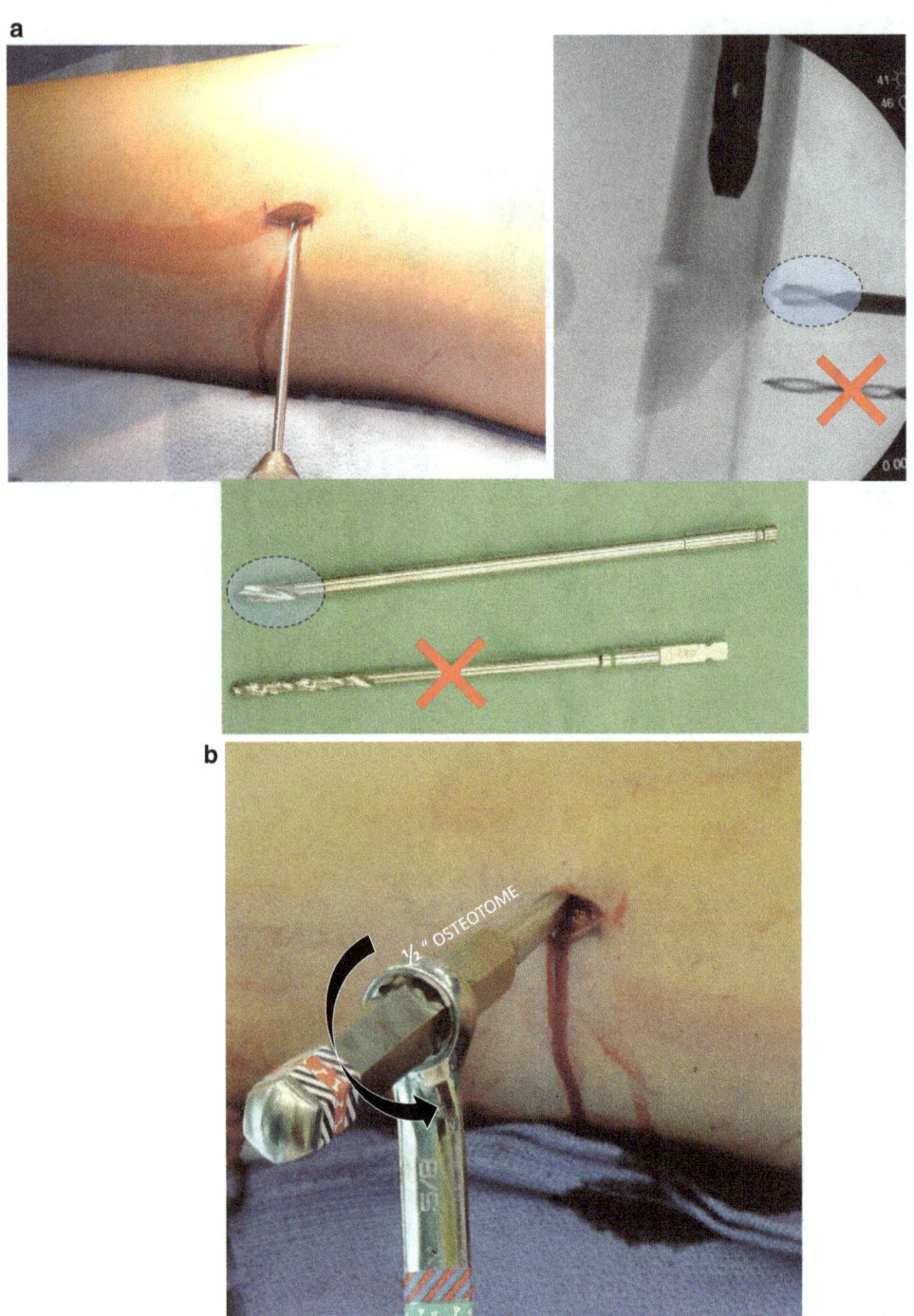

Fig. 4 a Through a 1-cm incision, a stout drill bit (*dotted oval*), with a self-centering tip and short flutes, is employed to drill several transverse holes to mark the osteotomy site and decompress the femur for reaming. **b** These holes are connected with a ½-inch Ilizarov wrench (*hexagonal handle*) that is then torqued with a wrench. Advance the guide pin and rod past the osteotomy site *before* correcting the anteversion. Insert the distal interlocking screw first (freehand), then the proximal (jig)

Hardware issues

There were 23 broken screws out of a total of 178 screws placed (including the two cases that underwent revision), giving a frequency of 12.5 %. This occurred typically between the second and fourth month postoperatively. The distal screw was more prone to failure by a ratio of 5:1. We surmise that, while both interlocking screws are subjected to the same vertical loading, the proximal screws are spared some of the rotational stresses due to the ball and socket nature of the hip. In contrast, the hinge action of the knee joint may impart more rotational stresses upon the

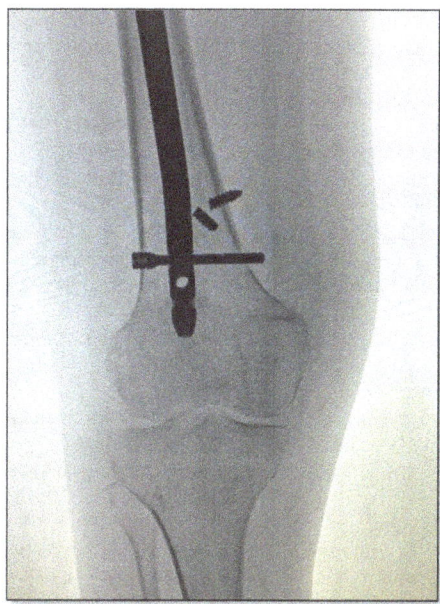

Fig. 5 The core diameter of 3.0 mm for the screw has been increased to 3.7 mm for the bolt. None of the bolts have broken

distal screws. This problem appears to have been resolved through the use of stronger bolts (Fig. 5).

We were not able to correlate the patient's BMI with the occurrence of broken screws. While early, protected weight-bearing was encouraged, we were unable to conclude that patient non-compliance or unauthorized activities were to blame for fatigue failure of the screws. None of the patients admitted to smoking tobacco. While this population may be at risk for dietary vitamin D deficiency, this was only documented on two patients (ages 13 and 15).

Discussion

Femoral anteversion, which is normal in infants and younger children, should reduce spontaneously with growth. This does not merit bracing or physical therapy; parental education and periodic follow-up are appropriate in most cases. The natural history leads to spontaneous resolution of the problem by the age of 8 years in most. However, some patients have persistence of anteversion, manifested by in-toeing, tripping, anterior knee pain and even patellar instability. Persistent femoral anteversion (PFA) is more prevalent in females and may be familial. There remains a false perception by some practitioners that persistent anteversion is merely a cosmetic concern and that osteotomies are aggressive and unnecessary. However, with the emerging field of "jump mechanics" that is available in Movement Analysis Laboratories, evidence is coming to light that femoral anteversion is not innocuous [3–5]. Persistent anteversion may compromise hip

kinematics and pose a rise of labral tears. At the knee, "dynamic valgus" puts increased stress on the patella and jeopardizes the integrity of the ACL. If unrecognized, the risks of failed knee surgery to correct these problems are increased [3].

In affected patients, a standard torsional profile (measured prone) will reveal both excessive inward femoral torsion (anteversion) and outward tibial torsion. If either (or both) reflects greater than 20° of malrotation, and when in a symptomatic child, corrective osteotomy may be warranted. This may be staged or performed simultaneously.

Radiographic evaluation should include a standing AP projection of the legs with the patellae facing forward. This will document the limb lengths and any deviation of the mechanical axis as well as revealing open physes. If the patello-femoral examination is abnormal or suspect, a sunrise view of the patella will reveal the sulcus along with lateral tilt and/or lateral subluxation of the patella. In specific patients, overt patellar mal-tracking or instability may warrant a lateral retinacular release or patellar tendon transfer at the time of the femoral rotational osteotomy. We no longer employ the "gunsight CT" scan due to concerns about radiation; gunsight MRI was briefly employed but subsequently was abandoned due to cost.

The optimal timing and staging of surgery must be individualized and is predicated upon thorough discussions with the parents regarding symptoms of tripping, anterior knee pain and, in some patients, patellar instability. While waiting until the age of 10 or older is preferable, some families prefer to intervene sooner. If there is pan genu torsion, due to concomitant tibial torsion, or overt patellar tilt or subluxation, these may be corrected simultaneously. Angular deviations (genu valgum or fixed knee flexion) may be addressed by simultaneous guided growth [6, 7].

The advantages of the percutaneous osteotomy are self-evident: the quadriceps and periosteum are spared from dissection; the osteotomy hematoma is contained within a closed space, expediting the formation of callus; the surgical scars are minimal, without the keloid formation seen sometimes with plates or blade plates [8].

With respect to the use of antegrade intramedullary rods in adolescent fractures (or osteotomies), the main concerns relate to the risk of iatrogenic osteonecrosis or disturbance of femoral neck growth [9]. Some authors have advocated against the use of antegrade rods in adolescents [10]. However, reported cases of osseous necrosis have been rare and subclinical, sometimes noted at the time of rod removal. Review of the literature implicates piriformis fossa entry techniques that were performed for introduction of straight rods [11, 12]. In an extensive meta-analysis of 1277 publications regarding locked antegrade rods in skeletally immature patients [13, 14], MacNeil et al. [15] extracted 19 relevant articles and concluded that the risk of necrosis was

2 % with piriformis entry, 1.4 % at the tip of the trochanter and 0 % utilizing a lateral trochanteric-entry site. This was the impetus for the development of the lateral trochanteric-entry point rods for trauma [1]. Stevens et al. [16] reported the use of the Philips intramedullary rod (Philips/Biomet) for 40 elective rotational osteotomies, with no observed growth disturbance in the femoral head or neck. The findings are consistent with recent trauma literature; in a series of 241 adolescent patients with 246 femoral fractures, Crosby et al. [17] reported only 2.2 % of clinically relevant growth disturbance and no femoral head osteonecrosis. We identified no clinically significant incidents of growth disturbance using the Pedi-Nail (Orthopediatrics, Warsaw, Indiana, USA) which is a lateral trochanteric-entry point device. We defined the threshold of "significant" as >5 mm change in the center of femoral head—tip of trochanter distance and >10 mm in relative femoral length as compared to the opposite side. Based upon our measurements of the center of femoral head to trochanteric tip distance, we concluded that the risk of causing proximal femoral growth disturbance in children and adolescent patients has been mitigated effectively by current implant designs that avoid the piriformis fossa perforation.

We describe the technique of percutaneous femoral rotational osteotomy of the femur, combined with an antegrade, trochanteric-entry intramedullary rod fixation. Despite the reported incidence of broken screws in this series, the outcomes were generally excellent with low morbidity. Since changing to a larger 3.7 mm unicortically threaded, interlocking bolts there have been no further incidences of fatigue failure. Problems experienced with extensile exposure and application of plate devices are averted, and osseous necrosis has not been observed with this technique.

References

1. Gordon JE, Khanna N, Luhmann SJ, Dobbs MB, Ortman MR, Schoenecker PL (2004) Intramedullary nailing of femoral fractures in children through the lateral aspect of the greater trochanter using a modified rigid humeral intramedullary nail: preliminary results of a new technique in 15 children. J Orthop Trauma 18(7):416–422 (**discussion 23-4**)

2. Kanellopoulos AD, Yiannakopoulos CK, Soucacos PN (2006) Closed, locked intramedullary nailing of pediatric femoral shaft fractures through the tip of the greater trochanter. J Trauma 60(1):217–222 (**discussion 22-3**)

3. Stevens P, Gilliland J, Anderson L, Mickelson J, Nielson J, Klatt J (2013) Success of torsional correction after failed surgeries for patellofemoral pain and instability. Strat Trauma Limb Reconstr 9(1):5–12

4. Kaneko M, Sakuraba K (2013) Association between femoral anteversion and lower extremity posture upon single-leg landing: implications for anterior cruciate ligament surgery. J Phys Ther Sci 25:1213–1217

5. Nguyen A, Schultz S, Schmitz R (2015) Landing biomechanics in participants with different static lower extremity alignment profiles. J Athl Train 50(5):498–507

6. Klatt J, Stevens PM (2008) Guided growth for fixed knee flexion deformity. J Pediatr4 Orthop 28(6):626–631

7. Stevens PM (2007) Guided growth for angular correction: a preliminary series using a tension band plate. J Pediatr Orthop 27(3):253–259

8. Bruce WD, Stevens PM (2004) Surgical correction of miserable malalignment syndrome. J Pediatr Orthop 24(4):392–396

9. Raney EM, Ogden JA, Grogan DP (1993) Premature greater trochanteric epiphysiodesis secondary to intramedullary femoral rodding. J Pediatr Orthop 3(4):516–520

10. O'Malley DE, Mazur JM, Cummings RJ (1995) Femoral head avascular necrosis associated with intramedullary nailing in an adolescent. J Pediatr Orthop 15(1):21–23

11. Miller DJ, Kelly DM, Spence DD, Beaty JH, Warner WC, Sawyer JR (2012) Locked intramedullary nailing in the treatment of femoral shaft fractures in children younger than 12 years of age: indications and preliminary report of outcomes. J Pediatr Orthop 32(8):777–780

12. Beaty JH, Austin SM, Warner WC, Canale ST, Nichols L (1994) Interlocking intramedullary nailing of femoral-shaft fractures in adolescents: preliminary results and complications. J Pediatr Orthop 14(2):178–183

13. Momberger N, Stevens P, Smith J, Santora S, Scott S, Anderson J (2000) Intramedullary nailing of femoral fractures in adolescents. J Pediatr Orthop 20(4):482–484

14. Buford D, Christensen K, Weatherall P (1998) Intramedullary nailing of femoral fractures in adolescents. Clin Orthop Relat Res 350:85–89

15. MacNeil JA, Francis A, El-Hawary R (2011) A systematic review of rigid, locked, intramedullary nail insertion sites and avascular necrosis of the femoral head in the skeletally immature. J Pediatr Orthop 31(4):377–380

16. Stevens PM, Anderson D (2008) Correction of anteversion in skeletally immature patients: percutaneous osteotomy and transtrochanteric intramedullary rod. J Pediatr Orthop 28(3):277–283

17. Crosby S, Kim E, Koehler D, Rohmiller M, Mencio G, Lovejoy S, Schoenecker J, Martus J (2014) Twenty-year experience with rigid intramedullary nailing of femoral shaft fractures in skeletally immature patients. J Bone Joint Surg Am 96:1080–1089

17

The outcome of treatment of chronic osteomyelitis according to an integrated approach

Leonard C. Marais[1] · Nando Ferreira[1] · Colleen Aldous[2] · Theo L. B. Le Roux[3]

Abstract Previous classification systems of chronic osteomyelitis have failed to provide objective and pragmatic guidelines for selection of the appropriate treatment strategy. In this study, we assessed the short-term treatment outcome in adult patients with long-bone chronic osteomyelitis prospectively where a modified host classification system was integrated with treatment strategy selection through a novel management algorithm. Twenty-six of the 28 enrolled patients were available for follow-up at a minimum of 12 months. The median patient age of was 36.5 years (range 18–72 years). Fourteen patients (54 %) were managed palliatively, and 11 patients (42 %) were managed through the implementation of a curative treatment strategy. One patient required alternative treatment in the form of an amputation. The overall success rate was 96.2 % (95 % CI 80.4–99.9 %) at a minimum of 12-months follow-up. Remission was achieved in all [11/11] patients treated curatively (one-sided 95 % CI 73.5–100.0 %). Palliative treatment was successful in 92.9 % [13/14] of cases (95 % CI 66.1–99.9 %). In patients with lower limb involvement, there was a statistically significant improvement of 28.3 (95 % CI 21.0–35.7; SD 17.0) in the AAOS Lower Limb Outcomes Instrument score (p value < 0.001). The integrated approach proposed in this study appears a useful guideline to the management of chronic osteomyelitis of long bones in adult patients in the developing world. Further investigation is required to validate the approach, and additional development of the algorithm may be required in order to render it useful in other clinical environments.

Keywords Osteomyelitis · Chronic · Classification · Outcome · Management

Introduction

Long-bone chronic osteomyelitis is challenging to treat in adult patients. The typical causative organisms possess characteristics that render greater resistance to the host's immune response and antibiotic therapy. Bacteria may persist in a biofilm-based colony or be intracellular, concealed within osteoblasts [1, 2]. While chronic haematogenous osteomyelitis is not associated with skeletal instability, it frequently involves a large segment of bone. In contrast, post-traumatic contiguous osteomyelitis is complicated often by the presence of instability or a compromised soft tissue envelope. Lastly, there are systemic risk factors present in the host that compromise the ability of the immune system to combat infection effectively.

Several classification systems have been proposed, but none has been accepted universally [3, 4]. Although the Cierny and Mader classification has been the most popular, the stratification of the physiological status of the host remains problematic [5, 6]. The definition of a C-host, according to this classification, is subjective in nature and is dependent on the treating surgeon's ability to predict the

✉ Leonard C. Marais
 maraisl@ukzn.ac.za

1 Tumour, Sepsis and Reconstruction Unit, Department of Orthopaedic Surgery, School of Clinical Medicine, Grey's Hospital, University of KwaZulu-Natal, Private Bag X9001, Pietermaritzburg 3201, South Africa

2 School of Clinical Medicine, College of Health Sciences, University of KwaZulu-Natal, Durban, South Africa

3 Department of Orthopaedics, 1 Military Hospital, University of Pretoria, Pretoria, South Africa

patient's response to a therapeutic intervention [7]. The differentiation between a type B- and C-host is important as it identifies patients who should be treated curatively or palliatively [3]. In addition, the lack of standardization in host classification has made comparison with results from different studies challenging [8].

There is no evidence-based guidance on the treatment of chronic osteomyelitis in adults [3]. There is no single-treatment regimen or surgical procedure that is appropriate for all patients [9]. Essentially, the choice is between a curative, a palliative or an alternative approach. Curative treatment usually involves surgical debridement with or without complex reconstructive procedures and short-term pathogen-directed antimicrobial therapy [10]. Palliative treatment on the other hand typically involves long-term chronic suppressive antibiotic therapy (CSAT) and rarely intralesional or minimally invasive surgical intervention [11]. An alternative treatment strategy is indicated occasionally and may comprise either of amputation of the limb or a combination of surgical intervention and chronic suppressive antibiotic therapy. The main difficulty lies in choosing the correct treatment strategy for each patient, a process further complicated by the aforementioned lack of standardization in host stratification.

The limitations of existing classification systems, as well as the lack of evidence-based guidelines, prompted us to develop a classification system and treatment algorithm that would assist in treatment strategy selection in a developing country. In this study, we investigate the short-term outcome of treatment in adult patients with long-bone chronic osteomyelitis where a modified host classification system was integrated, via a novel management algorithm, with treatment strategy selection.

Materials and methods

A prospective study was performed on 28 consecutive patients with long-bone chronic osteomyelitis treated at a tertiary-level tumour, sepsis, and reconstruction unit. All adult patients older than 18 years of age and with a minimum follow-up of 12 months were included in the series. Patients with infections involving the foot or hand, atypical organisms (including tuberculosis and fungal infections), arthroplasty-related periprosthetic infection, or early (within 90 days) post-operative surgical site infection with stable implants were excluded from the study. Data were collected with regard to patient demographics, the cause and site of infection, the initial and final impairment, causative organisms, management strategy employed, follow-up period, and outcome of treatment in terms of remission or suppression of infection. Impairment was assessed by means of the QuickDASH scoring system for

upper limbs or AAOS Lower Limb Outcomes Instrument (version 2.0) in the case of lower limb involvement [12, 13].

For the purposes of this study, chronic osteomyelitis was defined as an infection involving bone, with a duration of at least 10 days, where the causative organisms were thought to have persisted either intracellularly or in interactive biofilm-based colonies. Periprosthetic infections were excluded from the study based on the current trend of classifying and treating arthroplasty-related infections as a separate entity [14]. Following clinical, radiological, and biochemical evaluation, patients were classified according to a modified version of the original Cierny and Mader classification system (Table 1) [7]. In terms of the physiological status of the host, the Cierny and Mader classification system was modified in order to provide a more pragmatic and objective definition of a C-host. A patient was classified as a C-host if one major or more than two minor risk factors were present (Table 2). In order to remove any ambiguity during classification of the anatomical nature of the disease, this was performed prior to, rather than following, the debridement. The impairment resulting from the disease and the nidus of infection was added to the classification as these factors were to be considered during the treatment selection process.

Table 1 Modified version of the original Cierny and Mader classification system that served to guide treatment strategy selection

Classification	Characteristic
Physiological	
Type A-host	No risk factors
Type B-host	Less than three minor risk factors
Type C-host	One major and/or three or more minor risk factors
Pathoanatomy	
I—Medullary	No cortical sequestration
II—Cortical	Direct contiguous involvement in cortex only
III—Combined (stable)	Both cortex and medullary regions involved
IV—Combined (unstable)	As for III plus unstable prior to debridement
Nidus	
Sequestrum	Cortical sequestrum present
Implant	Biofilm-based infection in the presence of implant
No identifiable nidus	Minimal necrosis osteomyelitis
Impairment	
Minimal	Patient able to perform ADL (activities of daily living)
Severe	Unable to perform ADL

Table 2 Risk factors used to stratify the physiological status of the host

Major risk factors	Minor systemic risk factors	Minor local risk factors
CD$_4$ count <350 cells/mm^3	HIV infection	Poor soft tissues requiring flap
Albumin <30 g/l	Anaemia	Chronic venous insufficiency
HbA1C ≥8 %	Smoking	Peripheral vascular disease
Cellulitis or abscess formation	Diabetes mellitus	Previous radiation therapy
Malignancy at site of infection	Rheumatoid arthritis	Surgery will result in instability
Pathological fracture	Chronic lung disease	Adjacent joint stiff/arthritic
	Chronic cardiac failure	Heterotopic ossification
	Paraplegia/quadriplegia	Failed reconstruction elsewhere
	Drug or substance abuse	Foot involvement
	Chronic corticosteroid use	Pelvic involvement
	Active tuberculosis	Adjacent joint involved
	Ischaemic heart disease	Segmental resection of ≥6 cm
	Cerebrovascular disease	Required to achieve cure
	Compliance and motivation	
	Age > 65	

The modified classification system was integrated with treatment strategy selection through the implementation of a novel management algorithm (Fig. 1). All C-hosts, as well as A- or B-hosts with minimal impairment, no identifiable source and no skeletal instability, were managed palliatively. All remaining A- and B-hosts were treated curatively. Those C-hosts with severe impairment combined with skeletal instability were managed through the implementation of an alternative treatment strategy. This involved either amputation or chronic suppressive antibiotic therapy in combination with external fixation with or without intralesional debridement.

Curative treatment involved marginal or wide resection, dead space management, provision of bony stability, soft tissue reconstruction, and/or skeletal reconstruction, in conjunction with pathogen-directed adjuvant antibiotics for a period of 6 weeks. In cases without skeletal instability (Cierny and Mader anatomical type I, II and III lesions),

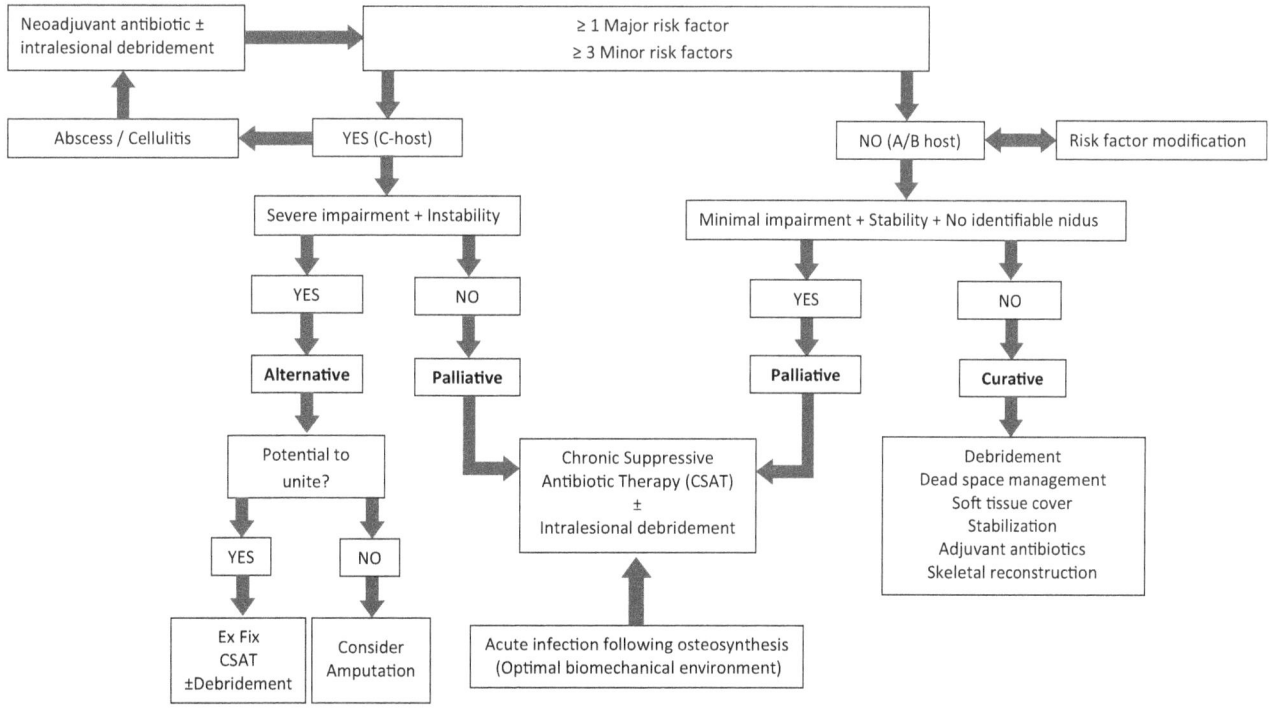

Fig. 1 Treatment selection algorithm

the aim was to maintain stability by marginal debridement through direct unroofing (tangential excision with high-speed burr) and/or indirect unroofing (medullary reaming). In cases involving skeletal instability, wide (segmental) resection was performed and stability provided by circular external fixation. Dead space management techniques were tailored to the anatomical nature of the pathology. A modified version of continuous irrigation, as proposed by Lautenbach, was used in type I (medullary) post-operative infections [15, 16]. A solution of 80 mg of gentamicin in 1000 ml 0.9 % NaCl was infused at 125 ml/h through a single perforated 6-mm drain tube that was placed intra-medullary through the nail entry site and a distal cortical window at the site of the previous locking screws. The irrigation was discontinued, and drain was removed once the effluent fluid was macroscopically clear. In type III lesions (stable combined medullary and cortical lesions), gentamicin-impregnated polymethylmethacrylate (PMMA) beads (Septopal® Merck, Darmstadt Germany) were used and removed at 6–8 weeks. Emphasis was placed on soft tissue reconstruction with the closure of soft tissue defects with well-perfused healthy tissue. Where direct primary closure was deemed unfeasible, a plastic surgeon performed closure with a tissue flap with preference given to muscular flaps. Post-operatively, all patients were treated with generic parenteral antibiotics in the form of cefazolin and imipenem until the 7-day microscopy, culture, and sensitivity (MCS) results became available. Oral antibiotic therapy, in the form of two agents that were tailored to the culture and sensitivity results, was commenced subsequently and continued for a period of 6 weeks.

Following this period, reconstruction of segmental bone defects in Cierny and Mader type IV lesions was undertaken if clinical and biochemical evaluation confirmed the absence of active infection. The treatment protocol dictated that the size of the bone defect would determine the nature of the subsequent skeletal reconstruction procedure. Defects less than 1–2 cm in magnitude were managed by acute shortening (Fig. 2). In long bones other than the tibia, defects between 2 and 4 cm in size were managed using the Masquelet technique, involving autogenous bone grafting into an induced membrane. Tibial defects larger than 2 cm and gaps in other long bones in excess of 4 cm were treated through the use of bone transport.

Palliative treatment involved the use of chronic suppressive antibiotic therapy (CSAT) in the form of trimethoprim–sulfamethoxazole (800 mg/160 mg twice daily) and rifampicin (600 mg daily). In cases where the general condition of the patient and local soft tissues allowed, an intralesional excision of discreet exposed sequestra was performed. In this series, all cases treated by an alternative treatment strategy required amputation of the limb.

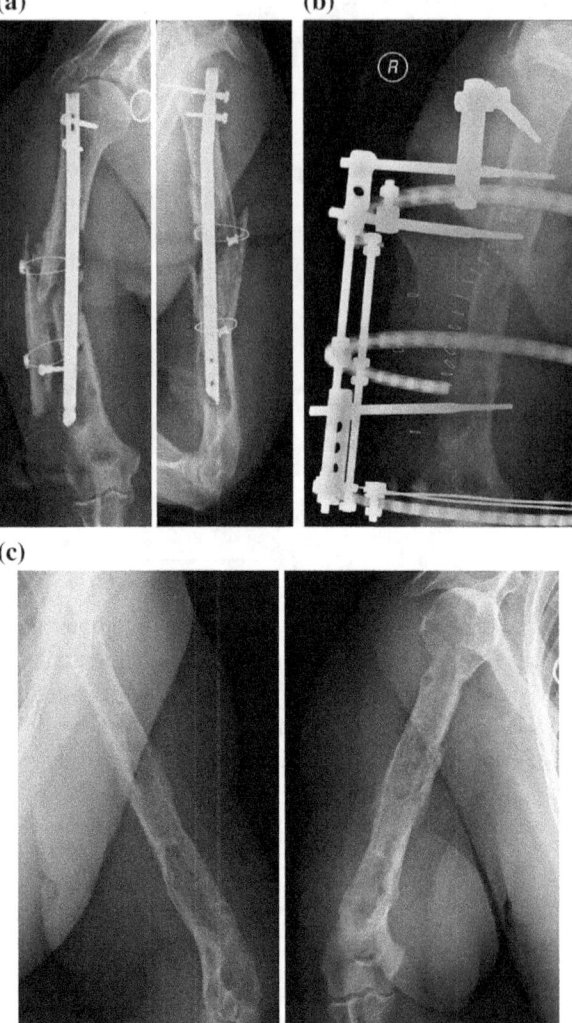

Fig. 2 X-ray images of a case involving pre-operative instability (anatomical type IV infection). **a** This 72-year-old diabetic patient presented with a septic non-union of the humerus following multiple previous surgeries. **b** Reconstruction of the post-debridement defect involved acute shortening, bone graft, and circular external fixation. **c** Radiological images following removal of external fixator

Following a minimum 12-month follow-up period treatment, success or failure was determined. Success was defined as achievement of remission through a curative treatment strategy or attainment of suppression in patients treated palliatively. Remission was defined as the absence of clinical signs of infection [8]. Suppression was defined as subjective resolution of infection symptoms and signs from the patient's point of view to the extent that the patient required no additional treatment. Treatment failure was defined as the failure to achieve the predetermined goal (remission or suppression). The outcome was also reported as failure if unplanned re-operation was required or if the patient was dissatisfied with the outcome.

Data were analysed using Stata 13.0 (StataCorp. 2013. Stata Statistical Software: Release 13. College Station, TX: StataCorp LP). Continuous variables were summarized using mean and standard deviation values. If the variable was skewed or outlier values were present, then the median and interquartile range were used. Categorical variables were summarized using frequency tables. Ninety-five per cent confidence intervals were constructed around sample point estimates. Changes in functional outcome score from initial assessment to final assessment were compared using a paired t test. A p value of <0.05 was considered statistically significant for all tests.

Ethical approval was obtained from the relevant ethics review boards prior to commencement of the study.

Results

Twenty-six of the 28 enrolled patients were available for follow-up at 12 months. One patient was excluded on the basis that he was diagnosed with a surgical site infection in association with stable fixation of a tibial plafond fracture in the early post-operative period. This infection was therefore not treated as chronic osteomyelitis. The second patient excluded was a 77-year-old male with post-operative chronic osteomyelitis following cephalomedullary nailing of a subtrochanteric fracture. The patient was lost to follow-up after the initial visit, and attempts to contact the patient were unsuccessful. The median age of the remaining patients was 36.5 years (range 18–72 years; interquartile range 24 years). Seven patients had chronic haematogenous osteomyelitis, eight had post-operative infections, nine developed chronic osteomyelitis after open fractures, and two patients developed contiguous chronic osteomyelitis as a result of direct local extension. The tibial diaphysis was the most commonly involved site (Table 3). Culture results, from tissue samples taken at the time of debridement in patients who were treated curatively, revealed a variety of causative organisms (Table 4).

Classification

Three patients (12 %) were classified as A-hosts, 11 patients (42 %) as B-hosts, and 12 (46 %) as C-hosts. Six patients classified as C-hosts had at least one major risk factor and six other patients on the basis of three or more minor risk factors. Of the 12 C-hosts, six had both a major and more than two minor risk factors present. Seven patients (27 %) were HIV-positive with a mean CD$_4$ count of 401 cells/mm^3 [range 220–986 cells/mm^3; standard deviation (SD) 238 cells/mm^3]. A variety of additional risk factors were identified amongst the patients enrolled (Fig. 3). Nine patients (35 %) were smokers, and three

Table 3 Site of infection

Site of infection	Number of patients
Tibia diaphysis	12 (46 %)
Femur diaphysis	8 (30 %)
Tibial plateau	2 (8 %)
Tibial plafond	1 (4 %)
Humerus diaphysis	2 (8 %)
Ulna shaft	1 (4 %)

Table 4 Micro-organism cultured from tissue samples taken during debridement in patients treated curatively

Micro-organisms	Number of patients
Staphylococcus aureus	3
Staphylococcus epidermidis	1
Enterobacter sp.	1
Streptococcus infantarius	1
Pseudomonas aeruginosa	1
Aeromonas hydrophila	1
Serratia sp.	1
Proteus mirabilis	1
Pantoea sp.	1
No growth	1
Multiple organisms	1

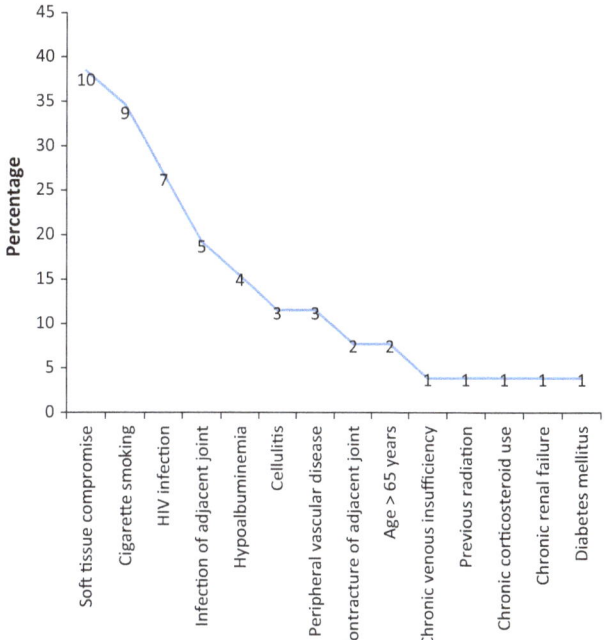

Fig. 3 Risk factors identified in the series of cases

patients (12 %) had hypoalbuminemia. The soft tissues in ten patients were considered to represent a significant risk factor for the development of complications following

Table 5 Functional outcome

Category	n	Mean	SD[c]	Range	p value[d]
Overall lower extremity[a]	23				
Initial		52	21.2	21–100	
Final		89	11.6	51–100	
Improvement		27	18.4	0–49	<0.001
Overall upper extremity[b]	3				
Initial		75	7.4	72.5–86.4	
Final		18.2	13.6	2.3–29.5	
Improvement		54.3	20.2	45.5–84.1	0.03
Palliative group[a]	14				
Initial		51.1	22.9	28–100	
Final		92.5	16.8	51–100	
Improvement		25.5	17.1	0–54	<0.001
Curative group[a]	8				
Initial		61	21.3	34–94	
Final		91	9.1	74–100	
Improvement		27.5	17.4	6–48	<0.01

[a] AAOS Lower Limb Outcomes Instrument
[b] QuickDASH
[c] Standard deviation
[d] Paired t test

surgery unless addressed by flap or other means. Cellulitis and abscess formation, precluding definitive surgery as the first line of treatment, were present in three patients. Peripheral vascular disease or chronic venous insufficiency with lipodermatosclerosis was present in three patients. The infection involved the adjacent joint in five cases, and there was significant loss in range of motion of the adjacent joint in the additional two patients. Other risk factors included previous radiation, chronic renal failure requiring dialysis and chronic corticosteroid use in one patient, diabetes mellitus in one patient, and age over 65 years in two patients. In terms of the anatomical extent of the disease, 20 patients had type III infection, five patients had preoperative instability, and in one patient, the infection was confined to the medullary cavity. The mean initial AAOS Lower Limb Outcomes score in patients with lower limb involvement was 58.2 (range 21–100; SD 22.9). In three cases, the upper limb was involved, with a mean initial QuickDASH score of 18.2 (range 2.3–29.5; Table 5).

Management

Fourteen patients (54 %) were managed palliatively, and 11 patients (42 %) were managed through the implementation of a curative treatment strategy. One patient required alternative treatment in the form of an amputation. This patient had infection and bone loss following a neglected open fracture and was classified as a C-host on the basis of the

presence of two major and two minor risk factors. The palliative treatment group comprised of 11 C-hosts and three B-hosts who had stable lesions with minimal impairment and no identifiable sequestra. All patients in the palliative treatment group received chronic suppressive antibiotic therapy—trimethoprim–sulfamethoxazole (800 mg/160 mg twice daily) and rifampicin (600 mg daily)—for a period of 3–6 months. One patient, who had an exposed sequestrum in the region of the tibial plateau, required an additional intralesional excision (simple sequestrectomy).

In the curative treatment group, surgical intervention involved marginal debridement (direct and/or indirect unroofing) in ten patients. Wide (segmental) resection of the ulna diaphysis, without subsequent reconstruction, was performed in one patient. Dead space management involved a modified Lautenbach continuous irrigation system in six cases, PMMA beads in four patients, and local muscle flap in one case. Primary soft tissue closure was obtained for all cases in the curative group. Direct primary closure of the wound was performed in ten cases, and in one instance, a local muscle flap was required. In the two patients, in whom skeletal stabilization and reconstruction were required, acute shortening and Ilizarov circular external fixation were performed. Union was achieved in both of these cases. All patients treated curatively received a combination of two oral antibiotics for a period of 6 weeks.

Outcome

The overall success rate was 96.2 % (95 % CI 80.4–99.9 %) after a minimum of 12 months of follow-up. Remission was achieved in all [11/11] patients treated curatively (one-sided 95 % CI 73.5–100.0 %). Palliative treatment was successful in 92.8 % of cases (95 % CI 66.1–99.9 %), with suppression in 46 % and remission in the remaining 54 % of these patients. The overall mean final AAOS Lower Limb Outcomes score was 86.6 (range 51–100; SD 14.5). This equated to a statistically significant (p value < 0.001) mean improvement of 28.3 (95 % CI 21.0–35.7, SD 17.0). In the upper limb, the mean final overall QuickDASH score was 75 (range 72.5–86.4), with a mean improvement of 54.3 (range 45.5–84.1). There was comparable improvement in the functional outcome scores in the palliative and curative treatment groups (Table 5).

One treatment failure occurred in the palliative treatment group in a patient who required regular dialysis as a result of Goodpasture syndrome. This patient had extensive involvement in the entire femoral diaphysis after irradiation for a sarcoma, peripheral vascular disease and avascular necrosis of the femoral head. A hip disarticulation was required when the palliative treatment protocol was abandoned.

Discussion

Chronic osteomyelitis management continues to pose a major challenge to orthopaedic surgeons [11]. The Mayo Clinic reported a 20 % failure rate in the management of chronic infections [17]. Twenty years later, the disease remains difficult to cure as was acknowledged in a recent Cochrane review on antibiotic therapy in chronic osteomyelitis [18]. The combined remission rate, in this analysis of four randomized controlled trials, was 78.8 % at 12 months. Specialized units have, however, been able to achieve superior results. Cierny, for example, achieved success in 84 % of patients managed curatively at 2-year follow-up [10]. The Bone Infection Unit in the UK reported an impressive cure rate of 90 % at 5-year follow-up [9]. While the multidisciplinary nature of the service offered by these specialized units is bound to improve outcomes, appropriate surgical candidate selection may also play a role.

Without a pragmatic and objective definition of a C-host (who should be palliated), the selection of a curative (surgical) treatment strategy, according to the Cierny and Mader classification system, is based on prior clinical experience [7]. By this approach, the expected outcome of a curative strategy should offer a distinct advantage over symptomatic treatment or amputation, in order to justify the potential morbidity and risks involved in limb salvage surgery [7, 10]. Selecting candidates for surgery on this basis requires considerable experience as it is based on a prediction of the patient's response to treatment. The experience gained in specialized units will therefore improve the success of curative treatment strategies due to, amongst other factors, improved surgical candidate selection. The approach followed in our study was developed to serve as a guideline for treatment of chronic osteomyelitis in a resource-poor clinical environment where treatment by specialized units is not always easily accessible.

In a previous retrospective series of 109 cases, we were able to achieve an overall success rate of 90 % at a mean 18-months follow-up through an approach which integrated the pragmatic host stratification with treatment strategy selection [19]. In this study, we aimed for a preliminary validation of a similar approach prospectively. After a minimum of 12-month follow-up, we achieved an overall success rate of 96.2 %, with 100 % remission in the curative group and 92.8 % suppression (or better) in the palliative group. These results are comparable to those achieved in our retrospective series, where curative and palliative treatments were successful in 93 and 87 %, respectively [19].

Although these results appear promising, caution is advised against widespread implementation of this approach. The proposed classification system and treatment algorithm were designed for use in the developing world. It is unlikely to be suitable in the developed world without further improvement or modification. Apart from the high incidence of HIV infection and hypoalbuminemia in our series, the pattern of causative organisms identified in our cases appears to differ somewhat from that seen in the developed world [20].

Additional problems may arise when the algorithm is tested on a wider range of patients. In one case in this series, the treatment algorithm was deemed to be inadequate as it prescribed chronic suppressive antibiotic therapy (CSAT) in a C-host (on the basis of the presence of skeletal stability), where amputation was inevitable. This algorithm error was, however, on the conservative side; in many C-hosts without skeletal instability, CSAT may suppress the disease to the extent that amputation may not be required. Furthermore, the proposed host stratification criteria could result in the initiation of palliative care in patients who may have been able to cope with curative treatment. This approach may hold some benefit as it emphasizes the importance of host factor modification prior to surgical intervention. Many high-risk cases who may initially be classified as C-hosts will become candidates for curative treatment (B-hosts) following implementation of the appropriate interventions aimed at risk factor reduction.

There are further limitations to this study. The heterogeneous nature of the disease demands a much larger series of cases to determine whether the algorithm is appropriate. The follow-up period in this series is too short to determine the ultimate success rate, and our results are likely to deteriorate over time due to relapse. While deterioration can be expected in both groups, it is bound to be more pronounced in the palliative group. Long-term follow-up will be required to shed more light on this subject. The lack of a control group is a further limitation. Randomizing high-risk patients to high- or low-risk interventions, in order to identify which factors are associated failure (amputation), presents obvious ethical concerns. Future comparative studies will, however, be facilitated by the fact that we have provided a standardized host stratification system.

Despite these limitations, preliminary results suggest that our proposed approach may be useful in certain clinical environments. Our modified classification system may be more relevant to clinicians inexperienced in the management of chronic osteomyelitis as it is less dependent on estimation of the response to treatment or the prediction of instability following debridement. Another important potential benefit of this approach is that standardized host stratification may enable the comparison of results from future studies. It may become possible to compare the outcome of different interventions or strategies if the physiological host status was classified using the same pre-defined pragmatic criteria. This may, in turn, allow us to answer many of the questions that remain regarding the management of adult chronic osteomyelitis [8].

Conclusion

The integrated approach proposed in this study appears to hold promise in the management of chronic long-bone osteomyelitis in adult patients in the developing world. Further investigation is required to validate the approach, and additional algorithm development may be required in order to render it useful in other clinical settings.

Acknowledgments The corresponding author has received a research grant from the South African Orthopaedic Association in support of this research project.

Informed consent Informed consent was obtained from all individual participants included in the study.

References

1. Galanakos SP, Papadakis SA, Kateros K, Papakostas I, Macheras G (2009) Biofilm and orthopaedic practice: the world of microbes in a world of implants. Orthop Trauma 23(3):175–179
2. Boyce BF, Xing L, Schwarz EM (2011) The role of the immune system and bone cells in acute and chronic osteomyelitis. In: Lorenzo J, Choi Y, Horowitz M, Takayanagi H (eds) Osteoimmunology: interactions of the immune and skeletal systems, 1st edn. Academic Press, Waltham, pp 369–390
3. Walter G, Kemmerer M, Kappler C, Hoffmann R (2012) Treatment algorithms for chronic osteomyelitis. Dtsch Arztebl Int 109(14):257–264
4. Marais LC, Ferreira N, Aldous C, Le Roux TLB (2014) Classification of chronic osteomyeltis. S Afr J Orthop 13(1):22–28
5. Roa N, Ziran BH, Lipsky BA (2011) Treating osteomyelitis: antibiotics and surgery. Plast Reconstr Surg 127(Suppl):177S–187S
6. Romanò CL, Romanò D, Logoluso N, Drago L (2011) Bone and joint infections in adults: a comprehensive classification proposal. Eur Orthop Traumatol 1:207–217
7. Cierny G, Mader JT, Penninck JJ (2003) A clinical staging system for adult osteomyelitis. Clin Orthop Relat Res 414:7–24
8. Lazzarini L, Lipsky BA, Mader JT (2005) Antibiotic treatment of osteomyelitis: what have we learned from 30 years of clinical trials? Int J Infect Dis 9:127–138
9. McNally M, Nagarajah K (2010) Osteomyelitis. Orthop Trauma 24(6):416–429
10. Cierny G (2011) Surgical treatment of osteomyelitis. Plast Reconstr Surg 127(Suppl 1):S190–S204
11. Lazzarini L, Mader JT, Calhoun JH (2004) Osteomyelitisin Long Bones. J Bone Jt Surg Am 86(10):2305–2318
12. Beaton DE, Wright JG, Katz JN, the Upper Extremity Collaborative Group (2005) Development of the QuickDASH: comparison of three item-reduction approaches. J Bone Jt Surg Am 87(5):1038–1046
13. Johanson NA, Liang MH, Daltroy L, Rudicel S, Richmond J (2004) American academy of orthopaedic surgeons lower limb outcomes assessment instruments. Reliability, validity, and sensitivity to change. J Bone Jt Surg Am 86(5):902–909
14. Cierny G, DiPasquale D (2002) Periprosthetic total joint infections. Staging, treatment, and outcomes. Clin Orthop Relat Res 403:23–28
15. Lautenbach E (1975) Chronic Osteomyelitis: irrigation and suction after surgery. J Bone Jt Surg Br 57(2):259
16. Hashmi MA, Norman P, Saleh M (2004) The management of chronic osteomyelitis using the Lautenbach method. J Bone Jt Surg Br 86:269–275
17. Hall BB, Fitzgerald RH, Rosenblatt JE (1984) Anaerobic osteomyelitis. J Bone Jt Surg Am 65:30–35
18. Conterno L, Turchi MD (2013) Antibiotics for treating chronic osteomyelitis in adults. Cochrane Database Syst Rev. doi:10.1002/14651858.CD004439.pub3
19. Marais LC, Ferreira N, Sartorius B, Aldous C, Le Roux TLB (2015) A modified staging system for chronic osteomyelitis. J Orthop 12:184–192. doi:10.1016/j.jor.2015.05.017
20. Sheehy SH, Atkins BA, Bejon P, Byren I, Wyllie D, Athanasou NA et al (2010) The microbiology of chronic osteomyelitis: prevalence of resistance to common empirical anti-microbial regimens. J Infect 60:338–343

18

Recognizing the elbow prosthesis on conventional radiographs

Kamilcan Oflazoglu[1] · Nienke Koenrades[2] · Matthijs P. Somford[2] ·
Michel P. J. van den Bekerom[3]

Abstract The objective of this study was to make an overview that can be useful in determining which type and brand of prosthesis a patient has when visiting the emergency department or outpatient clinic with a periprosthetic fracture, dislocation, or implant failure. The commonly used prostheses in Europe are opted for this list. The radiographs used for this list are obtained either from the company or from our own patients. This list contains the Coonrad/Morrey total elbow prosthesis, the Nexel total elbow prosthesis, the GSB III Elbow Prosthesis, the iBP Total Elbow System, the Discovery Elbow System, the NESimplavit Elbow System, the Latitude Elbow prosthesis, the Solar Elbow, and the Souter–Strathclyde total elbow. The characteristics of each prosthesis are described.

Keywords Elbow · Arthroplasty · Prosthesis · Radiograph

✉ Kamilcan Oflazoglu
k.oflazoglu@gmail.com

Nienke Koenrades
nienkekoen@hotmail.com

Matthijs P. Somford
mp_somford@hotmail.com

Michel P. J. van den Bekerom
bekerom@gmail.com

[1] Massachusetts General Hospital, 55 Fruit Street, 02114 Boston, United States

[2] Department of Orthopaedic Surgery, Medisch Spectrum Twente, Haaksbergerstraat 55, 7513 ER Enschede, The Netherlands

[3] Department of Orthopaedic Surgery, Onze Lieve Vrouwe Gasthuis Amsterdam, Oosterpark 9, 1091 AC Amsterdam, The Netherlands

Introduction

With the rising incidence of performing total elbow arthroplasties, orthopedic surgeons and radiologists will more often be confronted with elbow arthroplasty radiographs. The incline in the number of performed total elbow arthroplasties is mainly in acute and post-trauma cases, with probably a decline of the number in rheumatoid elbows because of the high-quality conservative treatment for this disease and, especially in cases of failure of an elbow arthroplasty, because the long-term follow-up of the elbow arthroplasty in general is not similar to the total hip prosthesis. In the Denmark arthroplasty register, an overall 10-year survival of 81 % (95 % CI 76–86 %) was reported [1].

When confronted with a periprosthetic fracture or (a)septic prosthesis failure, a basic knowledge of the implant and type of fixation is useful and probably essential in planning treatment. When no information is available concerning the first operation, the radiograph can guide in recognizing the type and brand of prosthesis. Also knowing whether it concerns a constrained or a non-constrained type helps in identifying hinge failure or recognizing a dislocation.

We present a list of commonly used elbow arthroplasties in Europe with their main features and a lateral radiograph to help the caregiver with identification and subsequent decision making.

Materials and methods

For this list of elbow prostheses, we opted for the commonly used prostheses in Europe. This list contains the prostheses of which we managed to collect conventional radiographs. The radiographs used for this list are obtained either from the company or from our own patients.

This list contains the next prostheses:

- Coonrad/Morrey total elbow
- Nexel total elbow
- GSB III Elbow Prosthesis
- Discovery Elbow System
- Kudo type-5 prosthesis
- iBP Total Elbow System
- NESimplavit Elbow System
- Latitude Elbow
- Solar Elbow
- Souter–Strathclyde total elbow

Results

Coonrad/Morrey total elbow

The Coonrad/Morrey total elbow is produced by Zimmer (Warsaw, IN, USA) as a prosthesis replacing the elbow. The prosthesis is made of Tivanium Ti–6Al–4V alloy and is a cemented prosthesis. The connection of the components is linked, but semi-constrained with a metal–polyethylene bushing. Length of humeral and ulnar components can be varied. The humeral stem is triangular and the ulnar stem is quadrangular. There are 12 different sizes for both the humeral and the ulnar stem. The Coonrad/Morrey total elbow has a 12-year survival of 92.4 % (Fig. 1) [2].

Nexel total elbow

The Nexel total elbow is also produced by Zimmer as a prosthesis replacing the elbow. It is built on the foundation

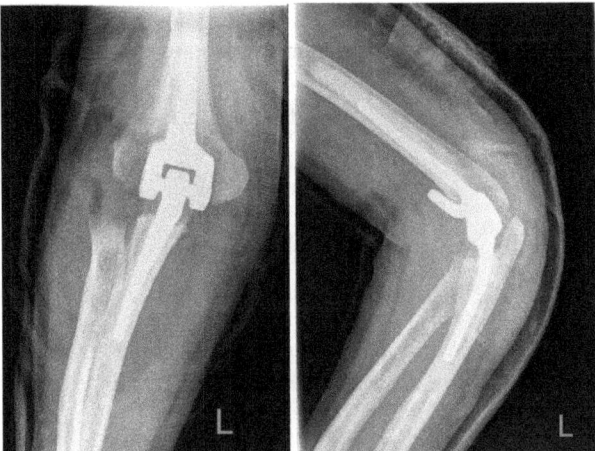

Fig. 1 Coonrad/Morrey total elbow; the humeral component of the prosthesis has a humeral anterior flange. The joint surface of the humeral component is quite angular, best seen on the AP view

of the Coonrad/Morrey total elbow. The prosthesis is made of Tivanium Ti–6Al–4V alloy and is cemented. The connection of the components is constrained with a different, thicker polyethylene bearing (Vivacit-E HXPE) compared with the Coonrad/Morrey total elbow. Therefore, it may reduce edge loading and stress and maximizes contact area to distribute joint reaction forces. Length of humeral and ulnar components can be varied similar to the Coonrad/ Morrey. The intramedullary stem geometry and anterior humeral flange are maintained from the Coonrad/Morrey total elbow (Fig. 2) [3].

GSB III Elbow Prosthesis

The GSB III Elbow Prosthesis is also produced by Zimmer. The prosthesis is made of titanium alloy and is cemented. The connection of the components between the humeral stem and the ulna component is "plug-in," non-constrained.

The GSB I Elbow Prosthesis was introduced in 1971. At that time, all rigid hinged arthroplasties showed a high rate of loosening. As a result, the GSB III Elbow Prosthesis was developed and is used since 1978. The humeral component has a large surface for support on the condyles and a wide stem for transference of rotational stress. All articulating surfaces are coated with polyethylene. The GSB III Elbow Prosthesis has three humeral sizes and four ulnar components all of which can be freely combined with each other (Fig. 3) [4].

Discovery elbow system

The Discovery Elbow System is produced by Biomet (Warsaw, IN, USA). The ulnohumeral prosthesis is made of CoCrMo alloy or titanium alloy, and both components are cemented. The connection of the components is constrained with an ultra-high molecular weight polyethylene (UHMWPE). Length and width of humeral and ulnar components can be varied (Fig. 4) [5].

Kudo type-5 prosthesis

The Kudo type-5 prosthesis is produced by Stryker Howmedica Osteonics (Limerick, Ireland) and is a non-constrained, unlinked prosthesis. Contrary to almost every prosthesis on this list, the Kudo type-5 does not require acrylic cement for fixation. The humeral component consists of cobalt–chromium alloy with half of the surface of the stem porous-coated with a plasma spray of titanium alloy. Porous coating of the stem with titanium alloy should achieve osseointegration at the bone–metal interface. The ulnar component either has a metal backing with a porous-coated stem or is either all-polyethylene. In the

Fig. 2 Nexel total elbow; this prosthesis also has a humeral anterior flange. As a result of the ticker bearing, there is more space between the two components on the X-ray compared with the Coonrad/ Murray total elbow. The joint surface of the humeral component of the Nexel is more circular shaped, in contrast to the Coonrad/Morrey total elbow, best seen on the AP view

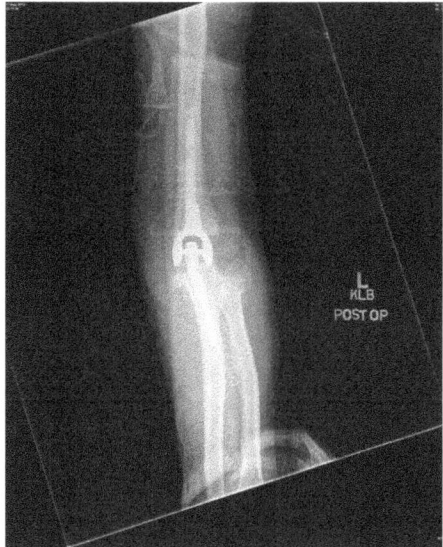
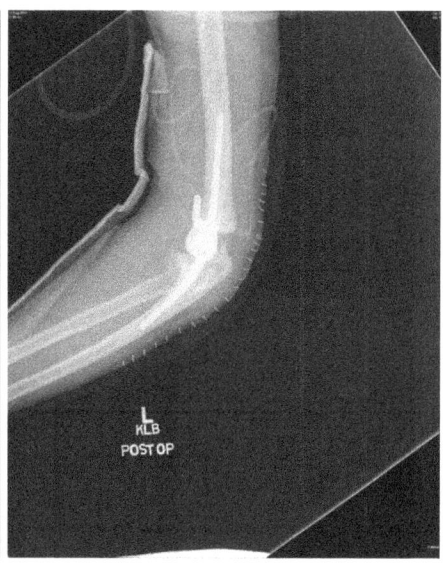

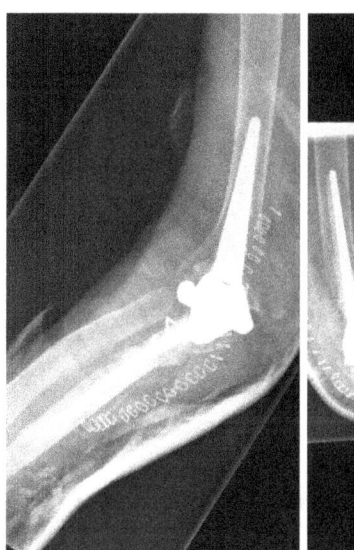
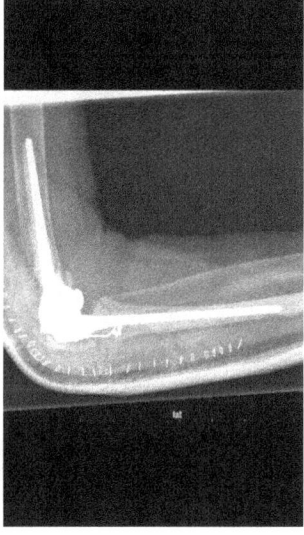

Fig. 3 GSB III Elbow Prosthesis; this prosthesis does not have a humeral anterior flange. On an anterior–posterior X-ray, the GSB III Elbow Prosthesis is recognizable because of the large joint surface of the humeral component

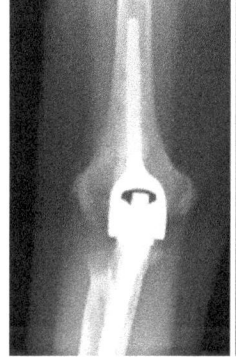
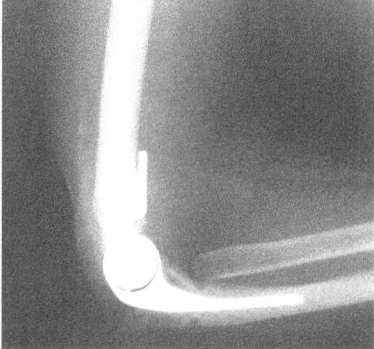

Fig. 4 Discovery elbow system; the humeral component of the prosthesis has a humeral anterior flange. It has a characteristic hinge, on de AP view, similar to shape of a horizontal hourglass

last case, cement is required for the fixation of the ulnar component. Both components articulate on a high-density polyethylene layer. The stem of both components, especially the ulnar component, are narrow and straight. The distal part of the humeral component is tube shaped (Fig. 5) [6].

iBP Total Elbow System

The iBP (instrumented bone preserving) Elbow System is also produced by Biomet (Warsaw, IN, USA). This is a modification of Stryker's Kudo elbow prosthesis, with more available sizes, improved humeral condyle requiring

less removal of humeral bone, and a more anatomical shape. This true unlinked prosthesis has four different humeral components (small, standard, large, and extra large) and three ulnar components (small, standard, and large). Both components are available in uncemented and cemented options. The humeral component is cobalt–chrome and the ulnar component is made of titanium. The articulation is ArCom polyethylene (Fig. 6) [7].

NESimplavit elbow system

The NESimplavit Elbow System, formerly known as the Norway elbow, is produced by Implant Cast (Buxtehude, Germany) as a prosthesis replacing the elbow. Ulnar and humeral components are made of cast CoCrMo alloy. The bobbin is made from UHMWPE. This is the cylinder part of the humeral component which articulates with the ceramic coated axle of the ulnar component. The axle is made from $TiAl_6V_4$ which is coated with TiN to reduce the

Fig. 5 Kudo type-5; both components have a straight and narrow humeral component on an AP view. The tube shape of the distal part of the humeral component, the 'oculus', is best seen on a lateral view

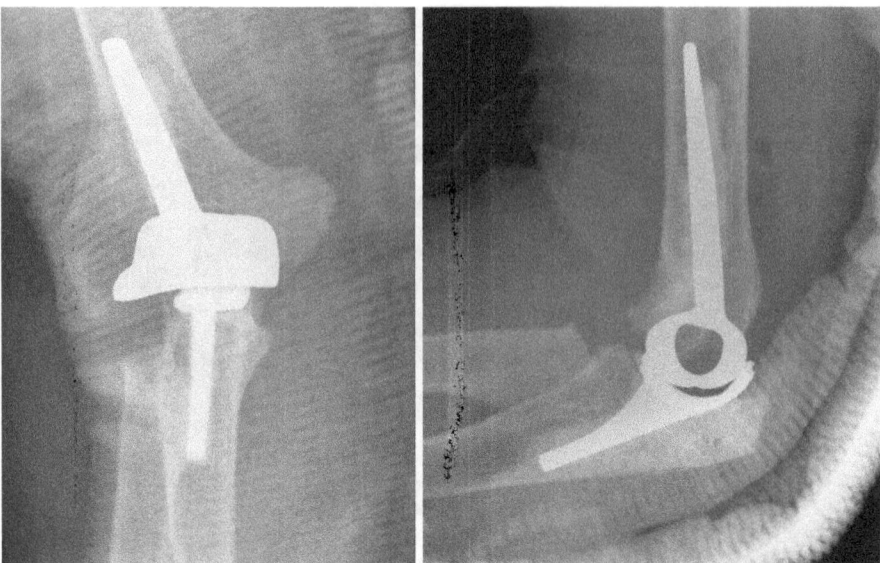

Fig. 6 iBP Total Elbow System; there is no humeral anterior flange. This prosthesis has a characteristic hook-shaped humeral component, best seen on the lateral viewed radiograph. The radial component is relatively short

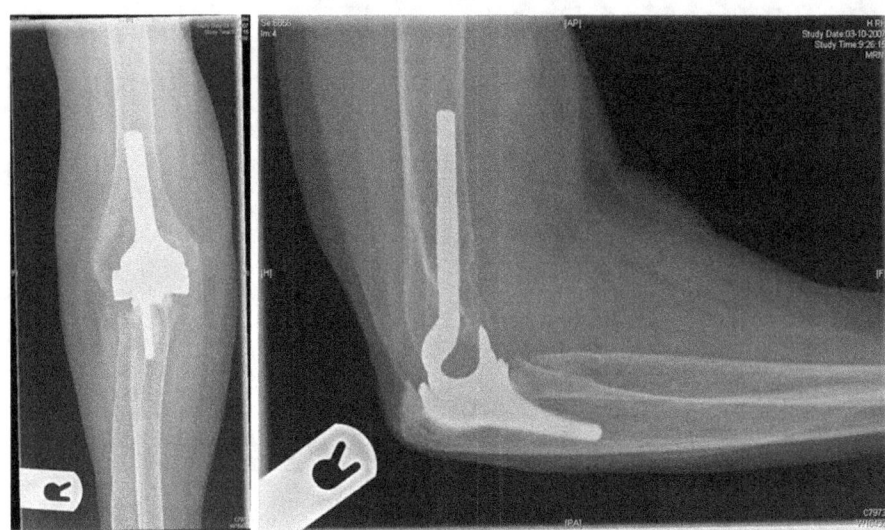

Fig. 7 *NES*implavit elbow system; the humeral component of the prosthesis does not have a humeral anterior flange. On the lateral view, the proximal part of the humeral component is smaller than the distal part. The ulnar component is relatively small

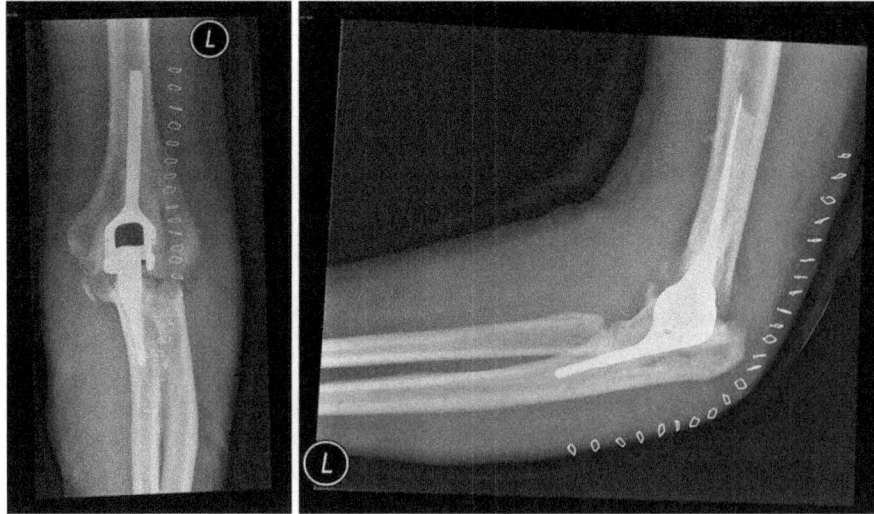

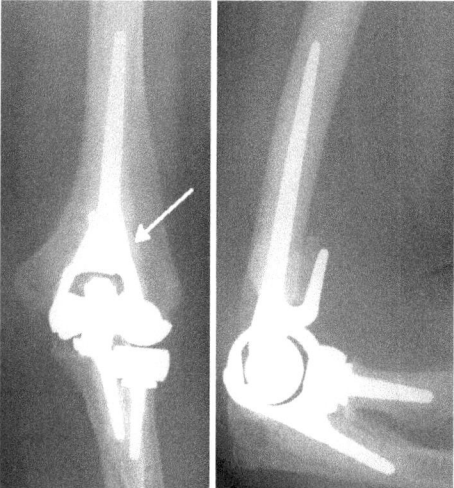

Fig. 8 Latitude Elbow; the humeral component of the prosthesis does not have a humeral anterior flange. The medial and lateral fins of the humeral component (best seen on AP view) make the distal part look pyramid-shaped. Noticeable is the radial head component

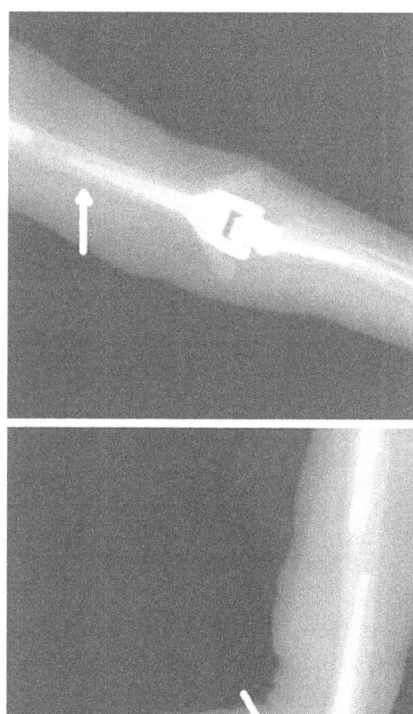

Fig. 9 Solar Elbow; the humeral component of the prosthesis does not have a humeral anterior flange. The hinge resembles the Coonrad/Murray on an AP view. However, the proximal paNESimplavit's humeral component. The subtle antrt of the humeral component is pointy, in contrast to that of the Coonrad/Morrey's and the erior fin of the ulnar component is seen on the lateral view

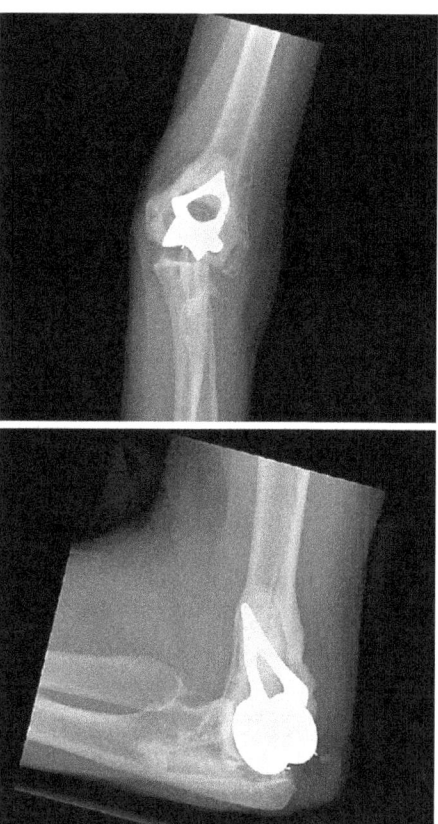

Fig. 10 Souter–Strathclyde; the humeral component differs from the other prostheses in this list. On an AP view, the proximal part of the humeral component has a pointed shape with a gap in the middle. It is relatively short. The ulnar component is less visible

polyethylene wear. This system is for cemented use only. The connection is semi-constrained. The intact ligaments and tendons are stabilizing the joint. Four different sizes are available for the humeral implants and can be combined independently with the three ulnar sizes (Fig. 7) [8].

Latitude Elbow

The Latitude Elbow is produced by Tornier (Montbonnot Saint Ismier, France) as a cemented cobalt–chrome prosthesis replacing the elbow with the possibility of placing a radial component. The Latitude ulnar stem is designed with an optional cap so that the components can be unlinked or linked, constrained, and non-constrained. The ulnar component, as well as the radial head component, articulates with a polyethylene layer. The humeral stem has medial and lateral fins to prevent intramedullary rotation. Humeral spools have been designed with a concave barrel shaped trochlea to preserve linear contact throughout 7 of valgus/varus movement with the ulnar component. In case of a humeral fracture, it is possible to replace solely the humeral component (Fig. 8) [9].

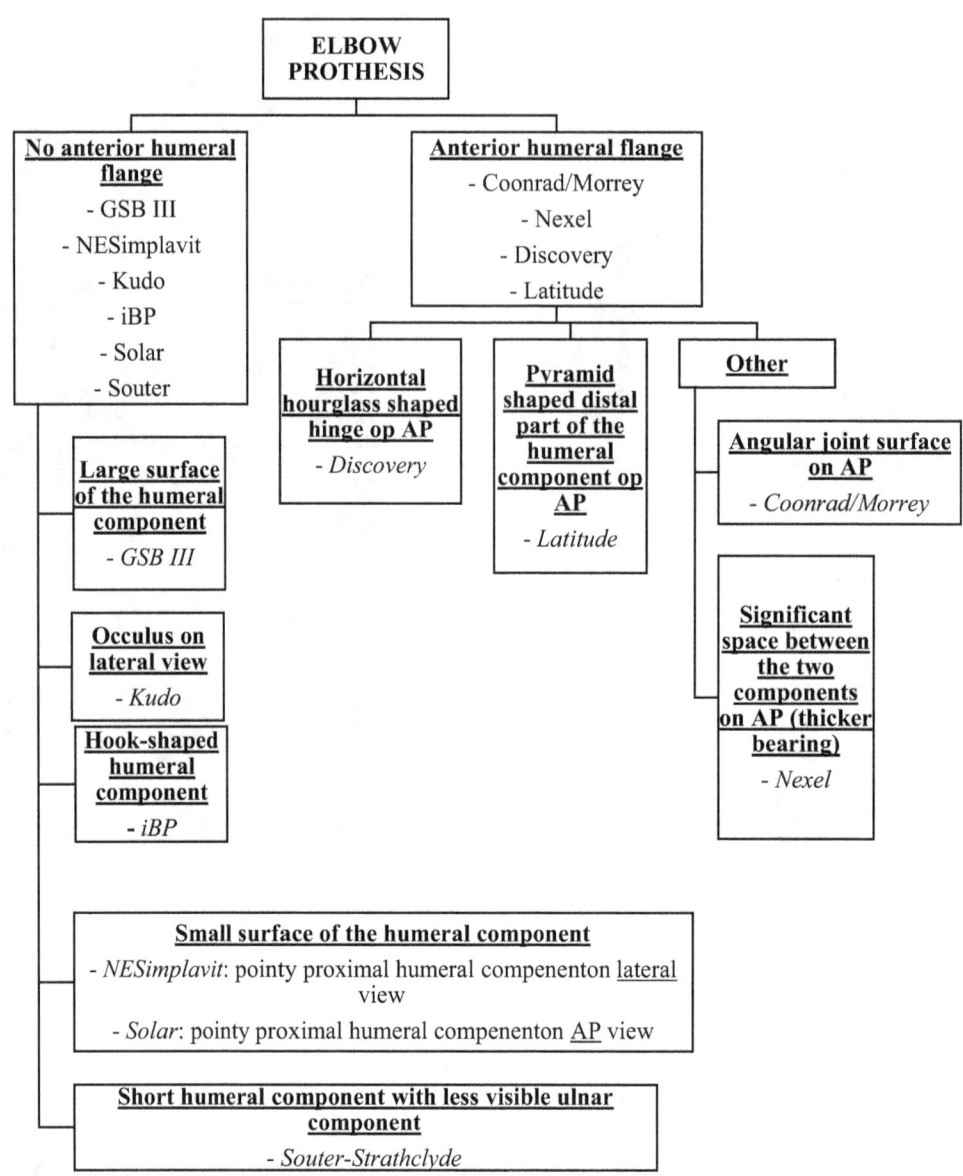

Fig. 11 Characteristics of each elbow prosthesis

Solar elbow

The Solar Elbow is produced by Stryker (Kalamazoo, MI, USA) as a cemented titanium alloy prosthesis replacing the total elbow. This linked prosthesis is semi-constrained. The humeral and ulnar component both articulate with a polyethylene layer. Similar to the Latitude Elbow, the humeral stem has medial and lateral fins to prevent intramedullary rotation. The ulnar component has a subtle anterior fin to help resist rotational forces placed across the joint. There are two sizes of humeral components, standard and large, along with three sizes of ulnar components, small, standard, and large (Fig. 9) [10].

Souter–Strathclyde total elbow

The Souter–Strathclyde total elbow is produced by Stryker Howmedica Osteonics (Limerick, Ireland) is a cemented unlinked and partially constrained elbow prosthesis. This elbow prosthesis differs from the other prostheses in this list because of the characteristic humeral component with humeral flanges projecting into the capitellum and the medial epicondyle. The relatively short humeral component is made of Vitallium is available in a small, medium, or large size. It is also available with long stems. The ulnar component has a keel and a small stem, and is made of ultra-high molecular weight polyethylene, which, at first sight, makes it less visible on a radiograph (Fig. 10) [11–13].

Discussion

The number of total elbow arthroplasties is growing in (post-) trauma cases. Although several imaging modalities are available, conventional radiography remains the mainstay of imaging evaluation of elbow replacements. The various types and brands of elbow replacements can be recognized on radiographs. In this article, an overview was provided of the most commonly used elbow arthroplasties in Europe and their specific characteristics.

This list contains the Coonrad/Morrey total elbow prosthesis, the Nexel total elbow prosthesis, the GSB III Elbow Prosthesis, the Discovery Elbow System, the Kudo type-5, the iBP Total Elbow System, the NESimplavit Elbow System, the Latitude Elbow prosthesis, the Solar Elbow, and the Souter–Strathclyde total elbow.

An important recognizable part of elbow prostheses on a lateral radiographic view is whether the humeral component of the elbow prosthesis has an anterior humeral flange. In this list, the Coonrad/Morrey total elbow prosthesis, the Nexel total elbow prosthesis, the Discovery Elbow System, and the Latitude Elbow prosthesis have a humeral anterior flange (Fig. 11).

Of all the prostheses on this list, only Tornier's Latitude Elbow prosthesis has a radial head component. All of the prostheses described in this overview are for cemented use, except for the Kudo type-5 and the iBP Total Elbow System (that provide both options). They all come in different sizes.

The Latitude Elbow can be used as a both constrained and non-constrained prosthesis, depending on the ability of the surrounding joint structures to provide stability to the joint.

The Souter–Strathclyde total elbow has a characteristic humeral component with a less visible ulnar component on a conventional radiograph.

Conclusion

This overview can be useful in determining which type and brand of prosthesis a patient has when visiting the emergency department or outpatient clinic with a periprosthetic fracture, dislocation, or implant failure.

Acknowledgments We appreciate the following people for providing us with radiographs of the prostheses: D. Hoornenborg, I. Kleinlugtenbelt, A. Bom, B. Ehrenburg, M. van Leeuwen, prof. L. Adolfsson.

Statement of human and animal rights All procedures performed in studies involving human participants were in accordance with the ethical standards of the institutional and/or national research committee and with the 1964 Helsinki declaration and its later amendments or comparable ethical standards. This article does not contain any studies with animals performed by any of the authors. This study did not involve human participants.

Informed consent This study did not include identifying information. For this type of study formal consent is not required.

References

1. Plaschke HC, Thillemann TM, Brorson S, Olsen BS (2014) Implant survival after total elbow arthroplasty: a retrospective study of 324 procedures performed from 1980 to 2008. J Shoulder Elb Surg Am Shoulder Elb Surg [et al]. 23(6):829–836
2. Zimmer's (2000) Coonrad/Murray Total Elbow product brochure. Available from the Zimmer website: http://www.zimmercom/content/dam/zimmer-web/documents/en-US/pdf/medical-profes sionals/elbow/Coonrad-Morrey-Total-Elbow-Brochure-97-8106-301-00-Rev-1-05-2009pdf. [updated in 2009]
3. Zimmer (2003) Nexel Total Elbow product brochure. Available from the Zimmer website: https://258413772373414384.s3.amazo naws.com/pdf/2014/6/NEXEL_brochureSNGL_7-2Final.pdf.pdf
4. Gschwend N, Scheier NH, Baehler AR (1999) Long-term results of the GSB III elbow arthroplasty. J Bone Joint Surg Br Vol 81(6):1005–1012
5. Biomet (2002) Discovery elbow system surgical technique brochure. Available from the Biomet website: http://www.rcsedacuk/fellows/lvanrensburg/classification/surgtech/biomet/manuals/dis covery%20total%20elbowpdf
6. Kudo H, Iwano K, Nishino J (1999) Total elbow arthroplasty with use of a nonconstrained humeral component inserted without cement in patients who have rheumatoid arthritis. J Bone Joint Surg Am Vol 81(9):1268–1280
7. Biomet (2004) iBP Total Elbow System product brochure. Available from the Biomet Company
8. Cast I. NESimplavit Elbow System product information. Available from the Implantcast website: http://www.implantcastde/indexphp?option=com_content&view=article&id=79%3Anesim plavitr-ellenbogen-system&catid=35%3Aendoprothetik-kleiner-gelenke&Itemid=24&lang=en
9. Tornier (2007) Latitude Elbow Surgical technique brochure. Available from the Tornier website: http://www.torniernl/images/upload/bloc_droite/Elleboog_-_Hand_-_Pols/Elleboog/fp_latitude_udlf092_eurpdf
10. Stryker (2004) Solar linked semi-constrained elbow system product brochure. Available from the Stryker company
11. Rozing P (2000) Souter–Strathclyde total elbow arthroplasty. J Bone Joint Surg Br Vol 82(8):1129–1134
12. Samijo SK, Van den Berg ME, Verburg AD, Tonino AJ (2003) Souter–Strathclyde total elbow arthroplasty: medium-term results. Acta Orthop Belg 69(6):501–506
13. Khatri M, Stirrat AN (2005) Souter–Strathclyde total elbow arthroplasty in rheumatoid arthritis: medium-term results. J Bone Joint Surg Br Vol 87(7):950–954

19

Comminuted supracondylar femoral fractures: a biomechanical analysis comparing the stability of medial versus lateral plating in axial loading

Nikolai Briffa[1] · Raju Karthickeyan[1] · Joshua Jacob[1] · Arshad Khaleel[1]

Abstract The aim of this study was to compare the biomechanical properties of medial and lateral plating of a medially comminuted supracondylar femoral fracture. A supracondylar femoral fracture model comparing two fixation methods was tested cyclically in axial loading. One-centimetre supracondylar gap osteotomies were created in six synthetic femurs approximately 6 cm proximal to the knee joint. There were two constructs investigated: group 1 and group 2 were stabilized with an 8-hole LC-DCP, medially and laterally, respectively. Both construct groups were axially loaded. Global displacement (total length), wedge displacement, bending moment and strain were measured. Medial plating showed a significantly decreased displacement, bending moment and strain at the fracture site in axial loading. Medial plating of a comminuted supracondylar femur fracture is more stable than lateral plating.

Keywords Supracondylar femur fracture · Medial versus lateral plating · Axial loading testing · Construct stability

Introduction

Whilst distal supracondylar femoral fractures have been treated with skeletal traction historically and this has healed well, there were some morbidity and mortality [1]. Operative fixation is the gold standard currently. Several stabilization modalities are used: a single lateral buttress plate; a fixed-angled plate; an antegrade or retrograde intramedullary nail; a combination of medial and lateral plates; fine-wire circular external fixators, hybrid fixation; or even a primary total knee arthroplasty [2–8]. The ideal fixation, in the presence of comminution, is unconfirmed.

A biomechanical study was designed utilizing a comminuted supracondylar femoral fracture sawbone model. Two single plating fixation methods were tested cyclically in axial loading.

Our null hypothesis was that no mechanical difference exists between lateral plating and medial plating in this simulated supracondylar femur fracture with medial comminution.

Materials and methods

Eight identical synthetic sawbone femurs (Synbone®) were utilized. These standard sawbones are made of polyurethane foam with a hollow canal. The femur is made of different densities of polyurethane at the epiphysis and diaphysis in order to simulate the native modulus of elasticity.

A standardized fracture pattern simulating a supracondylar femoral fracture with medial comminution was created. This was achieved by creating a 1-cm supracondylar gap osteotomy in the eight synthetic femurs 4 cm proximal and parallel to the epicondylar axis as depicted in Fig. 1. This was to simulate medial metaphyseal comminution where contact between bone fragments is minimal.

There were two groups. Group 1 ($n = 4$) had medial plate fixation and Group 2 ($n = 4$) had lateral plating, both with a contoured AO (Synthes) LC-DCP plate. One specimen from each group had five strain gauges placed on the fixing plate so that the strains in the plate could be recorded as a function of increasing load (Fig. 1c). Compressive loading was applied

✉ Nikolai Briffa
nukol@hotmail.com

[1] Trauma and Orthopaedic Department, Ashford and St. Peter's Hospital NHS Trust, London, UK

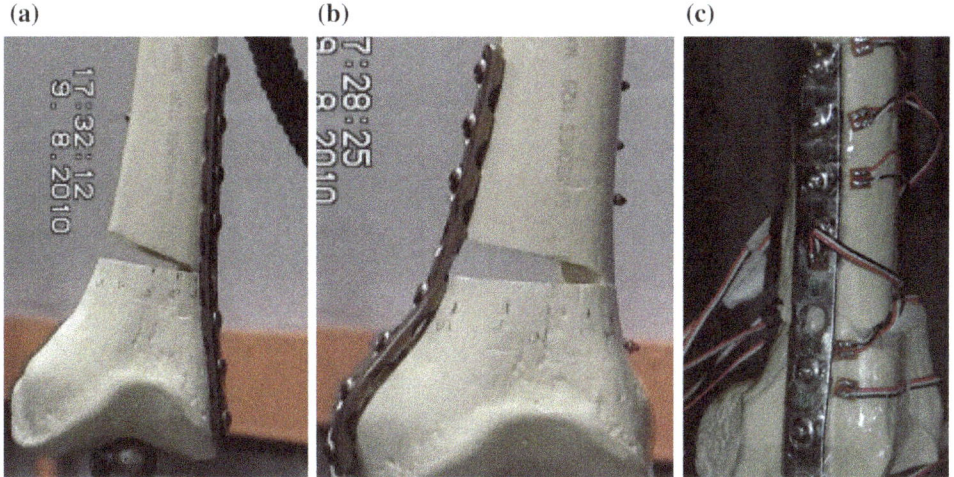

Fig. 1 a Femur with distal lateral fixation. **b** Femur with distal medial fixation. **c** Position of strain gauges 1–5

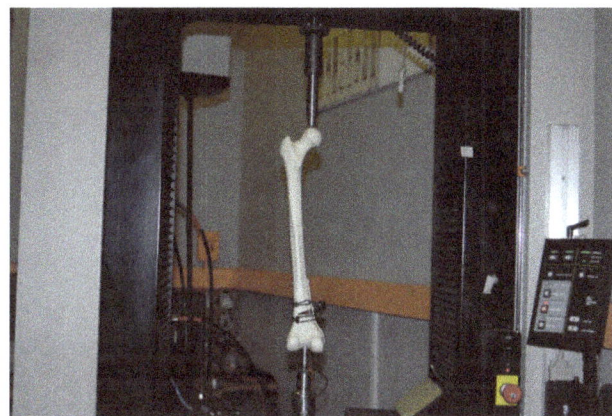

Fig. 2 Femur specimen loaded in the Instron test machine simulating in vivo loading with the extensometer straddling the open face of the wedge gap

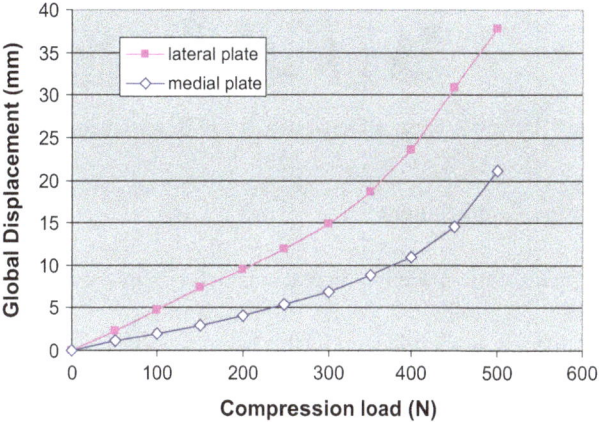

Fig. 3 Lateral and medial plated global femur displacements as a function of load

along the mechanical axis by an Instron® 5500R (Model 1185) test machine (Fig. 2). This simulated the normal in vivo loading. Each of the eight specimens experienced three cycles of loading up to 500 N followed by unloading. Global displacement (total length), wedge displacement, bending moment and plate strain were recorded.

Results

Global displacements

Typical plots of crosshead displacement as a function of load for a lateral plated and a medial plated femur are shown in Fig. 3. The medially plated femur is a much stiffer construct and deforms less than the laterally plated femur as shown in Fig. 4.

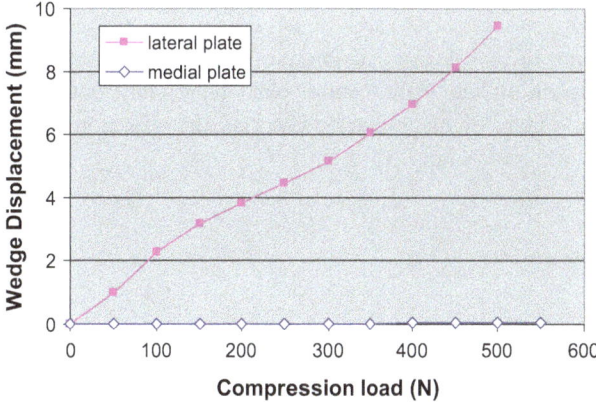

Fig. 4 Lateral and medial plated wedge displacements as a function of load

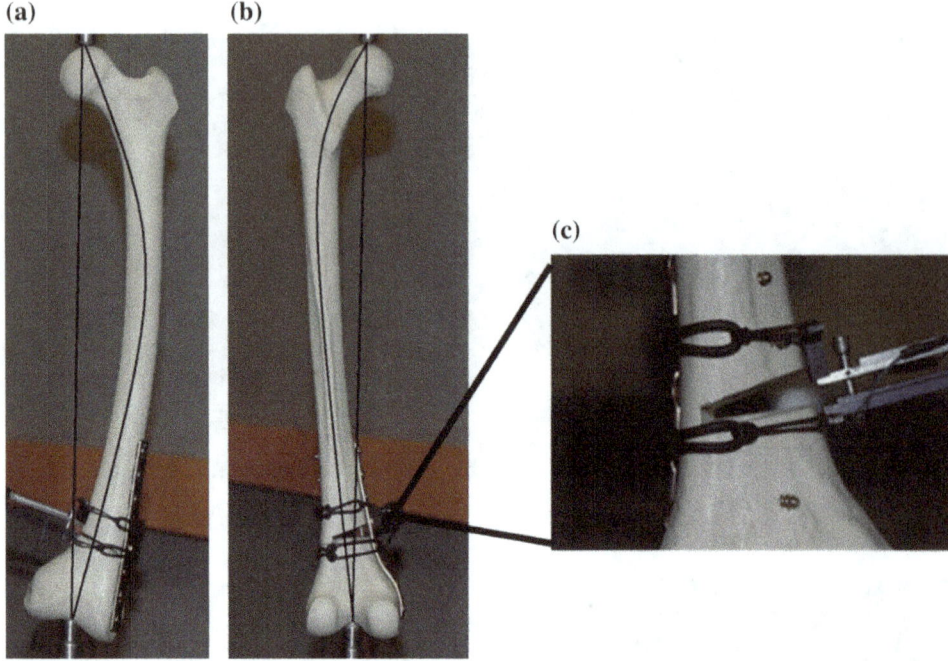

Fig. 5 Deformed femur **a** lateral plate at 250 N, **b** medial plate at 500 N, **c** extensometer

Wedge displacement

Typical plots of wedge displacement for both medial and lateral plates (Fig. 4) depict insignificant displacement on the medial side compared to the lateral construct.

Plate strains

Strains were measured at five different locations for both lateral and medial plated models (Fig. 1c) during both loading and unloading. Plate strains varied considerably between medial and lateral plating. The loading curve follows the line of steepest gradient for all gauges. It can be seen that there is no variation between cycles. Gauge 2 was found to have failed and so data from it were not utilized. The strains along the medial plate–bone construct are of two orders of magnitude lower than the strains recorded with lateral plating (Figs. 5, 6, 7).

Discussion

Open reduction and internal fixation is the treatment of choice for comminuted supracondylar fractures of the distal femur. Conventional plating, cable wiring, external fixators and, recently, low-profile contoured dynamic compression locking plating systems have been utilized [9–11]. New dedicated fixation systems merge conventional and locking screw technology, allowing the surgeon

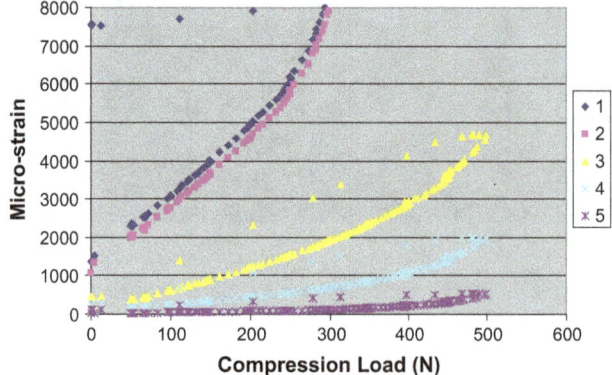

Fig. 6 Strains recorded with lateral plating with legends 1–5 depict the various gauges along the femur. Unloading data of gauge 2 are not available due to malfunction

to achieve angular stability and compression in tension with a small footprint (minimally invasive plate osteosynthesis technique). Despite this, the non-union rate is considerable. It was proposed that this was due to a fall in strain occurring within the zone of injury as bone healing progressed [9]. To overcome this, the dynamic locking screws pin–sleeve design that combines locking technology with dynamic motion was introduced. The play between the sleeve and pin determines the amount of micro-motion induced in the fracture gap, decreasing the construct stiffness; this was thought a beneficial feature when bridging is the chosen method of fracture treatment [10]. Modern fracture stabilization aims for mechanical stability whilst

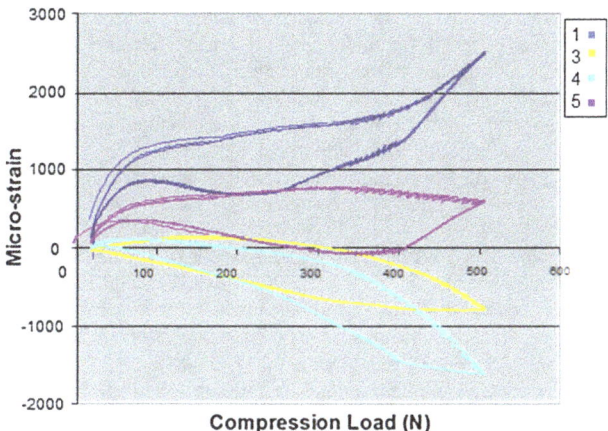

Fig. 7 Strains recorded with medial plating with legends 1, 3, 4, 5 depict the various gauges along the femur. Data from gauge 2 are discarded due to malfunction on unloading

protecting the biological environment of damaged bone and surrounding tissues, thereby optimizing the healing environment [12–15]. In supracondylar fractures of the femur which approach is best, direct lateral or medial?

This biomechanical study demonstrates that a plate placed medially is a more stable construct for this specific fracture simulation, namely medial comminution with the lateral cortex in contact to share load. These are conclusions drawn from an in vitro study, which emulates a clinical scenario. Anatomical reduction without undue biological disruption in metaphyseal comminuted fractures is rarely possible, leaving mechanical stability to be paramount. This has been shown to influence bony union positively [15]. Lateral plating alone supports the medial column indirectly and allows for a greater stress concentration on that side. Failure of fixation, through plate breakage, screw pull out and varus collapse, is a potential complication [16] and are more likely with lateral than medial plates. The biomechanical reasons are several. Firstly, there are reduced bending moments when using medial plates on the femur as the mechanical axis, which by definition runs from hip centre of rotation to ankle and falls slightly medial at the knee. This bending moment (load × moment arm) gives rise to the deformation; the moment arm of the load is the distance from the line of action of the load (mechanical axis) to the neutral axis of the bone and plate. The plate in turn draws the neutral axis from the centre of the femur towards the plate. Lateral plating increases the moment arm and hence increases the moment and deformation force. Conversely, with the medial plate the moment arm is smaller, and thus, deformation and plate strains would be lower. The total construct strain as recorded is much lower on the medial-sided plate, and there is no yielding. Thus, the lateral plate is more likely to undergo plastic deformation, resulting in

earlier failure of the bone–plate construct. The different strain patterns recorded along different points on the plates also differed; higher strains, and thus less stability, were recorded across the wedge in the lateral plate construct.

Secondly, there is lower wedge gap displacement in a medially plated femur when loaded. Medial plating supports the deficient medial column directly and reduces the stress environment. The medial plate becomes a load-bearing cantilever implant. In vivo, it has been shown that stable fixation in the presence of medial comminution was not achievable with lateral plates as varus collapse occurred [17]. Hence, double fixation, using medial and lateral plates, was suggested. This has been linked to an increased morbidity from knee contractures and delayed union, consequent to damage to the local biology from two exposures.

Lastly, medial and lateral plates produce different mechanical environments. A lateral plate has viscoelastic properties, going from elastic to plastic behaviour as the plate spans the wedge. The medial plate, conversely, acts like a buttress on axial loading, resulting in a stiffer stronger construct. Both effects annul each other.

There are limitations in our study. A laboratory-based study makes various assumptions and inferences. Forces on the plate and fracture site are a simplification of the in vivo loads, which are a combination of axial loading, torsion and muscle pull reaction forces. Our experimental construct tested axial load only, which we believe represents the major deforming force across this fracture pattern. The medial plate is more demanding technically due to practicalities of operating on the inner side of the thigh and the close proximity of vital anatomical structures, but medial femoral sub-muscular plating is an operative technique that can be performed safely with a judicious understanding of the relevant anatomy. Lastly, synthetic sawbones were utilized in the study. Although the properties of sawbones are not identical to human bone, they have a high degree of uniformity; as such, the changes noted during testing represent true differences in the mechanical properties of the implant placement rather than differences in bone quality [18].

Conclusion

The aim of this investigation was to determine the optimal side for plating, a comminuted supracondylar fracture of the femur. An investigation into stiffness, wedge displacement and plate strains between the lateral- and medial-sided plating was performed. The data indicate that medial-side plating is stronger and stiffer mechanically than lateral plating in this simulation.

Statement of human and animal rights This Research does not involve human participants and/or animals.

Informed consent It is not applicable.

References

1. Vallier HA, Immler W (2012) Comparison of the 95-degree angled blade plate and the locking condylar plate for the treatment of distal femoral fractures. J Orthop Trauma 26(6):327–332
2. Jazrawi LM, Kummer FJ, Simon JA, Bai B, Hunt SA, Egol KA, Koval KJ (2000) New technique for treatment of unstable distal femur fractures by locked double-plating: case report and biomechanical evaluation. J Trauma 48(1):87–92
3. Kummer FJ, Olsson O, Pearlman CA, Ceder L, Larsson S, Koval KJ (1998) Intramedullary versus extramedullary fixation of subtrochanteric fractures. A biomechanical study. Acta Orthop Scand 69(6):580–584
4. Koval KJ, Hoehl JJ, Kummer FJ, Simon JA (1997) Distal femoral fixation: a biomechanical comparison of the standard condylar buttress plate, a locked buttress plate, and the 95-degree blade plate. J Orthop Trauma 11(7):521–524
5. Koval KJ, Kummer FJ, Bharam S, Chen D, Halder S (1996) Distal femoral fixation: laboratory comparison of the 95 degrees plate, antegrade and retrograde inserted reamed intramedullary nails. J Orthop Trauma 10(6):378–382
6. Wähnert D, Hoffmeier KL, von Oldenburg G, Fröber R, Hofmann GO, Mückley T (2010) Internal fixation of type-C distal femoral fractures in osteoporotic bone. J Bone Joint Surg Am 92(6):1442–1452
7. Heiney JP, Barnett MD, Vrabec GA, Schoenfeld AJ, Baji A, Njus GO (2009) Distal femoral fixation: a biomechanical comparison of trigen retrograde intramedullary (i.m.) nail, dynamic condylar screw (DCS), and locking compression plate (LCP) condylar plate. J Trauma 66(2):443–449
8. Higgins TF, Pittman G, Hines J, Bachus KN (2007) Biomechanical analysis of distal femur fracture fixation: fixed-angle screw-plate construct versus condylar blade plate. J Orthop Trauma 21(1):43–46
9. Perren SM, Klaue K, Pohler O, Predieri M, Steinemann S, Gautier E (1990) The limited contact dynamic compression plate (LC-DCP). Arch Orthop Trauma Surg 109(6):304–310
10. DLS dynamic locking screw: boosting biological bone healing. http://www.synthes.com/sites/intl/Products/featured-products-solutions/Pages/DLS-Dynamic-Locking-Screw.aspx
11. Allgöwer M, Perren S, Matter P (1970) A new plate for internal fixation—the dynamic compression plate (DCP). Injury 2(1):40–47
12. Zlowodzki M, Williamson S, Zardiackas LD, Kregor PJ (2006) Biomechanical evaluation of the less invasive stabilization system and the 95-degree angled blade plate for the internal fixation of distal femur Fractures in human cadaveric bones with high bone mineral density. J Trauma 60(4):836–840
13. Zlowodzki M, Williamson S, Cole PA, Zardiackas LD, Kregor PJ (2004) Biomechanical evaluation of the less invasive stabilization system, angled blade plate, and retrograde intramedullary nail for the internal fixation of distal femur fractures. J Orthop Trauma 18(8):494–502
14. Oh JK, Sahu D, Ahn YH, Lee SJ, Tsutsumi S, Hwang JH, Jung DY, Perren SM, Oh CW (2010) Effect of fracture gap on stability of compression plate fixation: a finite element study. J Orthop Res 28(4):462–467
15. Perren SM (2002) Evolution of the internal fixation of long bone fractures. The scientific basis of biological internal fixation: choosing a new balance between stability and biology. J Bone Joint Surg Br 84(8):1093–1110 **(Review)**
16. Prayson MJ, Datta DK, Marshall MP (2001) Mechanical comparison of endosteal substitution and lateral plate fixation in supracondylar fractures of the femur. J Orthop Trauma 15(2):96–100
17. Sanders R, Swiontkowski M, Rosen H, Helfet D (1991) Double-plating of comminuted, unstable fractures of the distal part of the femur. J Bone Joint Surg Am 73(3):341–346
18. Cristofolini L, Viceconti M, Cappello A, Toni A (1996) Mechanical validation of whole bone composite femur models. J Biomech 29(4):525–535 **(Review)**

20

Stability at the half pin–frame interface on external fixation constructs

Alexios Dimitrios Iliadis[1] · Parag Kumar Jaiswal[1] · Jay Meswania[2] ·
Gordon Blunn[2] · David Goodier[1] · Peter Calder[1]

Abstract A mechanical study investigating the use of two different methods (grub and bolt screws) to secure external fixation half pins to circular frames. A four part experiment: (1) Grub and bolt screws were used to secure half pins in Taylor Spatial frames. Loosening torques were measured using a calibrated torque wrench. (2) Using universal testing machine (UTM), axial loading was applied to establish thresholds for loosening in grub and bolt screw constructs. (3) We established the application torque to produce failure at the head–driver interface using these two methods. (4) Grub and bolt screw constructs were created controlling torque. Using UTM, axial loading was applied to establish thresholds for loosening. Statistical analysis was conducted using SPSS v20.0.0. (1) Higher torque is employed when bolt rather than grub screws is used to secure half pins on Rancho cubes ($p < 0.05$). (2) Loading threshold for loosening is higher in bolt screw constructs when the torque applied to secure the constructs is not controlled ($p < 0.05$). (3) Torque required for failure at the head–driver interface was 5.3 Nm for grub screws and 9.9 Nm for bolts. (4) Loading threshold for loosening is higher in grub screw constructs when the same torque was applied to secure them ($p < 0.05$). Bolt screws can be employed to secure the half pin–frame interface. They offer good stability and reduce failure at the head–driver

interface. Further research is needed to determine the mechanical properties of such constructs in vivo.

Keywords Half pin–frame interface · External fixation constructs · Grub screws · Bolt screws · Stability

Introduction

The Ilizarov method has proved successful in the treatment of a wide spectrum of orthopaedic disorders [1]. The success of this method is to be attributed to the combination of the biomechanics of the external fixation apparatus and the biological principles of distraction osteogenesis [1]. The stability of the external fixation apparatus is critical in preventing excessive movement which could increase morbidity and compromise bone healing [2, 3].

Half pins were introduced to address some of the disadvantages of the conventional apparatus which consisted of fine wires only. There are contested benefits in reducing soft tissue transfixation so allowing for less morbidity and increased mobility [4]. Furthermore, there is simplicity with regard to insertion in anatomically challenging areas, a reduction in fixation time and lower risk of complications [5].

High stresses at the pin–bone interface contribute to micro-motion and failure resulting in unicortical loosening. Experimental models have demonstrated far higher pressures are generated under loading conditions at the bone interface from half pins as compared to fine wires [5]. The pin–bone interface has therefore been regarded as the weakest link in the mechanical stability of external fixation systems and has been investigated extensively [6–8]. In contrast, no studies have looked at the interface between the half pin and frame assembly. Loss of stability here

✉ Alexios Dimitrios Iliadis
alexiliadis@mail.com

[1] Limb Reconstruction Unit, Royal National Orthopaedic Hospital NHS, Brockley Hill, Stanmore, Middlesex HA7 4LP, UK

[2] University College London - Institute of Orthopaedics and Musculoskeletal Science, Royal National Orthopaedic Hospital (RNOH), Brockley Hill, Stanmore HA7 4LP, UK

compromises the bone remodelling process through a change in the biomechanics of the construct. In the systems of Ilizarov and Taylor Spatial frames (TSF) external fixation by Smith and Nephew, grub screws are used to secure half pins on Rancho cubes. The aim of this study is to investigate 2 different methods used (grub screw or 10 mm stainless steel hexagonal headed bolt [M6 A2-70]) to secure external fixation half pins to circular frames. This is to determine whether use of bolts is appropriate and could reduce the potential for loosening at this interface.

Materials and methods

All participating clinicians were members of the Limb Reconstruction Unit at the Royal National Orthopaedic Hospital with experience in the assembly and application of external fixation systems. Two of the authors participated. The remaining participants were blinded as to the purposes of the study.

In an attempt for mounting conditions to resemble those in the operating room, hybrid external fixation frames (Taylor Spatial frames (TSF)—Smith and Nephew, Memphis, TN) were constructed and mounted on saw bones (Fig. 1a), and appropriate instruments available from the TSF set were utilized exclusively. They consisted of two 180-mm rings connected by fast struts and secured with two tensioned wires and one half pin per ring. A universal testing machine at the University College London Institute of Orthopaedics and Musculoskeletal Science was used, under the supervision of an experienced technician, to apply axial loading on the constructs.

The experiment was conducted in four parts:

Part 1

We sought to determine whether there was a difference in the torque applied for securing half pins to Rancho cubes when employing these two methods; the mounting conditions were similar to those encountered in clinical practice. Five participants were asked to secure half pins on Rancho cubes using 5 grub (set) screws and 5 standard 10-mm bolts (Fig. 1b) in an alternating fashion to account for fatigue. They were instructed to apply as much torque as they

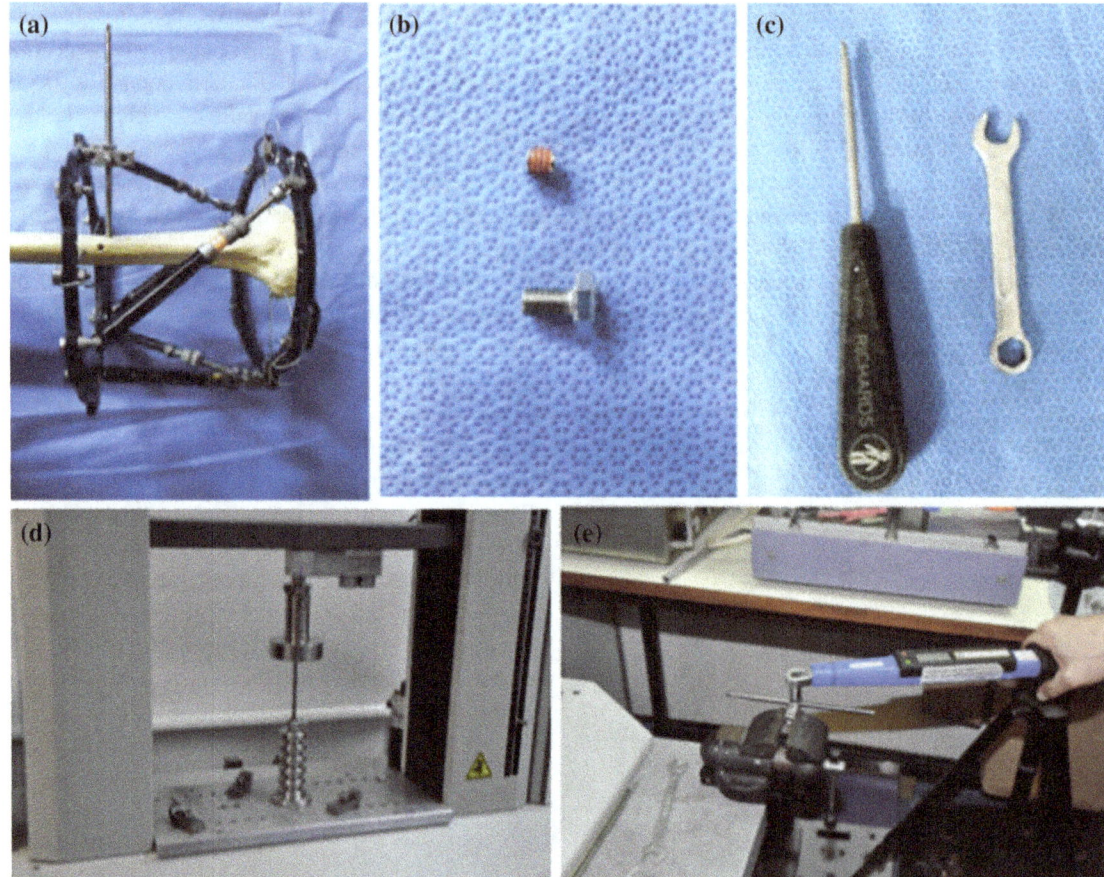

Fig. 1 Form *top left clockwise*: **a** TSF mounted on saw bone, **b** set and bolt screws, **c** wrench and straight hex driver, **d** universal testing machine and **e** calibrated torque wrench

would in clinical practice to the point they were satisfied that the half pin has been secured adequately in the Rancho cube. New Rancho cubes and screws were used on each occasion to avoid threads cutting out and altering the results. Wrenches were used to tighten the standard 10-mm bolts and straight hex drivers for the grub screws as would be the case when done intra-operatively (Fig. 1c).

Using a calibrated torque wrench (Torqueleader TWD20 Torque Wrench—MSK/EQ/40 Calibration 03/02/2012), the torque (Nm) required to loosen; the screws was measured for each construct.

Part 2

We sought to examine which of the two methods held the half pin better; this was tested in loading similar to those encountered in clinical practice. Two participants were each asked to secure 5 half pins using grub screws and 5 half pins using standard 10-mm bolts in the same manner as the first part of our experiment. The Rancho cubes were released from the rings, and the whole half pin–Rancho cube construct was removed from the saw bone using T-handles. The constructs were then placed on a universal testing machine—UTM (Fig. 1d), and increasing axial loading was applied to determine loosening points. This was determined as mechanical failure on the load deformation curve and was associated with loosening at the interface between the pin and Rancho cube.

Part 3

We sought to determine the tightening torque that can be applied safely (prior to breakage) at the head–driver interface when using these two methods. Twenty grub screws and twenty bolts were used to secure half pins on Rancho cubes using a calibrated torque wrench to determine the point at which breakage at the driver–head interface occurs (Fig. 1e).

Part 4

We sought to examine, when a controlled torque was applied for securing all half pins, the loosening points of these constructs when subjected to axial loading. From the investigation in part 3, it was established that 5 Nm was a safe amount of torque to be applied on grub screws prior to breakage at the driver–head interface. Ten constructs using grub screws and ten using bolts were secured applying 5 Nm with a calibrated torque wrench. The constructs were then placed on a universal testing machine—UTM (Fig. 1d), and increasing axial loads were applied to determine points of loosening as determined as mechanical failure on the load deformation curve.

The same process was followed for ten bolt constructs secured using 9.5 Nm torque which, in part 3, was found to be a safe amount of torque prior to breakage at the driver–head interface.

Statistics

SPSS 20 was used to perform statistical analysis. Our data distribution was assessed for normality using the Shapiro–Wilk test. The t test was used for parametric data and Mann–Whitney U test for nonparametric data. Statistical significance was determined as p values of <0.05.

Results

Part 1

Figure 2 demonstrates the loosening torque values obtained in the first part of our experiment. The values obtained for bolts were higher (median 6.3 SD 1.1) than grub screws (median 1.84 SD 0.4). The Shapiro–Wilk test confirmed both our data sets are normally distributed. A t test confirmed the statistical significance ($p < 0.05$).

Part 2

Table 1 demonstrates the loads required to produce loosening at the half pin–Rancho cube interface when ten constructs with grub screws and ten constructs with bolts were subjected to increasing axial loading on UTS. The Mann–Whitney test was employed for statistical analysis as determined appropriate by Shapiro–Wilk test of our data distribution. Significantly higher loads were required for loosening to occur on the construct using bolts ($p < 0.05$).

Part 3

The mean torque applied for breakage to occur at the driver–head interface when using grub screws was 5.31 Nm (SD 0.19). In every case, breakage occurred at torque values >5 Nm when using bolts this was 9.92 Nm (SD 0.15). In every case, breakage occurred at torque values >9.5 Nm (Fig. 3).

Part 4

When comparing axial loads to loosening in grub screw constructs secured with a 5-Nm torque and those on the bolt constructs secured without torque control, there was a statistically significant difference in favour of bolt constructs (Mann–Whitney U test, $p < 0.05$). This is shown in Table 2. When comparing the values obtained for grub

Fig. 2 *Box plot* demonstrating loosening torque values (Nm) for bolt and grub screw constructs

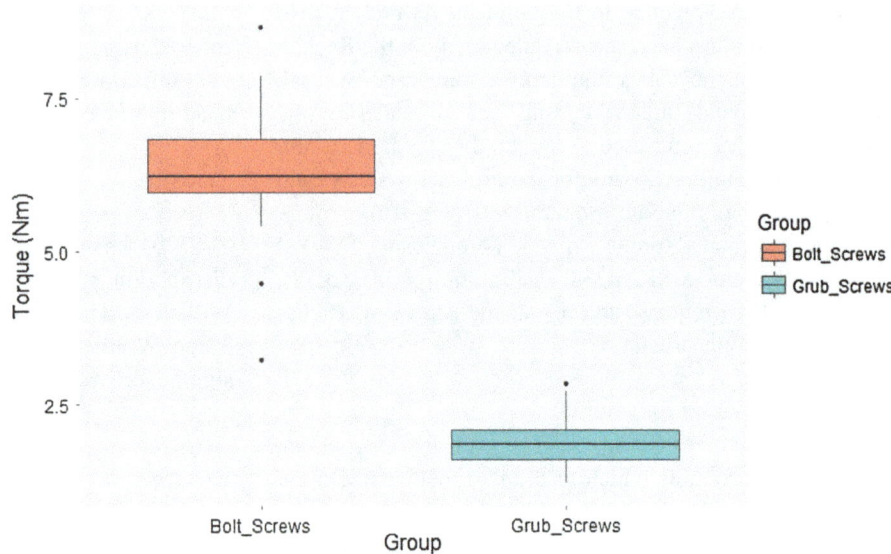

Table 1 Loads required on UTS for loosening at the half pin–Rancho cube interface for grab screw and bolt screw constructs mounted without controlling torque

Group	N	Min (N)	Q25 (N)	Median (N)	Mean (N)	Q75 (N)	Max (N)	SD (N)
BS	10	1799.9	2010	2102.8	2032.7	2103.6	2104.4	122.5
GS	10	949	1084.6	1368.4	1281.6	1393.8	1674.6	226.3

Fig. 3 Axial loads (N) required on UTM for loosening at the half pin–Rancho cube interface for bolt screw (BS) and grub screw (GS) constructs secured with a torque of 5 Nm

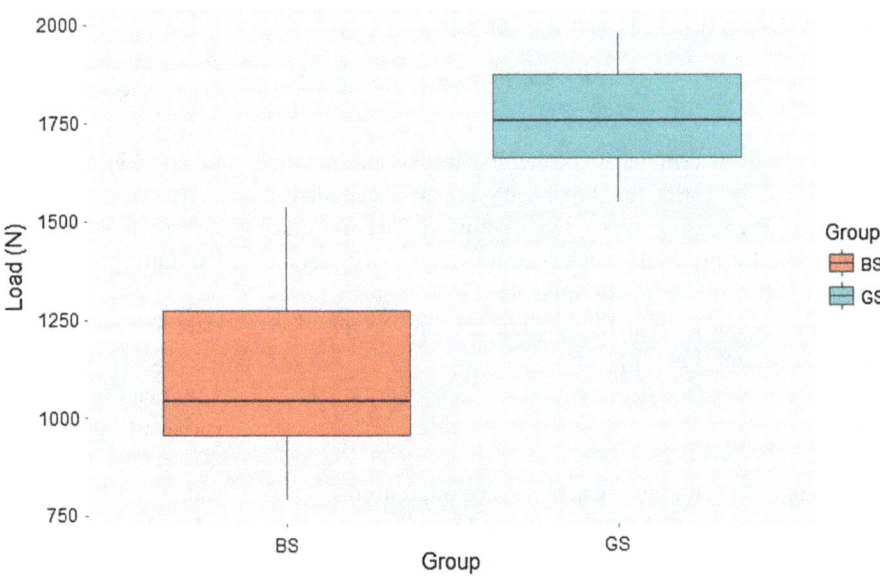

Table 2 Axial loads required for loosening at the half pin–Rancho cube interface for grab screw constructs using 5-Nm torque to secure and bolt screw constructs mounted without controlling torque

Group	N	Min (N)	Q25 (N)	Median (N)	Mean (N)	Q75 (N)	Max (N)	SD (N)
BS	10	1799.9	2010	2102.8	2032.7	2103.6	2104.4	122.5
GS	10	1547.9	1662.9	1757	1766.4	1871.9	1979.9	148.9

screws tightened with a torque of 5 Nm with those obtained for bolts tightened at torque of 9.5 Nm, significantly higher axial loads can be applied before loosening on the bolt constructs (Mann–Whitney test). This is shown in Fig. 4.

Discussion

We have simulated clinical conditions by use of saw bone models; we recruited subjects with experience in mounting frames and instructed them to assemble these constructs in a manner similar to their clinical practice. In the first part of the experiment, loosening torque values were determined. These are not the same as the tightening torque values as different forces are involved (static vs dynamic). Values obtained demonstrate statistically significant higher loosening torque values when bolts are used to secure half pins. This suggests a higher torque is applied when half pins are secured with bolts. We surmise the difference is due to a wrench (spanner) being used in contrast to the straight hex driver for grub screws. The axial compression force (clamp force) applied through either bolt or grub screw would determine the security of hold at the half pin–Rancho cube interface. This clamp force is affected by many other variables too: the bolt diameter. The type and number of threads on the bolt, the bolt material and the torque applied. The last variable is that under control by the surgeon and may influence the likelihood of these constructs to failure.

In the second part of the experiment, we demonstrated that, under such mounting conditions, significantly higher axial loading forces are required for loosening to occur at the half pin–Rancho cube interface when bolts are used instead of grub screws. Failure in our experiments was defined as mechanical failure on the load deformation curve, and this was associated with loosening at the half pin–Rancho cube interface. Based on these results, we can demonstrate that bolts hold the half pins equally or better than grub screws in experimental conditions of loading to failure.

The results obtained in the first two parts of the experiment suggest that higher stability is offered by bolts; this may be from the use of wrenches for securing the half pins with higher torques and clamp forces applied.

Hex wrenches and Allen keys are available in the supplied instrument sets for mounting half pins in Rancho cubes. In our experience, they are associated with a risk of breakage at the head–driver interface, causing difficulties should the fixator assembly need to be dismantled. The third part of the experiment showed that higher torques can be applied safely when using bolts.

In the fourth part, we controlled the torque applied when securing these fixator constructs. The results suggested that, when equal torque is applied, grub screws are superior in providing stability in axial loading. The grub screw point profile may produce a better grip on the half pin than that on the bolt when the same torque is used, but when both types of screws are mounted applying maximum torque, bolts demonstrate a significantly higher threshold for loads

Fig. 4 Axial loads (N) required on UTM for loosening at the half pin–Rancho cube interface for bolt screw (BS) and grub screw (GS) constructs secured with a torque of 9.5 and 5 Nm, respectively

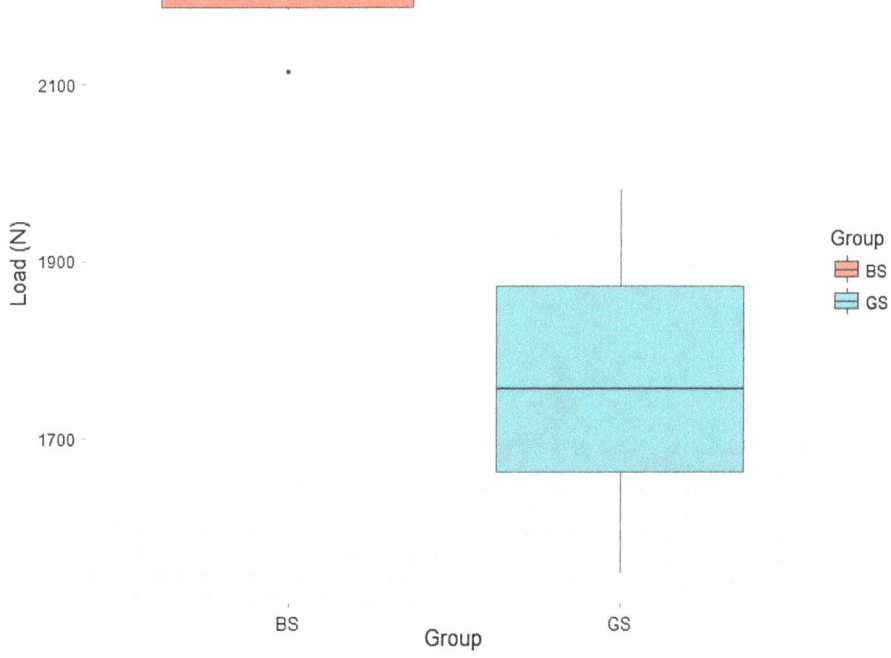

prior to loosening. This reinforces the clinical practice to increase tightening torque in application so that an increase in clamp force is achieved and correspondingly the tolerance to load to failure.

These results demonstrate that bolts achieve good stability at the half pin–Rancho cube interface by tolerating higher axial loads than grub screws before loosening. This is a result from the greater torque that can be produced using a spanner or wrench. Whilst the point profile of the grub screw secures a better hold of the half pin when the torque used is equal, the driver used to insert the grub screw is limited in delivery of a high maximum torque before breakage; this appears to be the limiting factor for the security of hold on the half pin by grub screws.

We conclude that bolts can be employed safely to secure half pins in Rancho cubes and, if tightened maximally, provide as good or better security of hold on the pin to grub screws.

Statement of human and animal rights This article does not contain any studies with human participants or animals performed by any of the authors.

Informed consent For this type of study formal consent is not required.

References

1. Marsh DR, Shah S, Elliot J, Kurdy N (1997) The Ilizarov method in nonunion, malunion and infection of fractures. J Bone Joint Surg Br 79(2):273–279
2. Noordeen MHH, Lavy CBD, Shergill NS, Tuite JD, Jackson AM (1995) Cyclical micromovement and fracture healing. J Bone Joint Surg Br 77(4):645–648
3. Bronson DG, Samchukov ML, Birch JG, Browne RH, Ashman RB (1998) Stability of external circular fixation: a multivariable biomechanical analysis. Clin Biomech 13:441–448
4. Board TN, Yang L, Saleh M (2007) Why fine wire fixators work: an analysis of pressure distribution at the wire-bone interface. J Biomech 40(1):20–25
5. Green SA, Harris NL, Wall DM, Ishkanian J, Marinow H (1992) The Rancho mounting technique for the Ilizarov method. A preliminary report. Clin Orthop Relat Res 280:104–116
6. Calhun JH, Li F, Bauford WL, Lehman T, Ledbetter BR, Lowery R (1992) Rigidity of half pins for the Ilizarov external fixator. Bull Hosp Jt Dis 52(1):21–26
7. Aro HT, Markel MD, Chao EY (1993) Cortical bone reactions at the interface of external fixation half pins under different loading conditions. J Trauma 35(5):776–785
8. Green SA (1991) The Ilizarov method: Rancho technique. Orthop Clin North Am 22(4):677–688

21

The callus fracture sign: a radiological predictor of progression to hypertrophic non-union in diaphyseal tibial fractures

S. Salih[1] · C. Blakey[1] · D. Chan[1] · J. C. McGregor-Riley[1] · S. L. Royston[1] ·
S. Gowlett[2] · D. Moore[2] · M. G. Dennison[1]

Abstract We report a radiological sign which predicts progression to hypertrophic non-union for fractures of the tibial diaphysis. Radiographs of 46 tibial fractures were reviewed independently by four orthopaedic trauma surgeons and two musculoskeletal radiologists. Patients were identified from a database of tibial fractures managed with Ilizarov frame fixation. There were 23 fractures that progressed to non-union requiring further surgery. The controls were 23 fractures that had united without need for further surgery at 1-year follow-up. Radiographs selected were the first images taken following frame removal. All radiographs were anonymised and randomized prior to review. Presence of the callus fracture sign was identified in 16 radiographs of the fractures that progressed to non-union, and 7 of the united fracture group. Sensitivity is 69.6 %. Specificity is 91.4 %. Positive and negative predictive values are 88.9 and 75.0 %, respectively. These results compare favourably with computerised tomography for predicting non-union. Intra- and inter-observer reliability was good ($\kappa = 0.68$), and moderate ($\kappa = 0.57$), respectively. The callus fracture sign is a useful radiological predictor of progression to non-union and may represent insufficient mechanical stability at the fracture site.

Keywords Ilizarov technique · Tibial fracture · Fracture healing · Radiography · X-ray · Hypertrophic non-union

Introduction

Fracture union is dependent on the biological environment and the mechanical properties of the fracture site [1]. Hypertrophic non-union can occur in the presence of an appropriate biological response but inadequate mechanical stability. In the context of the Ilizarov method, fractures heal by secondary or indirect bone healing, i.e. in the presence of relative stability provided by the circular fine-wire fixator, the fracture heals by periosteal bony callus (intramembranous ossification) at the periphery of the fracture and fibrocartilaginous bridging callus (endochondral ossification) between bone ends [1, 2]. Here the term 'bridging callus' is used to describe the appearance of calcified tissue between the ends of a fracture. Several authors define union as the radiological presence of bridging callus at 3 out of 4 cortices on AP and lateral views [3, 4]. The classic elephant's foot appearance of a hypertrophic non-union (Fig. 1) results from instability preventing ossification with further cartilaginous material continued to be laid down [1].

The incidence of aseptic non-union for fractures of the tibial shaft is 1.5 % in this unit. The senior author has identified a radiological sign in a series of fractures thought to have united but which progressed to established non-union after removal of fixation. In these cases, bridging callus, as defined above, was seen to join the bone ends across the fracture site in more than one view but, on closer examination, the fracture cleavage can be seen to extend beyond the original cortical boundary of the bone but not to the boundary of the bridging callus (Fig. 2). This detail in

✉ S. Salih
saifsalih@hotmail.com

M. G. Dennison
Mick.Dennison@sth.nhs.uk

[1] Department of Trauma and Orthopaedics, Northern General Hospital, Herres Rd, Sheffield S5 7AU, UK

[2] Department of Radiology, Northern General Hospital, Sheffield, UK

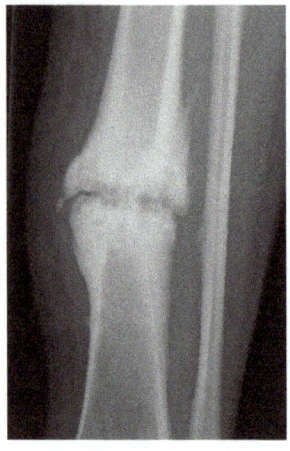
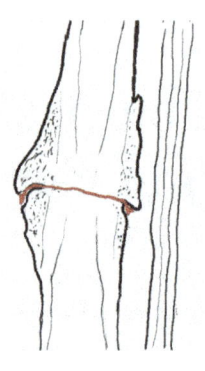

Fig. 1 A hypertrophic non-union in a diaphyseal tibial fracture. The line drawing depicts the extension of the fracture line to the periphery of the callus

Callus fracture sign

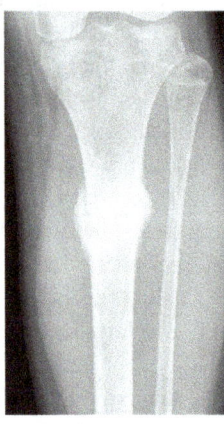

The callus fracture sign is the extension of the fracture line beyond the cortex into the callus but NOT to the edge of the callus. As shown below:

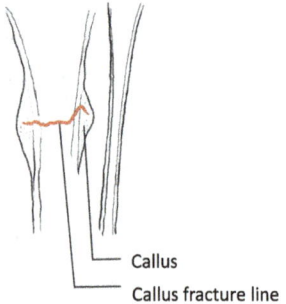

Callus
Callus fracture line

Fig. 2 An example of the callus fracture sign. The line drawing highlights the extension of the fracture line beyond the original cortical boundary but not to the periphery of the fracture callus

interpretation of the characteristics of bridging callus has not been identified previously. We have labelled this the 'callus fracture sign' and recognise it to be predictive for progression to non-union. The study aims to establish the validity of this radiological sign and its reliability for clinical use.

Materials and methods

This study was registered with the local audit and research department as a service evaluation, and ethical approval was not required. The study was performed by retrospectively reviewing patients on the Ilizarov database. This database is data prospectively collected from all patients treated by the Ilizarov method.

Between October 2000 and January 2011, a total of 1533 fractures of the tibia treated by the Ilizarov technique were recorded in the database. Fractures of the tibia treated by the Ilizarov technique but went on to an established hypertrophic non-union needing revision frame fixation were included. We excluded patients with confirmed or suspected infection, internal fixation metalwork remaining in situ, atrophic non-unions, and patients with an incomplete set of medical notes or radiographic images. A total of 23 suitable cases were identified; all were closed injuries. A same number of age- and sex-matched patients were identified as controls; these patients had successful union after the same treatment with an Ilizarov frame and had a minimum of 12 months in follow-up. This provided 46 pairs of radiographs.

Radiographs studied were the first images obtained after removal of the Ilizarov all-wire circular fixator. The vast majority of the Ilizarov fixators are removed in an outpatient clinic with the post-removal AP and lateral radiographs taken immediately after. Both AP and lateral views were reviewed in all cases with the 46 pairs of images anonymised and randomised prior to being assessed by six assessors. Three were trauma consultants, two were specialist musculoskeletal radiology consultants, and one was a trauma and limb reconstruction fellow. An example of the 'Callus Fracture' sign (Fig. 2) was given with clear written instructions to the assessors for identifying it. An example of an established hypertrophic non-union (Fig. 1) was also provided, and the assessors were permitted to acknowledge whether they felt this was present but it did not count as the 'Callus Fracture' sign being present. We have used the term callus fracture sign to describe the extension of the fracture cleavage beyond the limits of the cortex but within the boundary of the callus.

Reviewers were asked to identify the presence or absence of a 'callus fracture sign' in either view. The instructions given to the reviewers are shown in Fig. 3. Four or more reviewers had to agree on the presence of the sign in order for it to be considered a positive finding. The senior author was asked to review the radiographs on two separate occasions, after a 6-month interval, to allow for analysis of intra-observer reliability.

Statistics

A contingency table summarising the results was constructed. Pearson's Chi-square values were calculated using SPSS v17.0 (IBM). True positives (TP) were defined as those with the callus fracture sign who developed a non-union. True negatives (TN) were defined as those without the callus fracture sign who united successfully. False negatives (FN) were those who did not have the callus

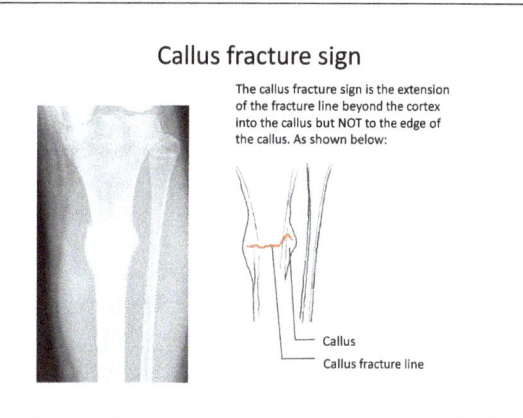

Instructions

- Please look at the following radiographs and decide whether the 'callus fracture sign' is present or not.
- An example of the sign is on the next slide.

Callus fracture sign

The callus fracture sign is the extension of the fracture line beyond the cortex into the callus but NOT to the edge of the callus. As shown below:

Callus

Callus fracture line

Not this.

Here the fracture line extends to the edge of the fracture callus.

If you feel the radiograph shows this then the callus fracture sign is not present. If you feel that it is a non-union that does not display the fracture callus sign then record this on the form.

Radiographs

- All the radiographs are in one folder with file names as numbers xxxxxxx_yy (1/2)
- yy corresponds to the number on the response sheet. The first bank of numbers can be ignored.
- For each radiograph mark whether you feel the sign is present or not.
- If you wish you can predict whether the fracture progressed to union or not too but this is not essential.

THANK YOU!

Fig. 3 Instructions were provided to the authors as a powerpoint presentation. The slides are shown

fracture sign and developed a non-union. False positives (FP) were those who had the sign and united. From this sensitivity (SN), specificity (SP), positive predictive value (PPV), negative predictive value (NPV) and accuracy (AC) were calculated using the following formulas:

$$SN = TP/(TP + FN), \quad SP = TN/(TN + FP),$$
$$PPV = TP/(TP + FP), \quad NPV = TN/(TN + FN)$$
$$AC = (TP + TN)/(TP + FP + TN + FN)$$

The κ statistic was calculated using Fleiss' modification for multiple observers using SPSS v17.0 (IBM, USA) [5] A κ value of <0.2 was considered poor, 0.21–0.40 fair, 0.41–0.60 moderate, 0.61–0.80 good, 0.81–1.00 very good [6]. Categorical data were analysed using the Chi-square test. A p value of <0.05 was considered statistically significant.

Results

Table 1 shows the results of the senior author alone. Table 2 shows the results when four or more of the assessors considered the callus fracture sign to be present.

Table 1 Contingency tables summarising results for the senior author

	Senior author review	
	Union	Non-union
Callus fracture sign present	4	14
Callus fracture sign absent	19	9
χ^2	9.127	
p value	0.006	

Table 2 Contingency table summarising results when four or more of the reviewers independently assessed the callus fracture sign to be present

	Agreement of four or more reviewers	
	Union	Non-union
Callus fracture sign present	2	21
Callus fracture sign absent	16	7
χ^2	17.889	
p value	<0.001	

Presence of the callus fracture sign was agreed in 16 radiographs of the fractures that had progressed to non-union, and 2 of the united fracture group. Using the combined results, sensitivity is 69.6 %, specificity is 91.3 %, positive and negative predictive values are 88.9 and 75.0 %, respectively. Accuracy is 80.6 %. Overall, intra-observer reliability was good ($k = 0.68$) and inter-observer reliability was at the high end of the moderate range ($k = 0.58$).

Discussion

Perren's strain theory of fracture healing suggests that the degree of inter-fragmentary strain dictates the type of tissue formed between the fracture ends [1]. It has been demonstrated that the tissue within a non-union site contains mesenchymal progenitor cells that are capable of transforming into cartilage and bone forming cells [7]. When a non-union is deemed to be hypertrophic, increasing stability, for example by fracture distraction, can lead to bony union [8]. Treatment is aimed at increasing mechanical stability and thereby initialising mineralisation of fibrocartilage.

The point at which a tibial fracture is united is a key step in management but is of particular importance in those treated with an Ilizarov frame as it determines when the fixator can be removed. In our unit, like others, this is done when a collection of clinical features are present: bridging callus on the radiographs; the patient is weight-bearing

painlessly; and there is no clinically detectable movement at the fracture site. Once deemed a fracture has united, the frame is dynamised then disconnected. If there is no movement between the rings on manual stressing, it is likely no movement has occurred at the fracture site and the frame then removed. These criteria are similar to those described by Sarmiento [9].

These results demonstrate a significant relationship between the callus fracture sign and a requirement for revision surgery. If the callus shows a defect, there may be the tendency for this to break down rather than consolidate if greater stability is not provided. The callus fracture sign is thought to represent a prognostic sign where the visible fracture line on the radiograph evolves into a cleavage plane which would eventually form a hypertrophic non-union when the plane reaches the outer surface of the callus.

Determining fracture union is not straightforward. The original work done on rabbit tibias demonstrated that callus strength peaks when three cortices are bridged by callus [4]. However, in humans radiological union and mechanical strength do not correlate well [10, 11]. As a result, attempts have been made to devise scoring criteria to determine fracture union. Although these scoring criteria have good inter- and intra-observer reliability [12], they correlate poorly with union [10] or have not been validated [13]. Furthermore, these have been designed to assess union in a tibia treated with intramedullary nailing; this is a scenario where the implant is not normally removed after union unlike a circular frame. If these scoring systems are applied to fractures treated with Ilizarov circular frames, there is a risk the fixation may be removed before fracture union is complete then prompting the need for revision surgery. It is unlikely that the callus fracture sign can be applied to fractures treated by internal fixation as, unlike in Ilizarov treatment, it is difficult to subsequently alter the construct to affect the overall rigidity.

CT has been used to diagnose non-union in such cases. The callus fracture sign is similar to CT with respect to sensitivity, specificity and accuracy [14]. Furthermore, one-seventh of the patients in this study underwent unnecessary surgery because of a false-positive CT result. The callus fracture sign has a lower negative predictive value. This may be explained by those with a NPP included cases that had a line across the fracture but not beyond the cortex, and a small number of non-union cases which the assessors felt displayed signs of an established non-union but not the callus fracture sign. If these cases were removed from the analysis, the false-negative rate would be lower and sensitivity, negative predictive value and accuracy would all be improved.

We suggest that those patients demonstrating the callus fracture sign, i.e. the cleavage plane of the fracture extending beyond the original cortical boundary of the bone but remaining within the boundary of the callus as in Fig. 2, should undergo a period of increased fracture stabilization prior to removal of their fixators. In our unit this is done by distraction across the fracture site to place the callus under tension [8].

The limitations of this study include the retrospective design and relatively small number of cases. All the non-unions identified for this study were diaphyseal fractures and the findings cannot be extrapolated to other regions of the tibia. Whilst it may seem logical to extend this clinical sign to metaphyseal and epiphyseal fractures, we do not have the data to confirm this.

The usual progression of treatment with circular fixation is progressive destabilisation of the frame prior to removal. These results suggest the callus fracture line is an indicator that stability may be inadequate and the reversal of this standard protocol to a period of increased stability from the frame, prior to further testing of fracture stability, should reduce the risk of development of hypertrophic non-union.

Acknowledgments The authors wish to thank Maria Vincent who manages the database and interrogated it to allow identification of the cases used in this study.

References

1. Perren SM (2002) Evolution of the internal fixation of long bone fractures. The scientific basis of biological internal fixation: choosing a new balance between stability and biology. J Bone Joint Surg Br 84:1093–1110
2. Bucholz RW (2005) Rockwood and green's fractures in adults. Lippincott Williams and Wilkins, Philadelphia
3. Whelan DB et al (2002) Interobserver and intraobserver variation in the assessment of the healing of tibial fractures after intramedullary fixation. J Bone Joint Surg Br 84:15–18
4. Panjabi MM, Walter SD, Karuda M, White AA, Lawson JP (1985) Correlations of radiographic analysis of healing fractures with strength: a statistical analysis of experimental osteotomies. J Orthop Res 3:212–218
5. Fleiss JL (1971) Measuring nominal scale agreement among many raters. Psychol Bull 76:378
6. Hubert L (1977) Kappa revisited. Psychol Bull 84:289–297
7. Iwakura T et al (2009) Human hypertrophic nonunion tissue contains mesenchymal progenitor cells with multilineage capacity in vitro. J Orthop Res 27:208–215
8. Saleh M, Royston S (1996) Management of nonunion of fractures by distraction with correction of angulation and shortening. J Bone Joint Surg Br 78:105–109
9. Sarmiento A, Sobol P (1984) Prefabricated functional braces for the treatment of fractures of the tibial diaphysis. J Bone Joint Surg Am 66:1328–1339
10. Hammer RR, Hammerby S, Lindholm B (1985) Accuracy of radiologic assessment of tibial shaft fracture union in humans. Clin Orthop Relat Res (199):233–238
11. Eastaugh-Waring SJ, Joslin CC, Hardy JRW, Cunningham JL (2009) Quantification of fracture healing from radiographs using the maximum callus index. Clin Orthop 467:1986–1991
12. Kooistra BW et al (2010) The radiographic union scale in tibial fractures: reliability and validity. J Orthop Trauma 24(Suppl 1):S81–S86
13. Whelan DB et al (2010) Development of the radiographic union score for tibial fractures for the assessment of tibial fracture healing after intramedullary fixation. J Trauma 68:629–632
14. Bhattacharyya T et al (2006) The accuracy of computed tomography for the diagnosis of tibial nonunion. J Bone Joint Surg Am 88:692–697

22

Inter- and intra-observer agreement of the AO classification for operatively treated distal radius fractures

Jesse M. van Buijtenen[1] · Mischa L. C. van Tunen[1] · Wietse P. Zuidema[1] ·
Emile A. Heilbron[2] · Jeroen de Haan[3] · Henrica C. W. de Vet[4] · Robert J. Derksen[5]

Abstract The reproducibility of the AO classification for distal radius fractures remains a topic of debate. Previous studies showed variable reproducibility results. Important treatment decisions depend on correct classification, especially in comminuted, intra-articular fractures. Therefore, reliable reproducibility results need to be undisputedly determined. Hence, the study objective was to assess inter- and intra-observer agreement of the AO classification for operatively treated distal radius fractures. A database of 54 radiographs of all AO types (A, B and C) and groups (A$_{2-3}$, B$_{1-3}$, and C$_{1-3}$) of distal radius fractures was assessed in twofold. Likewise, a subset of 152 radiographs of solely C-type groups (C$_{1-3}$) was assessed. All fractures were classified by six observers with different experience levels: three consultant trauma surgeons, one sixth-year trauma surgery resident, a consultant trauma radiologist, and an intern with limited experienced. The inter-observer agreement of both main types and groups was moderate ($\kappa = 0.49$ resp. $\kappa = 0.48$) in combination with a good intra-observer agreement ($\kappa = 0.68$ resp. $\kappa = 0.70$). The inter-observer agreement of the subset C-type fractures group was fair ($\kappa = 0.27$) with moderate intra-observer agreement ($\kappa = 0.43$). According to these results, the reproducibility of the AO classification of main types and groups of distal radius fractures based on conventional radiographs is insufficient ($\kappa < 0.50$), especially at group level of C-type fractures.

Keywords Distal radius fracture · Surgical procedures · Intra-observer agreement · Inter-observer agreement · AO classification · C-type fractures

Introduction

The lifetime risk of sustaining a distal radius fracture is 15 % for women and 2 % for men [1]. Through the years, many different classification systems were developed for distal radius fractures [2]. Nowadays, the most frequently used classification system is that of the Arbeitsgemeinschaft für Osteosynthesefragen (AO). This system, based on an alphanumeric system, was developed by Müller and colleagues in 1986 and was slightly modified in 1990 [3]. Starting point was that the classification needed to be logical and consistent, reflect fracture complexity, easy to reproduce, and internationally comprehensive making it eligible for data processing [4]. The correct classification in combination with the AO surgical reference tool may guide clinicians in decision-making with regard to the treatment of these fractures.

The AO system allocates a code to the fracture based on its location and morphology. Distal radius fractures are referred to as "AO-23" fractures, in which "2" means forearm and "3" stands for distal. As for morphology, the fracture is divided into three types: extra-articular (A), unicondylar or combined metaphyseal (B), and intra-articular fractures (C). Each fracture type is subdivided into

✉ Jesse M. van Buijtenen
jessevb@gmail.com; j.vanbuijtenen@vumc.nl

[1] Department of Surgery, VU University Medical Centre,
1007 MB Amsterdam, The Netherlands

[2] Department of Radiology, VU University Medical Centre,
Amsterdam, The Netherlands

[3] Department of Surgery, Westfriesgasthuis, Hoorn,
The Netherlands

[4] Department of Epidemiology and Biostatistics and the
EMGO Institute for Health and Care Research, VU
University Medical Centre, Amsterdam, The Netherlands

[5] Department of Surgery, Zaandam Medical Centre, Zaandam,
The Netherlands

three groups (1, 2, or 3) based on fracture location and fracture morphology (complexity of the fracture) [3–5].

Since the new millennium, the diagnostic performance of the system was investigated and yielded variable results. The inter- and intra-observer agreement of these studies varied from fair to good [6–9]. These results are not consistent and raise questions on clinical usefulness in daily practice.

Classification systems should have acceptable inter- and intra-observer agreement since reproducibility is a key clinimetric property of a diagnostic test. Differently classified fractures may lead to different treatment options resulting in suboptimal outcomes.

The need for this study was deemed clear due to the inconsistent reproducibility results from existing literature on the AO distal radius classification system. Therefore, the study objective was to assess inter- and intra-observer agreement of the AO classification for operatively treated distal radius fractures.

Materials and methods

All consecutive patients between 18 and 60 years of age who had been operatively treated for a distal radius fracture between January 1, 2007 and December 31, 2010 were included in this study. Eligible patients were identified by cross-referencing hospital diagnostic codes. A database of 54 digitized radiographs of all types (A, B and C) of distal radius fractures could be constructed. Since C-type fractures are the most complex and unstable fractures, operative treatment is often necessary to stabilize the fracture. Therefore a group of 152 radiographs consisting of solely C-type fractures was assessed separately at group level (C_{1-3}).

Sample-size estimation was based on the rule of thumb that 50–100 patients are needed in order to obtain adequate power for a study on reproducibility [10]. Exclusion criteria were bone abnormalities, previous distal radius fractures, isolated ulna fractures (AO A_1), and incomplete radiograph series.

Both radiographs of acute distal radius fractures and radiographs directly after closed reduction were used since decision-making is largely based upon these two series. The observers were blinded for patient characteristics and for each other's answers. All radiographs were assessed twice by six different observers: three consultant trauma surgeons (WZ, JH, RJD), a consultant trauma radiologist (EH), a sixth-year trauma surgery resident (JB), and an intern with limited experienced (MT). A handout depicting the AO classification was used during all assessments. Each of the observers classified the radiographs in the same order, independently and at their own pace. The observers assessed all radiographs twice; the second assessment was

shuffled and repeated after 3 weeks to avoid recall bias. The overall group was analyzed both at the level of distinction between main types (A, B and C) and at group levels (A_{2-3}, B_{1-3} and C_{1-3}). The agreement of main types and groups was calculated using the data from the assessment of the overall classification.

Cohen's Kappa and 95 % confidence interval were calculated to render inter- and intra-observer agreement. It was assumed that misclassifications between two categories close to each other are less severe (i.e., A_2 vs. A_3) than misclassifications between categories which are further apart (i.e., A_2 vs. C_3), and therefore a weighted kappa was used [11]. Quadratic weights were used since these are usually applied in these instances. Since the weighted quadratic kappa equals the intra-class correlation coefficient of agreement and intra-class correlation can be calculated for groups of observers, calculation of intra-class correlation coefficient was used to obtain a value for the group kappa coefficient [11].

The kappa coefficients of the inter- and intra-observer agreement were classified according to the Landis and Koch classification: $\kappa = 0.00$ 'Poor', 0–0.20 'Slight', 0.21–0.40 'Fair', 0.41–0.60 'Moderate', 0.61–0.80 'Substantial', and 0.81–1.00 'Near 'perfect' [12]. In general, kappa values of <0.5 are considered unsatisfactory [13]. The inter- and intra-observer agreement of the types and groups were assessed using SPSS v16.0 (IBM, Armonk, New York).

Results

In total, 54 radiographs of all types (A, B and C) and groups (A_{2-3}, B_{1-3} and C_{1-3}) of operated distal radius fractures and 152 radiographs of exclusively C-type fractures (C_{1-3}) were assessed in twofold.

Inter-observer agreement

All types (ABC) and groups (A_{2-3}, B_{1-3} and C_{1-3})

For all six observers, the mean Cohen's kappa for both types and groups was moderate ($\kappa = 0.49$ and 0.48) (Table 1). As for the three consultant trauma surgeons in particular, the mean kappa coefficient of the main types and that of their groups were both fair ($\kappa = 0.39$).

C-type fractures (C_{1-3})

The kappa coefficient concerning all observers for the separate C- type fractures group was fair ($\kappa = 0.27$). In the consultant trauma surgeon group, the inter-observer agreement was fair ($\kappa = 0.31$).

Table 1 Inter-observer agreement

Classification	All observers			Trauma surgeons		
	κ First assessment (95 % CI)	κ Second assessment (95 % CI)	Mean κ value	κ First assessment (95 % CI)	κ Second assessment (95 % CI)	Mean κ value
Main AO types ABC	0.47	0.50	**0.49**	0.32	0.45	**0.39**
($N = 54$)	(0.35–0.60)	(0.38–0.63)		(0.16–0.50)	(0.28–0.60)	
Groups	0.46	0.50	**0.48**	0.32	0.47	**0.39**
A_{2-3}, B_{1-3}, C_{1-3}	(0.32–0.60)	(0.37–0.63)		(0.14–0.50)	(0.30 –0.62)	
($N = 54$)						
Group	0.30	0.24	**0.27**	0.31	0.30	**0.31**
C_{1-3}	(0.21–0.40)	(0.14–0.34)		(0.21–0.42)	(0.13–0.46)	
($N = 152$)						

Kappa value and 95 % confidence interval for the inter-observer agreement of all observers and the trauma surgeons separately

Table 2 Intra-observer agreement

	ABC	A_{2-3}, B_{1-3}, C_{1-3}	C_{1-3}
Assessor 1 resident	0.87	0.88	0.25
	(0.79–0.92)	(0.80–0.93)	(0.09–0.39)
Assessor 2 intern	0.60	0.64	0.52
	(0.40–0.75)	(0.45–0.77)	(0.39–0.62)
Assessor 3 radiologist	0.77	0.80	0.48
	(0.63–0.86)	(0.67–0.86)	(0.35–0.59)
Assessor 4 trauma surgeon	0.54	0.56	0.47
	(0.29–0.71)	(0.32–0.73)	(0.32–0.59)
Assessor 5 trauma surgeon	0.68	0.69	0.43
	(0.49–0.80)	(0.49–0.81)	(0.29–0.55)
Assessor 6 trauma surgeon	0.60	0.65	0.45
	(0.40–0.75)	(0.47–0.78)	(0.31–0.56)
Mean kappa value	0.68	0.70	0.43

Kappa value of intra-observer agreement and 95 % confidence interval for main groups (A–C), subgroups (A_{2-3}, B_{1-3}, C_{1-3}) and type C fractures

Intra-observer agreement

All types (ABC) and groups (A_{2-3}, B_{1-3} and C_{1-3})

The kappa values of the intra-observer agreement for all main types and groups for all observers were both found to be good ($\kappa = 0.68$ and 0.70) (Table 2). For the three trauma surgeons, the mean kappa value of the main types was moderate ($\kappa = 0.60$) and at group level was good ($\kappa = 0.63$).

C-type fractures (C_{1-3})

The mean kappa value for the intra-observer agreement of C-type fractures is both moderate for all observers ($\kappa = 0.43$) and the group of trauma surgeons ($\kappa = 0.45$).

Discussion

A classification should have good validity and reproducibility [11]. The reproducibility depends on inter- and intra-observer agreement. The mean kappa value for inter-observer agreement of the main types (A, B and C) and that of its groups (A_{2-3}, B_{1-3} and C_{1-3}) were both found to be moderate but with a good kappa value for the intra-observer observer agreement. For the trauma surgeon group in particular, the mean kappa value of the inter-observer agreement was moderate in both main types and groups in combination with a moderate (types) and good (groups) intra-observer agreement.

For the exclusive C-type fracture group, the mean kappa coefficient of the inter-observer agreement for groups (C_{1-3}) was fair, with a moderate intra-observer agreement for all observers and for the consultant trauma surgeons in particular.

Previous literature

The results of this study of the inter-observer agreement of the eight groups ($\kappa = 0.48$) were comparable with the results of Kreder et al. [7] (SAV = 0.48). The SAV value is a kappa value for multiple assessors. Other studies which date from 1996 and 2001 showed a lower agreement: Both studies recorded a kappa of 0.30 [6, 8]. However, more recent studies showed comparable results: After reviewing 98 cases in 2008, Belotti et al. concluded that the inter-observer agreement was moderate ($\kappa = 0.49$) in the AO/ASIF classification system [14]. In 2015, Plant et al. classified 456 patients and also found a moderate ($\kappa = 0.56$) inter-observer agreement for AO types. They concluded that inclusion of groups and subtypes reduced the agreement to fair ($\kappa = 0.29$ and 0.28) [15]. However, in our study the addition of groups to the type of fracture did not show any significant decrease in the mean kappa value ($\kappa = 0.49$ resp. $\kappa = 0.48$). This might be explained by the fact that we used both pre- and post-reduction radiographs yielding more detailed information at the group level.

The result from our study ($\kappa = 0.49$) is at the lower end of the 'moderate' spectrum. Andersen, Oskam, and Kreder found higher kappa values, respectively, 0.64, 0.68 (SAV), and 0.65 [6, 7, 9]. Only the study of MacDermid showed a lower kappa value ($\kappa = 0.35$) [8]. The inter-observer agreement of C-type fractures in our study at group level ($\kappa = 0.27$) approaches the agreement found by Illarramendi ($\kappa = 0.37$) [16] and is considered to be too low for reliable prognostic evaluation, research purposes, or fracture planning management.

We included only patients with pre- and post-reduction radiographs in contrast to the study of MacDermid [8]. Where available, pre- and post-reduction radiographs were used in the study of Andersen [6]. The availability of two radiograph series instead of only one could very well have led to a higher kappa coefficient. However, since reduction is commonly performed before surgery, it was deemed appropriate in our present study to include post-reduction radiographs for the assessments as well. Also, in contrast to our study, Andersen excluded radiographs of poor quality. Poorer-quality radiographs are more difficult to classify and could have led to a lower kappa coefficient in our study [6]. A higher agreement in the study of Oskam et al. might have been caused by the fact that fractures that could not be attributed to a particular AO main group (ABC) were classified as type D. Therefore, a separate category for undisplaced distal radius fractures in the AO classification was recommended by them [9].

Illarramendi et al classified distal radius fractures in five categories: group I included AO type A fracture, group II included AO type B fractures, group III, IV, and V were type C1, C2, and C3 fractures, respectively [14]. The inter-observer agreement in this study was $\kappa = 0.37$ (0.25–0.48). Their classification into two main groups A and B and the three subtypes for C fractures might be an explanation for their higher inter-observer kappa value compared to our study since the agreement of the three main groups in our study is also higher ($\kappa = 0.49$) than the agreement of C-type fractures. Another explanation is that the radiographs that were not classified in one of the pre-specified groups of fractures were excluded by Illarramendi et al.

Limitations

While the kappa values were calculated by marginals, reasonable agreement could possibly have resulted in a low kappa value if the marginals contained small amounts. Since our study population contained relatively few type B fractures, this might have resulted in a skewed distribution and therefore a lower kappa value [11]. In order to prevent assessment bias, clinical information was not available for the observers despite the fact that all patients had been operatively treated. However, this patient-related information is of great importance on decision-making in daily practice, and it could be argued that patient information should have been added. However, our aim was to assess the reproducibility of radiograph interpretation as 'lean' as possible, and therefore, patient details were left out.

Also, fracture analysis could have been complicated in the post-reduction series by the applied cast although this was considered the most realistic method since it exactly resembles clinical practice. Moreover, the initial radiograph series showed unreduced fractures without a cast. Knowing that all patients were treated operatively, severity of the fracture might be overrated by the observers leading to bias.

In conclusion, the overall inter-observer agreement of the main AO types and their groups was moderate with good intra-observer agreement. Among the consultant trauma surgeons, the inter-observer agreement was fair with moderate intra-observer agreement for the main types and good intra-observer agreement for the groups. For C-type fractures in particular, the overall inter-observer agreement was fair with moderate intra-observer agreement. These results show that the AO classification for distal radius fractures requiring operative treatment does not have an adequate reproducibility. Classification of distal radius fractures with both pre- and post-reduction radiographs might lead to a higher inter-observer agreement although the agreement is still not sufficient. A simplified classification system may improve agreement among clinicians.

References

1. Koval KJ, Harrast JJ, Anglen JO, Weinstein JN (2008) Fractures of the distal part of the radius. The evolution of practice over time. Where's the evidence? J Bone Joint Surg Am 90:1855–1861

2. Ploegmakers JJW, Mader K, Pennig D, Verheyen CCPM (2007) Four distal radial fracture classification systems tested amongst a large panel of Dutch trauma surgeons. Injury 38:1268–1272

3. Kural C, Sungur I, Kaya I, Ugras A, Erturk A, Cetinus E (2010) Evaluation of the reliability of classification systems used for distal radius fractures. Orthopedics 33:801

4. Colton CL (1991) Telling the bones. J Bone Joint Surg Br 73:362–364

5. Johnstone DJ, Radford WJ, Parnell EJ (1993) Interobserver variation using the AO/ASIF classification of long bone fractures. Injury 24:163–165

6. Andersen DJ, Blair WF, Steyers CMJ, Adams BD, El-Khouri GY, Brandser EA (1996) Classification of distal radius fractures: an analysis of interobserver reliability and intraobserver reproducibility. J Hand Surg Am 21:574–582

7. Kreder HJ, Hanel DP, McKee M, Jupiter J, McGillivary G, Swiontkowski MF (1996) Consistency of AO fracture classification for the distal radius. J Bone Joint Surg Br 78:726–731

8. MacDermid JC, Richards RS, Donner A, Bellamy N (2001) Reliability of hand fellows' measurements and classifications from radiographs of distal radius fractures. Can J Plas Surg 9:51–58

9. Oskam J, Kingma J, Klasen HJ (2001) Interrater reliability for the basic categories of the AO/ASIF's system as a frame of reference for classifying distal radial fractures. Percept Mot Skills 92:589–594

10. Terwee CB, Mokkink LB, Knol DL, Ostelo RW, Bouter LM, de Vet HCW (2012) Rating the methodological quality in systematic reviews of studies on measurement properties: a scoring system for the COSMIN checklist. Qual Life Res 21:651–657

11. de Vet HCW, Terwee CB, Mokkink LB, Knol DL (2011) Measurement in medicine. Practical guides to biostatistics and epidemiology. Cambridge University Press, Cambridge, pp 96–146

12. Landis JR, Koch GG (1977) The measurement of observer agreement for categorical data. Biometrics 33:159–174

13. Martin JS, Marsh JL, Bonar SK, DeCoster TA, Found EM, Brandser EA (1997) Assessment of the AO/ASIF fracture classification for the distal tibia. J Orthop Trauma 11(7):477–483

14. Belloti JC, Tamaoki MJ, Franciozi CE, Santos JB, Balbachevsky D, Chap Chap E, Albertoni WM, Faloppa F (2008) Are distal radius fracture classifications reproducible? Intra and interobserver agreement. Sao Paulo Med J 126(3):180–185

15. Plant CE, Hickson C, Hedley H, Parsons NR, Costa ML (2015) Is it time to revisit the AO classification of fractures of the distal radius? Inter- and intra-observer reliability of the AO classification. J Bone Joint Surg Br 97-B:818–823

16. Illarramendi A, González Della Valle A, Segal E, De Carli P, Maignon G, Gallucci G (1998) Evaluation of simplified Frykman and AO classifications of fractures of the distal radius. Assessment of interobserver and intraobserver agreement. Int Orthop 22(2):111–115

23

The use of recombinant morphogenic protein-2 (rhBMP-2) in children undergoing revision surgery for persistent non-union

Madhavan C. Papanna[1] · K. A. Saldanha[1] · Binu Kurian[1] · James A. Fernandes[1] · Stan Jones[1]

Abstract The purpose of the study was to evaluate the safety and efficacy with the use of BMP-2 for treating persistent non-unions in children with underlying complex conditions. Between October 2006 and November 2010 in our unit, 15 patients were treated with rhBMP-2 to enhance bone union. There were nine females and six males with a mean age of 9.5 years (range 4–15) at time of surgery. Seventy-five per cent of the patients required revision of internal fixation with insertion of rhBMP-2 to the non-union site, and the reminder had freshening of the non-union site with rhBMP-2 application. Patients had undergone a mean of 2 (1–5) operations prior to implantation of rhBMP-2. All the patients in the study group were available for review with mean follow-up of 44 months (range 21–70). The mean time to union was 16 weeks (range 10–28 weeks). No adverse events related to BMP-2 application were noted in our study group. Healing occurred clinically and radiographically in 16 of the 17 sites. Our study demonstrates that BMP-2 enhances healing of the persistent non-unions without any adverse events

Keywords Bone · Congenital abnormalities non-union · rhBMP-2

✉ Madhavan C. Papanna
drmadhavan@hotmail.com

James A. Fernandes
james.fernandes@sch.nhs.uk

Stan Jones
stanjoness80@hotmail.com

1   Department of Trauma and Orthopaedics, Sheffield Children Hospital, Sheffield S10 2TH, UK

Introduction

Autologous bone grafting (ABG) has osteogenic, osteoinductive and osteoconductive properties and is the gold-standard biological treatment for non-union [1, 2]. However, limited availability and donor site morbidity limit its use [3, 4]. In 1965, Marshal R Urist discovered a substance within the extracellular matrix of bone that induced new bone formation when implanted into extraskeletal sites in a host. This substance triggers a proliferation of undifferentiated mesenchymal cells and the formation of osteoprogenitor cells to form bone. It was called bone morphogenic protein (BMP). By 1988, molecular clones had been characterised and the amino acid sequence from a highly purified bovine bone preparation was derived. This led to the isolation of human complimentary DNAs, recognised subsequently as a member of the superfamily of transforming growth factor β. At least 20 human variants of BMPs that possess varying degrees of osteoinductive activity have been identified since [5].

Two (BMP-2 and BMP-7) have been the subject of intense research for treatment of non-union and are available currently as recombinant protein molecules of human genes [5]. The Food and Drug Administration (FDA) and the European agency for the evaluation of medical products have approved the use of BMP-2 as bone graft substitute in adults with open tibial fractures and those undergoing anterior lumbar inter-body spinal fusion as an adjunct to standard care by internal fixation [6–10].

In addition to the approved use, there have been reports of use in an off-label fashion in children undergoing surgery for spinal and orthopaedic conditions [11–13, 18, 19]. However, there are limited published data on the use and outcomes of BMP-2 in revision non-union surgery in the paediatric population.

In children, fractures and corrective osteotomies heal well mostly. However, union may be difficult to achieve in patients with skeletal dysplasias, congenital deficiencies of the limbs and some complex fractures. This is our experience with the use of BMP-2 in children undergoing revision surgery for persistent non-union.

Materials and methods

We undertook a retrospective review of all the patients who received rhBMP as a part of their treatment at the Sheffield Children's Hospital between October 2006 and November 2010. This review was approved by the research and development department of our institution. In all patients, the decision to use rhBMP-2 was made at a multidisciplinary team meeting. We had approval from the hospital pharmacy department and also obtained informed consent from the parents of our patients for the use of rhBMP-2.

Clinical data for each patient were gathered from the medical records and included demographics, anatomical site, diagnosis, initial treatment, number and type of previous operations, operative details at the time of rhBMP-2 use, time to union and the length of follow-up (see Table 1).

Nineteen patients (21 surgical procedures) received rhBMP-2 as a part of their treatment during the study period. Four patients were excluded as they were either older than 18 years, had autologous bone graft in addition to rhBMP-2 or had a spinal fusion procedure. The final sample was comprised of 15 patients (17 surgical procedures). Case 4 required two episodes of rhBMP-2 application to a femoral non-union site and case 10 had bilateral application of rhBMP-2 to tibial non-union sites at different stages. The mean age of these patients at the time of rhBMP-2 use was 9.5 years (range 4–15 years). Nine were female and six male (Table 1).

All the patients had a persistent non-union or pseudoarthrosis despite previous surgery to achieve union. With the exception of one case (case 8) that was an atrophic non-union, the remainder had radiographic features of oligotrophic non-union (Table 1).

The patients had undergone a mean of 2 (range 1–5) previous surgical procedures prior to the use of rhBMP-2. The surgical procedures included resection of pseudoarthrosis and autologous bone grafting in 10 patients (62 %), intramedullary fixation with rods, fixation with a plate and screws or application of external fixator.

The predominant primary diagnosis was osteogenesis imperfecta (5 patients). The other diagnoses were proximal femoral focal deficiency (2 patients), neurofibromatosis with pseudoarthrosis of the tibia (2 patients), non-union after comminuted fractures (2 patients), achondroplasia,

arthrogryposis, Coats' plus disease and a femoral fracture in a patient with both Down's syndrome and Perthes disease.

The senior authors (JAF and SJ) evaluated patients for clinical evidence of healing by pain and tenderness at the non-union site and the ability to weight bear on the affected limb with the orthosis. The radiographs were evaluated independently for any complications and signs of healing. Friedlander's criterion (the presence of bone bridging at the site of non-union in at least one view) was used [20]. The non-union was considered healed if it fulfilled radiological and clinical criteria.

Operative technique

All the surgical procedures were performed under general anaesthetic. Prophylactic antibiotic was administered at the time of induction and two further doses given at 8 and 16 h postsurgery. Using a tourniquet, the non-union site was exposed through a longitudinal skin incision. Fibrous tissue and avascular bone were excised until healthy bone ends were exposed. In some cases of tibial non-union, it was necessary to undertake a fibular osteotomy, done through a separate lateral skin incision.

The next stage of the surgery involved a revision of the fixation device if required. For intramedullary nails, the medullary canal of the proximal and distal segments was drilled with increasingly larger drill bits to accommodate the larger nails. In those patients with external fixators in situ, these were adjusted accordingly and some compression applied.

BMP-2 was reconstituted with sterile water to a concentration of 1.5 mg/ml and a bovine collagen sponge used as delivery matrix. After at least 15 min of soak time and just before closure of the surgical wound, the BMP-2-impregnated sponge was cut into rectangular pieces and implanted directly over the bone ends. Demineralised bone matrix (DBX) was placed over the BMP-2 in patients with large defects. The amount of BMP-2 used was determined by the size of the bone cavity or defect. Autologous bone graft was not used in any of the cases.

All the patients were allowed to commence partial weight bearing once the surgical wound had healed. Clinical and radiological follow-up was undertaken at regular intervals until union was achieved.

Results

None of the patients was observed to have a septic non-union. At the time of revision surgery with rhBMP-2, 75 % of the patients required revision of the previous fixation device. Twelve patients required revision fixation at the

Table 1 Demographics and clinical profile of the patients

Case number	Age (years)/gender	Diagnosis	Anatomical site	Type of non-union	Previous surgical treatment	Number of previous surgeries	Revision surgical procedure	Number of application sites	Time to healing (weeks)	Outcomes	Follow-up (months)
1	M,4	PFFD	Femur	Oligotrophic	Hybrid frame application	1	Revision IF	1	22	Healed	26
2	F,4	PFFD	Femur	Oligotrophic	Proximal femoral osteotomy and acetabuloplasty	1	Revision IF and debridement of non-union site	1	24	Healed	30
3	F,11	OI type 3	Femur	Oligotrophic	Growing rod insertion	2	Revision IM nail	1	16	Healed	42
4	F,12	(Perthes disease/down's syndrome)	Femur	Oligotrophic	Pelvic supportive osteotomy + femoral lengthening with hybrid frame application	3	Freshening non-union site	2	28	Healed	25
5	F,10	Non-union achondroplasia	Femur	Oligotrophic	Intramedullary nail insertion	2	Revision fixation	1	20	Healed	22
6	M,13	OI type 4	Tibia	Oligotrophic	Growing rod insertion	3	Revision growing rod	1	10	Healed	21
7	M,12	CPT	Tibia	Oligotrophic	Growing rods +bone grafting application	5	Revision to growing rod	1	14	Healed	33
8	M,15	Fracture nonunion (coats plus disease)	Tibia	Atrophic	Taylor spatial frame application	3	Freshening non-union site	1	N/A	No (awaiting revision surgery)	44
9	F,4	CPT	Tibia	Oligotrophic	Nancy nails insertion	4	Revised to growing rod	1	12	Healed	70
10	F,12	OI type 3	Bilateral tibia	Oligotrophic	Growing rods insertion	2	Revision growing rod	2	18	Healed	34
11	F,13	OI type 3	Tibia	Oligotrophic	Growing rod insertion	1	Revision growing rod	1	26	Healed	24
12	F,14	Non-union (closed fracture)	Tibia	Oligotrophic	Taylor spatial frame application	1	Freshening non-union site	1	12	Healed	41
13	M,15	OI type 4	Ulna	Oligotrophic	Corrective osteotomy and intramedullary nail	2	Revision IM nail	1	12	Healed	36
14	M,12	Malunited monteggia fracture with radial head dislocation	Ulna	Oligotrophic	Intramedullary nail insertion	1	Corrective ulna osteotomy + TSF Application	1	10	Healed	38
15	F,9	Arthrogryposis with fixed equinus	Ankle	Oligotrophic	Arthrodesis of the ankle with screws	1	Freshening of non-union site	1	8	Healed	46

OI osteogenesis imperfecta, *PFFD* proximal femoral focal deficiency, *CPT* congenital pseudoarthrosis of the tibia, *TSF* Taylor spatial frame, *IM* intramedullary nail, *IF* internal fixation

time of BMP-2 insertion that included Sheffield telescopic rods for the tibia and femur in five and two patients, respectively, whereas Fassier–Duval telescopic rods were used in the tibia of two patients. In two patients with femoral non-unions, plates were used, and in one patient, an Ilizarov ring fixator was used to stabilise the femur.

All the patients in the study group were available for review at a mean follow-up of 44 months (range 21–70). The mean time to union was 16 weeks (range 10–28 weeks) (Fig. 1a, c). Clinical and radiological healing was observed in 16 of the 17 sites at the last follow-up. One patient (case 8) with Coats' plus disease was treated with BMP-2 and an Ilizarov fixator for tibial non-union 10 months after the index surgery and failed to heal. Further autologous bone grafting was performed, and at 6 months postoperatively the bone has failed to unite and the patient is awaiting further surgery.

No local or systemic complications attributable to BMP-2 were noted in any of our patients. In particular, none of our patients had a wound breakdown, local soft tissue calcification or heterotrophic ossification.

Discussions

Bone morphogenic proteins possess good osteoinductive properties that enhance healing and are used in the treatment of adult patients with recalcitrant non-unions and spinal fusion procedures successfully to facilitate union/fusion [7, 8, 20]. The manufacturers of commercially available recombinant human BMP-2 have stated that it is contraindicated for use in the paediatric population because they have not been able to provide data that establish the safety and efficiency of BMP-2 in children below 18 years of age. There have been reports of use of BMPs in the paediatric population [11–19] with most as case reports [13, 14] and small case series [15, 17–19]; the prevalent clinical condition for its use was congenital pseudoarthrosis of the tibia [12, 15–19].

In comparison, use of rhBMP-7(OP-1) for treating non-union and congenital pseudoarthrosis of the tibia in the paediatric population [14–17] had mixed success. Lee et al. reported on five patients with congenital pseudoarthrosis of the tibia treated using bone graft, rhBMP-7 and fixation. Union was achieved in only one of the five cases, and it was felt that variables in the surgical technique contributed to the poor outcome [15]. Other authors have reported reasonable outcomes [14, 16–18]. The results of these studies suggest that rhBMP-7 should be combined with autologous bone graft and optimum fixation of the pseudoarthrosis is required.

The current literature describes rhBMP-2 used mostly for the treatment of congenital pseudoarthrosis of tibia in

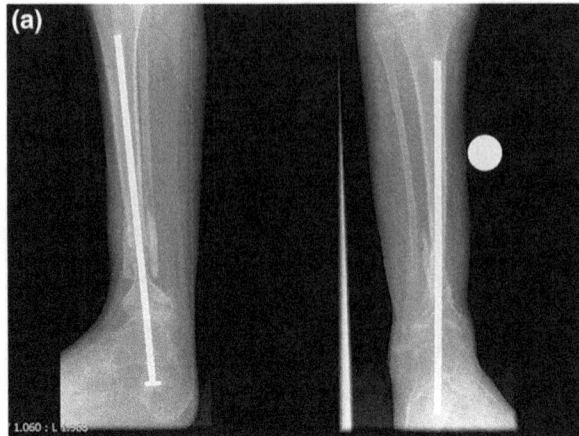
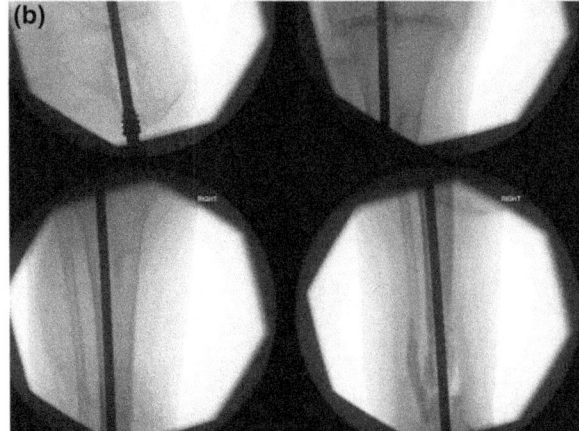
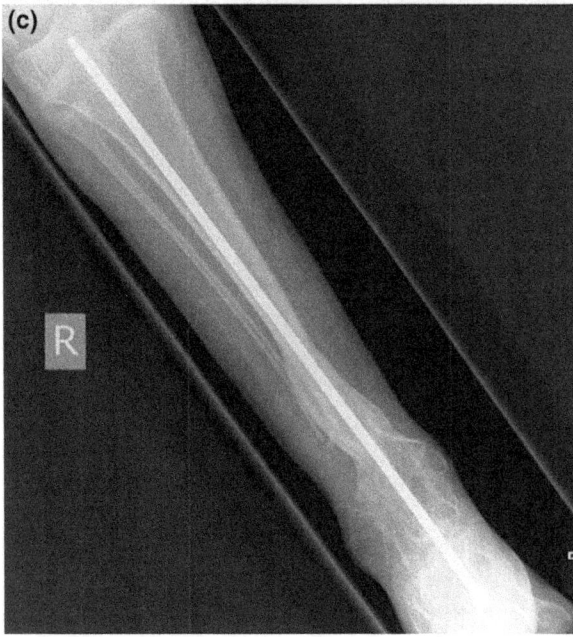

Fig. 1 This 12-year-old patient with congenital pseudoarthrosis of the tibia had multiple surgical procedures to enhance the healing of non-union. **a** Preoperative radiograph showing the non-union of the pseudoarthrosis with growing rod in situ. **b** Intraoperative images illustrating the revision intramedullary nailing and BMP-2 insertion. **c** Anteroposterior view radiograph at 14 weeks after initial surgery showing healing at the pseudoarthrosis site

the paediatric population [18, 19]. Spiro et al. [18] reported four children with congenital pseudarthrosis of the tibia treated with intramedullary stabilisation, Ilizarov external fixators and rhBMP-2. Only one out of four had previous failed surgery. Radiological union was achieved at a mean of 3.5 months postoperatively with a mean follow-up of 31 months. They concluded that the initial rate of union may be improved and the time to union reduced with this strategy. Richards et al. [19] reported on seven children with CPT treated using rhBMP-2, autologous bone graft and intramedullary rodding. Two patients had failed previous surgery. Radiological union was achieved in five patients at a mean of 6.4 months. The average follow-up was 72 months, and no adverse effect of BMP was observed. They also noted an improvement in the time to initial union. Their average of 6.4 months compared favourably with 16 months reported by Dobbs et al. [22] who treated a similar group of patients using autologous bone graft and intramedullary rodding but without BMP.

In this series, we observed a mean time to union of 16 weeks. This compares favourably with the reports of Spiro et al. (14 weeks) and Richards et al. (26 weeks). This may be because most of our cases were not congenital pseudoarthroses of the tibia. The time to union of the two cases of CPT in this study was 12 and 14 weeks, respectively. The non-unions in this series were due to multiple factors, viz. biology and stability. RhBMP-2 is not effective in the presence of instability at the non-union site. The one patient in this study who failed union despite using rhBMP-2 and an Ilizarov fixator was a case of Coats' plus disease with a tibial non-union (case 8). Further autologous bone grafting failed, and further surgery is being planned. We believe the failure to achieve healing is related to the underlying diagnosis and not surgical technique. It is established that congenital defects decrease fusion rates [1].

This report contains the second largest number of patients (15 patients) but with a longer follow-up than that published by Oetgen et al. Fifty-three of 81 patients in their series were skeletally immature, and BMP-2 was used mostly as part of spinal surgery. The report was focussed on the complications associated with the use of BMP-2 [12], citing an overall complication of 17.5 % in 81 patients. The complications included excessive wound discharge and swelling, wound dehiscence, deep infection, enlargement of optic glioma, compartment syndrome, progressive myelopathy and dural fibrosis. They believed that only one of the complications may have been directly related to the use of BMP-2; this was dural fibrosis associated with motor weakness after exposure of the spinal cord to rhBMP-2 [12].

Ritting et al. [13] reported a case of massive inflammatory reaction following the use of rhBMP-2 to treat an ulnar non-union in a child. Circulating antibodies against type 1 collagen and anti-BMP-2 antibodies have been detected in a smaller number of patients treated with BMP, but these studies have concluded that there is insufficient evidence to establish a relationship between these antibodies and the absence of ossification [6, 20, 21].

Although there is a theoretical risk of adverse events in association with the use of BMP in skeletally immature patients, this is not confirmed in the literature. In the follow-up period of this study, we did not observe any local or systemic adverse events related directly to the use of BMP-2. The patients and the families in this study were warned of the risk of developing adverse effects and complications such as deep infection, a severe inflammatory reaction, neuralgia, resorption of bone, compartment syndrome, heterotrophic ossification and local nerve compression.

There are limitations to this study. This is a retrospective review of a small sample described by the common feature of having had failed attempts to treat a non-union. The sample was heterogeneous and without a control group for comparison. Alteration to the biomechanics (adjustment of fixation method) across the non-union would have influenced the results as would have use of the rhBMP.

In conclusion, this review describes successful use of rhBMP-2 as a part of a treatment strategy for persistent non-unions in children who have failed to achieve bone healing despite standard methods of treatment.

Informed consent Informed consent was obtained from all the individual participants included in the study.

References

1. Megas P (2005) Classification of non-union. Injury 36(Supp 4):S30–S37
2. Phieffer LS, Goulet JA (2006) Delayed unions of the tibia. JBJS [Am] 88(1):206–216
3. Goulet JA, Senunas LE, DeSilva GL, Greenfield ML (1997) Autogenous iliac crest bone graft. Complications and functional assessment. CORR 339:76–81
4. Schnee CL, Freese A, Weil RJ (1997) Analysis of harvest morbidity and radiographic outcome using autograft for anterior cervical fusion. Spine 22:222–227
5. De Biase P, Capanna R (2005) Clinical applications of BMPs. Injury 36(Suppl 3):S43–S46
6. Govender S, Csimma C, Genant HK, Valentin-Opran A, Amit Y, Arbel R (2002) BMP-2 Evaluation in Surgery for Tibial Trauma (BESTT) Study Group. Recombinant human bone morphogenetic protein-2 for treatment of open tibial fractures: a prospective, controlled, randomized study of four hundred and fifty patients. J Bone Joint Surg Am 84:2123–2134
7. Boden SD, Kang J, Sandhu H, Heller JG (2002) Use of recombinant human bone morphogenetic protein-2 to achieve posterolateral lumbar spine fusion in humans: a prospective, randomized clinical pilot trial: 2002 Volvo Award in clinical studies. Spine 27:2662–2673

8. Burkus JK, Transfeldt EE, Kitchel SH, Watkins RG, Balderston RA (2002) Clinical and radiographic outcomes of anterior lumbar interbody fusion using recombinant human bone morphogenetic protein-2. Spine 27:2396–2408

9. Jones AL, Bucholz RW, Bosse MJ, Mirza SK, Lyon TR, Webb LX (2006) Recombinant humanBMP-2 and allograft compared with autogenous bone graft for reconstruction of diaphyseal tibial fractures with cortical defects. A randomized, controlled trial. J Bone Joint Surg Am 88:1431–1441

10. Krause F, Younger A, Weber M (2008) Recombinant human BMP-2 and allograft compared with autogenous bone graft for reconstruction of diaphyseal tibial fractures with cortical defects. J Bone Joint Surg Am 90:1168

11. Abd-El-Barr MM, Cox JB, Antonucci MU, Bennett J, Murad GJ, Pincus DW (2011) Recombinant human bone morphogenetic protein-2 as an adjunct for spine fusion in a pediatric population. Pediatr Neurosurg 47(4):266–271

12. Oetgen ME, Richards BS (2010) Complications associated with the use of bone morphogenetic protein in pediatric patients. J Pediatr Orthop 30:192–198

13. Ritting AW, Weber EW, Lee MC (2012) Exaggerated inflammatory response and bony resorption from BMP-2 use in a pediatric forearm non-union. J Hand Surg Am 37(2):316–321

14. Dohin B, Dahan-Oliel N, Fassier F, Hamdy R (2009) Enhancement of difficult nonunion in children with osteogenic protein-1 (OP-1): early experience. Clin Orthop Relat Res 467(12):3230–3238

15. Lee FY, Sinicropi SM, Lee FS, Vitale MG, Roye DP Jr, Choi IH (2006) Treatment of congenital pseudarthrosis of the tibia with recombinant human bone morphogenetic protein-7 (rhBMP-7). A report of five cases. J Bone Joint Surg Am 88(3):627–633

16. Birke O, Schindeler A, Ramachandran M, Cowell CT, Munns CF, Bellemore M (2010) Preliminary experience with the combined use of recombinant bone morphogenetic protein and bisphosphonates in the treatment of congenital pseudarthrosis of the tibia. J Child Orthop 4(6):507–517

17. Fabeck L, Ghafil D, Gerroudj M, Baillon R, Delincé P (2006) Bone morphogenetic protein-7 in the treatment of congenital pseudarthrosis of the tibia. J BoneJoint Surg Br 88:116–118

18. Spiro AS, Babin K, Lipovac S, Stenger P, Mladenov K, Rupprecht M (2011) Combined treatment of congenital pseudarthrosis of the tibia, including recombinant human bone morphogenetic protein-2: a case series. J Bone Joint Surg Br 93(5):695–699

19. Richards BS, Oetgen ME, Johnston CE (2010) The use of rhBMP-2 for the treatment of congenital pseudarthrosis of the tibia: a case series. J Bone Joint Surg [Am] 92-A:177–185

20. Friedlaender GE, Perry CR, Cole JD, Cook SD, Cierny G, Muschler GF (2001) Osteogenic protein-1 (Bone morphogenetic protein-7) in the treatment of tibial nonunions. J Bone Joint Surg Am 83-A(suppl 1):S151–S158

21. Geesink RG, Hoefnagels NH, Bulstra SK (1999) Osteogenic activity of OP-1 bone morphogenetic protein (BMP-7) in a human fibular defect. J Bone Joint Surg Br 81(4):710–718

22. Dobbs MB, Rich MM, Gordon JE, Szymanski DA, Schoenecker PL (2005) Use of an intramedullary rod for the treatment of congenital pseudarthrosis of the tibia. Surg Tech Suppl 1(Pt 1):33–40

24

External fixation of paediatric subtrochanteric fractures using calcar rather than neck pins

Sherif Galal[1]

Abstract Subtrochanteric femoral fractures in children are uncommon and have received limited attention in the literature. Its treatment is controversial, and different options are available: traction, spica casting, internal fixation and external fixation. The aim of this study is to present our results with external fixation of subtrochanteric femoral fractures in children using Ilizarov frame. Between January 2012 and January 2014, 14 patients with closed subtrochanteric femoral fractures were treated in Cairo University School of Medicine Teaching Hospital. The average age at the time of injury was 6.4 years (range 3.8–11.5 years). Pathological fractures and fractures associated with neuromuscular diseases were excluded from this study. Two patients were multiply injured with abdominal injuries (as ruptured spleen). In all cases, a low profile Ilizarov frame was inserted using two half pins inserted proximally from greater to lesser trochanters parallel to the hip joint orientation line (line between tip of greater trochanter and femoral head centre) and secured to an arch, and another three half pins were inserted distally perpendicular to the femoral shaft and secured to an arch that was connected by three rods to the proximal arch. No post-operative spica was used. Average follow-up was 18 months (range 12–36 months). All fractures united with anatomical alignment within an average of 8 weeks (range 6–12 weeks). There were no deep infections and no significant limb length discrepancies. At the latest follow-up, no patient had any restriction of activities. External fixation with a low profile Ilizarov frame appears as a good treatment option for subtrochanteric femoral fractures in children.
Level of evidence: Level IV.

Keywords External fixator · Paediatric · Subtrochanteric · Fracture

Introduction

Subtrochanteric femoral fractures in children are a special type starting 1–2 cm below the lesser trochanter [1]. There is difficulty maintaining fracture reduction due to the strong deforming muscle forces displacing the proximal fragment into a flexed, abducted and externally rotated position [1, 8, 9]. These forces make it difficult to maintain reduction using traction or spica casting [3]. There are increasing reports in the literature, suggesting operative treatment leads to better results than non-operative methods [13]. Methods of fixation include intramedullary nails, compression plating and external fixation [2, 10].

The aim of the study was to evaluate the results of a new configuration of the Ilizarov fixator for stabilising subtrochanteric femoral fractures in children.

Patients and methods

Between January 2012 and January 2014, fourteen children (14 hips, 10 boys and 4 girls) with an average age of 6.4 years (range 3.8–11.5 years) sustained closed subtrochanteric femoral fractures and were treated operatively at Cairo University Hospital. Injury was caused by a fall from a height in 2 patients and through motor vehicle

✉ Sherif Galal
Sherif.Galal@kasralainy.edu.eg

[1] Department of Orthopaedic Surgery and Traumatology, Faculty of Medicine, Kasr AL-Ainy School of Medicine, Cairo University, Cairo 11559, Egypt

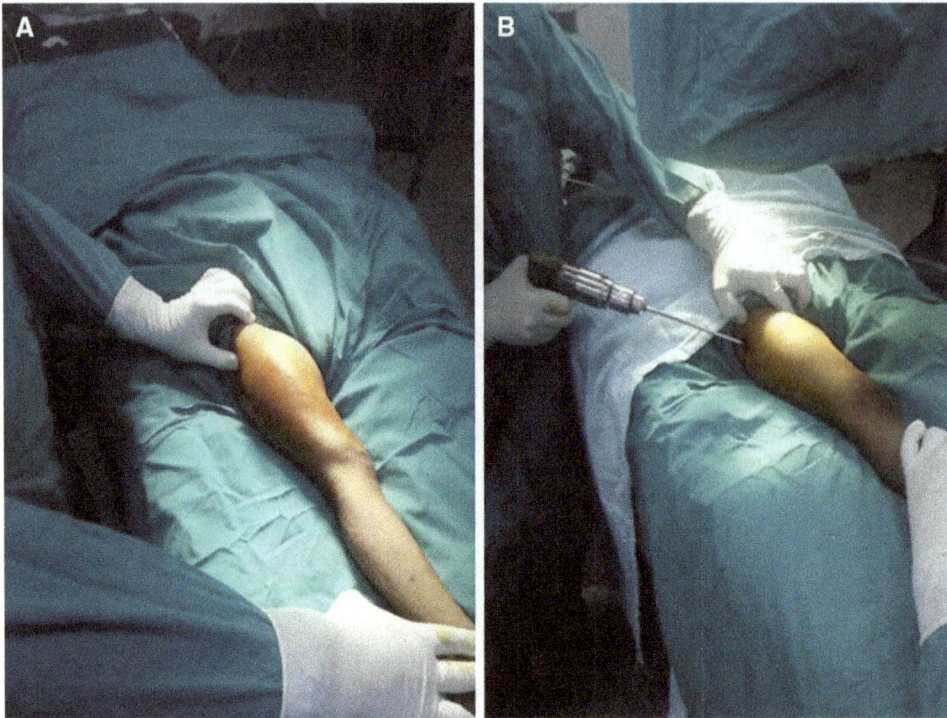

Fig. 1 **a** Hip neutral position with leg internally rotated; **b** first proximal half pin introduced

incidents in 12 patients. Two patients had abdominal injuries, and the remaining had isolated subtrochanteric femoral fractures. Radiographs revealed the most common fracture pattern to be a transverse fracture (in 8 patients); 3 had a spiral pattern, 2 patients a short oblique fracture, and one a fracture with a butterfly fragment. Surgery was performed 2–5 days after injury under general anaesthesia in the supine position and under fluoroscopic control. With leg internally rotated (hip neutral) (Fig. 1a), one half pin was inserted from anterolateral to posteromedial starting at the base of greater trochanter aiming at the lesser trochanter parallel to hip joint orientation line (line between tip of greater trochanter and femoral head centre, Fig. 1b). Using this pin to joystick the proximal fragment to correct flexion and external rotation, another half pin was inserted from posterolateral to anteromedial at a 90° angle to the first pin in the axial plane and parallel to hip joint orientation line (Fig. 2). With patella forward (knee neutral, Fig. 3a), three half pins were inserted perpendicular to the shaft (Fig. 3b) in the distal segment of the fracture with another half pin added in another plane in some cases. Proximal and distal pins were secured to Ilizarov arches that were then connected to one another by three threaded rods that were used for further improvement of the reduction in frontal plane (using the lateral rod) or in the sagittal plane (using the anterior and posterior rods, Fig. 4). Weight bearing was allowed as tolerated after surgery, and patients were followed up until union. The fixator was

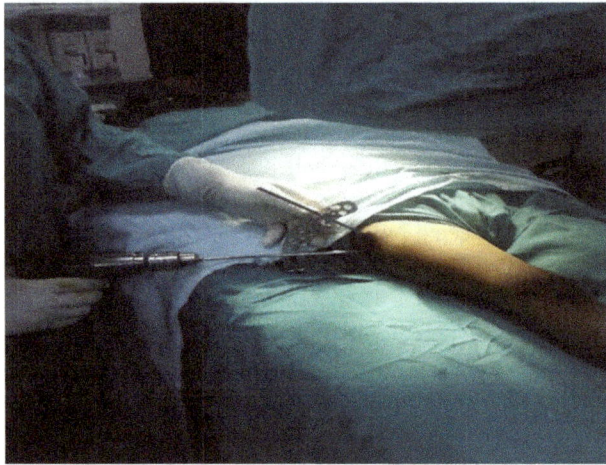

Fig. 2 Second proximal half pin introduced

removed after complete union with no need for a spica cast or brace. The average follow-up was 18 months (range 12–24 months).

Results

All patients stayed in hospital for 2 days post-operatively except for those with abdominal injuries who were hospitalized for a longer period. All fractures united with anatomical alignment (Fig. 5) within an average of

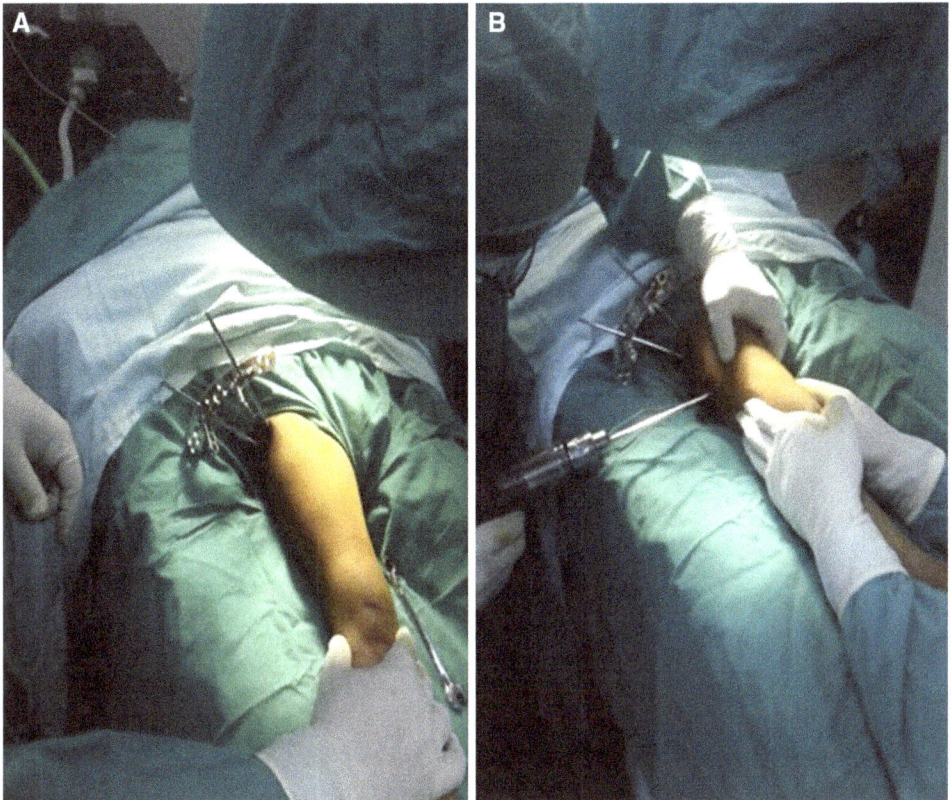

Fig. 3 **a** Knee neutral position; **b** first distal half pin introduced

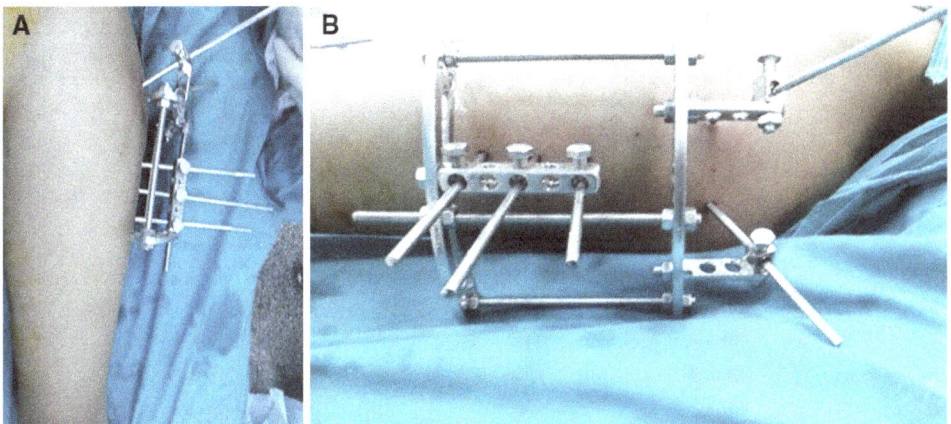

Fig. 4 Proximal and distal arches are connected by 3 threaded rods, frontal (**a**) and side (**b**) views of the frame

8 weeks (range 6–12 weeks). Clinical evaluation at final follow-up revealed a full range of motion at both the hip and knee joints in all patients. There were no deep infections, but four patients had pin site infections that responded to oral antibiotics and pin site care. There were no incidences of refracture or avascular necrosis of the femoral head (Table 1).

Discussion

Paediatric subtrochanteric femoral fractures are an unstable fracture type with little published in the literature [3]. Several studies have documented superior results with internal fixation compared to non-operative treatment [13]. According to Kregor et al. [10], the indications for opera-

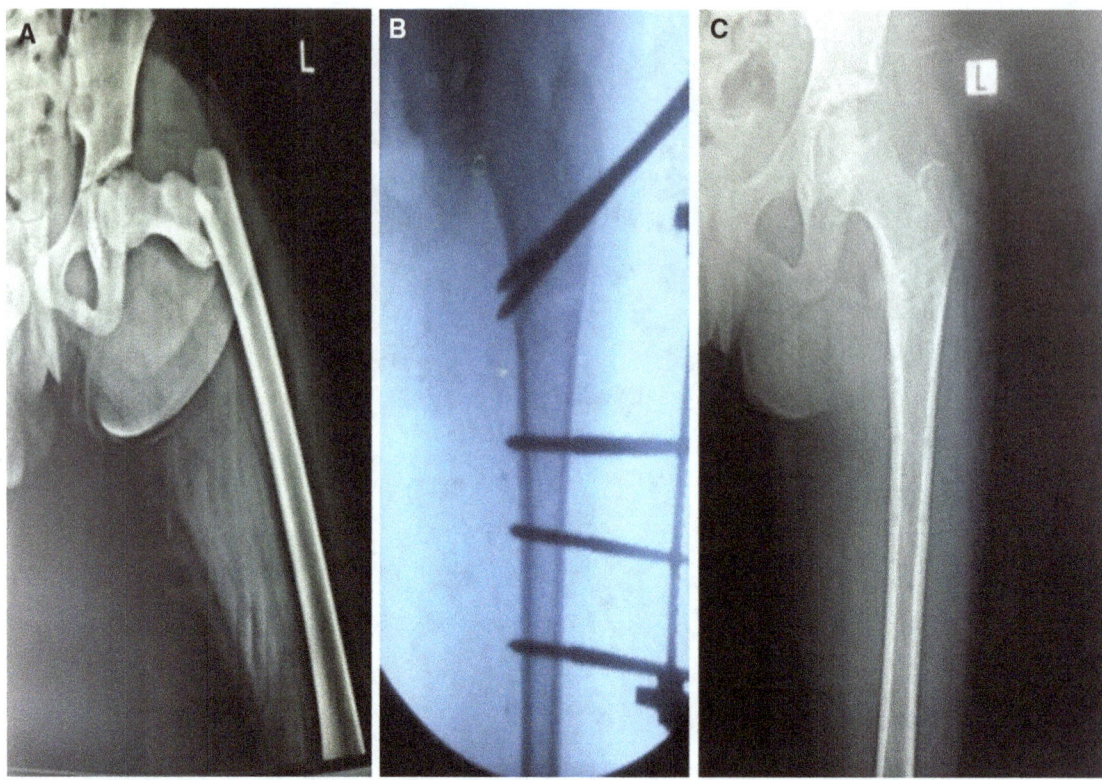

Fig. 5 Preoperative AP X-rays (**a**) of 10-year-old female patient who sustained subtrochanteric fractures, intraoperative imaging after fixation (**b**). Anteroposterior (**c**) X-rays after complete union (11 weeks) and frame removal

Table 1 Patients data

	Age	Sex	Mechanism of injury	Complications	Fracture pattern	Time to union (week)
Case 1	6.4	M	Fall from height	–	Butterfly	8
Case 2	6.2	M	Motorcar accident	Pin site infection	Transverse	9
Case 3	7.4	F	Motorcar accident	–	Spiral	8
Case 4	6.1	M	Motorcar accident	–	Transverse	7
Case 5	3.8	M	Motorcar accident	–	Short oblique	6
Case 6	7	M	Motorcar accident	Pin site infection	Transverse	9
Case 7	7.3	M	Motorcar accident	–	Spiral	9
Case 8	7.1	F	Motorcar accident	–	Transverse	7
Case 9	7.6	M	Motorcar accident	Pin site infection	Transverse	9
Case 10	4.5	M	Motorcar accident	–	Short oblique	7
Case 11	4.1	F	Fall from height	–	Spiral	7
Case 12	4.7	M	Motorcar accident	–	Transverse	7
Case 13	6.4	M	Motorcar accident	–	Transverse	8
Case 14	11.5	M	Motorcar accident	Pin site infection	Transverse	12

tive fixation of paediatric femoral fractures were presence of an associated closed head injury and/or multiple injuries, open fractures and failure of conservative treatment. We applied the same indications for this study but extended the indications to include isolated subtrochanteric femoral fractures as we felt it difficult to maintain such fractures in an accepted position by non-operative means.

Aronson et al. [1] studied 54 children who had been treated with distal femoral 90/90 traction for an average of 24 days before being placed in a 1 1/2 hip spica cast. At an average follow-up of 4.3 years, all children were functionally normal and showed a symmetric range of motion of hip and knee. This method requires a long period of hospitalization and accurate control of fracture alignment with frequent radiographs and adjustments in traction as needed. The external fixation method proposed in this study requires less hospitalization time no major adjustment after application.

Hughes et al. [7] evaluated 23 children ranging in age from 2 through 10 years who had femoral fractures treated with early spica casting to determine the impact of treatment on the patients and their families. The greatest problems encountered by the family in caring for a child in a spica cast were transportation, cast intolerance by the child and hygiene. Although most children did not attend school while in the cast, no child was required to repeat a grade and the parents reported no permanent psychological effects. The researchers found treatment in a spica cast was much easier overall for families having pre-school children rather than for those with school-age children. Such data should inform the decisions of orthopaedic surgeons and families who are trying to choose among the many options for young school-age children. In this study, transportation did not pose an issue as the child was allowed to weight-bear as tolerated and the after-care was easier.

Ferguson and Nicol [4] conducted a prospective study of early spica casting for children <10 years of age. They found that age >7 years was a variable predictive of a higher risk of failure of this technique for achieving satisfactory alignment. Martinez et al. [11] reported excessive shortening and angular deformity in 26 of 51 patients after immediate spica casting. In comparison, the small sample in this study showed an outcome without shortening or angular deformity for all ages treated with this configuration of Ilizarov external fixation.

Ward et al. [14] reported the use of a 4.5-mm AO dynamic compression plate for the treatment of femoral shaft fractures in 25 children, 6–16 years of age, 22 of whom had associated fractures or multisystem injury. The average time to fracture union was 11 weeks. Kregor et al. [10] reported on 12 patients who had 15 femoral fractures treated with compression plating with an average union time of 8 weeks. The average healing time in this study was comparable to that reported by Kregor et al.

Fyodorov et al. [6] reported hardware failure in 2 of 23 femoral fractures treated with dynamic compression plating. Hardware failure occurred at 6 weeks with one patient treated by revision plating and the other with spica casting; both fractures healed uneventfully. Ward et al. [14] reported one broken plate post-operatively in a boy who began full weight bearing a few days post-operatively. Implant failure did not occur in any patient in this series.

Good results have been reported using external fixators for femoral shaft fractures [2, 12], but the problem using external fixation in subtrochanteric femoral fractures was the limited room for application of the pins into the proximal femoral fragment. This problem is avoided by adopting the calcar fixation (rather than neck fixation) technique. There is better control of the proximal fragment, especially for correcting rotation and varus; this can be difficult to achieve or maintain with other minimally invasive internal fixation techniques, e.g. flexible intramedullary nails [5].

Conclusions

We describe a new configuration of half pin insertion for subtrochanteric femoral fractures in children. Although the case series is of a small sample, the benefits have been shown to include avoidance of a large surgical exposure, decreased blood loss, risk of deep infection, an accurate and sustained reduction in the fracture displacement, early mobilization with a short hospital stay and avoiding the need for another open procedure for implant removal. Drawbacks include familiarity with the use of the Ilizarov fixator, the inconvenience to the patient of using the external fixator and the possibility of pin site-related problems.

Informed consent Written informed consent was signed by all patients.

References

1. Aronson DD, Singer RM, Higgins RF (1987) Skeletal traction for fractures of the femoral shaft in children. A long-term study. J Bone Joint Surg 69-A:1435–1439
2. Blaiser RD, Aronson J, Tursky EA (1997) External fixation of femur fractures in children. J Pediatr Orthop 17:342–346
3. DeLee JC, Clanton TO, Rockwood CA Jr (1981) Closed treatment of subtrochanteric fractures of the femur in a modified cast brace. J Bone Joint Surg 63-A:773–779
4. Ferguson J, Nicol RO (2000) Early spica treatment of pediatric femoral shaft fractures. J Pediatr Orthop 20:189–192
5. Flynn JM, Hresko T, Reynolds RA et al (2001) Titanium elastic nails for pediatric femur fractures: a multicenter study of early results with analysis of complications. J Pediatr Orthop 21:4–8
6. Fyodorov I, Sturm PF, Robertson WW Jr (1999) Compression-plate fixation of femoral shaft fractures in children aged 8–12 years. J Pediatr Orthop 19:578–581
7. Hughes BF, Sponseller PD, Thompson JD (1995) Pediatric femur fractures: effects of spica cast treatment on family and community. J Pediatr Orthop 15(4):457–460
8. Ireland DC, Fisher RL (1975) Subtrochanteric fractures of the femur in children. Clin Orthop 110:157–166
9. Kasser JR, Beaty JH (2006) Femoral shaft fractures. In: Beaty JH, Kasser JR (eds) Rockwood and Wilkins, fractures in children, vol 3, 6th edn. Lippincott Williams and Wilkins, Philadelphia, pp 894–936

10. Kregor PJ, Song KM, Routt MLC et al (1993) Plate fixation of femoral shaft fractures in multiply injured children. J Bone Joint Surg 75-A:1774–1780

11. Martinez AG, Carrol NC, Sarwark JF et al (1991) Femoral shaft fractures in children treated with early spica cast. J Pediatr Orthop 11:712–716

12. Miner T, Carrol KL (2000) Outcomes of external fixation of pediatric femoral shaft fractures. J Pediatr Orthop 20:405–410

13. Reeves RB, Ballard RI, Hughes JL (1990) Internal fixation versus traction and casting of adolescent femoral shaft fractures. J Pediatr Orthop 10:592–595

14. Ward WT, Levy J, Kaye A (1992) Compression plating for child and adolescent femur fractures. J Pediatr Orthop 12:626–632

25

Femoral locking plate failure salvaged with hexapod circular external fixation: a report of two cases

N. Ferreira[1] · L. C. Marais[2]

Abstract Femoral non-unions are difficult to treat even for the experienced orthopaedic trauma surgeon. If the non-union follows failure of modern stable internal fixation, the complexity of the management is further increased. We report two cases of stiff hypertrophic femoral non-unions after failed locking plate fixation that were successfully treated with a new hexapod circular external fixator. In addition to providing the necessary stability for functional rehabilitation and union, the hexapod circular fixator software allows gradual correction of deformities in order to restore the normal mechanical alignment of the limb.

Keywords Locking plate · Non-union · Hexapod · Circular external fixator · Reconstruction

Background

The use of locking plate technology for orthopaedic trauma has increased in the past 10 years. Their use has a considerable learning curve and is governed by strict biomechanical principles that have to be adhered to [1–3]. Failing to do so can result in a biomechanical environment that is not conducive to fracture healing and may potentially lead to mechanical failure and non-union development [1, 4, 5].

✉ N. Ferreira
nferreira@sun.ac.za

[1] Present Address: Department of Orthopaedic Surgery, Tygerberg Hospital, University of Stellenbosch, Cape Town 7505, South Africa

[2] Tumour, Sepsis and Reconstruction Unit, Department of Orthopaedic Surgery, Greys Hospital, Nelson R. Mandela School of Medicine, University of KwaZulu Natal, Pietermaritzburg, South Africa

Managing non-unions after internal fixation can be challenging for even the most experienced orthopaedic trauma surgeon [6–10]. There is significant morbidity for the patient in terms of immobility, time away from work, narcotic dependency, and emotional impairment as patients are disillusioned often with medical services [11, 12]. Femoral non-unions in particular have profound influence on quality of life often leading to early retirement and unemployment [13]. The optimal management strategy to promote rapid consolidation of the non-union while simultaneously allowing functional rehabilitation remains unclear.

We report two cases of femoral non-unions associated with failure of locking plate fixation which were successfully treated with the TL-Hex (Orthofix, Verona, Italy) circular external fixator.

Case 1

A 36-year-old man was referred after failure of internal fixation to an open fracture (Gustilo–Anderson IIIA) of the distal meta-diaphysis of the left femur 5 months earlier. This initial injury was managed by emergency debridement, irrigation and distal femoral locking plate fixation. At presentation with the non-union, the patient had healed scars with no evidence of sepsis. The painful non-union was evident clinically and associated with a varus deformity of the femur in the region of the fracture site.

Local and systemic staging confirmed the patient to be smoker with no other co-morbidities. Radiographs displayed a broken locking plate and a femoral non-union with a 12° varus and 5° procurvatum deformity (Fig. 1). Knee motion was reduced, with a passive range of motion from full extension to 50° flexion. No evidence of infection

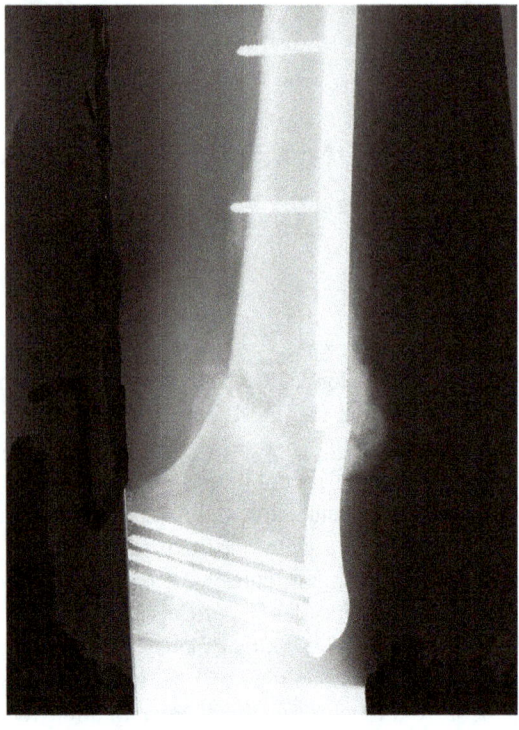

Fig. 1 Anteroposterior radiograph of the distal femur demonstrating angulation, nonunion and failed locking plate at the fracture site

was found after routine biochemical investigation and confirmed after intra-operative sampling.

Surgery consisted of plate and screw removal through an exposure along the entire length of the plate followed by circular external fixator application (TL-Hex, Orthofix SRL, Verona, Italy) using the 'rings first' method. Proximal fixation consisted of three hydroxyapatite coated half pins secured to a 5/8th ring and an arch. Distal fixation consisted of one 1.8 mm tensioned transverse wire and two hydroxyapatite half pins secured to a full ring (Fig. 2). The non-union site was left undisturbed, and no bone graft used.

After a latency period of 7 days, gradual correction was achieved over 6 days. This included 5 mm of distraction at a rate of 1 mm per day to facilitate reduction. Final anatomical alignment in the coronal and sagittal plane was confirmed on radiographs. Functional rehabilitation was encouraged with the assistance of a physiotherapist during the correction and consolidation phases. Full weight bearing was allowed from the first post-operative day. Pin track care followed our standard protocol and included twice daily cleaning with an alcoholic solution of chlorhexidine [14, 15].

The only complications encountered during the treatment period were minor pin track infections. One half pin developed a Checketts and Otterburn stage II infection that responded to oral antibiotics [16]. The tensioned wire developed a stage III infection at a late stage of treatment. The wire was removed without further complications.

Radiographs confirmed solid union with exuberant callus formation after 13 weeks. The external fixator was removed when painless weight bearing on a dynamized frame was achieved. At last follow-up, 9 months after frame removal, no deformity had occurred at the union site and knee range of motion had improved at full extension to 90° flexion (Fig. 3).

Case 2

The second patient had two failed attempts at locking plate fixation of a left femur fracture. This 22-year-old male sustained a closed fracture of the diaphysis treated with a femoral locking plate. After failure at the screw-plate interface, a repeat of the locking plate fixation was performed. This second plate fractured at the femoral non-union site (Fig. 4).

Local and systemic staging confirmed the patient to be a smoker with no other co-morbidities. Radiographs revealed a broken locking plate and a femoral non-union with a 3°

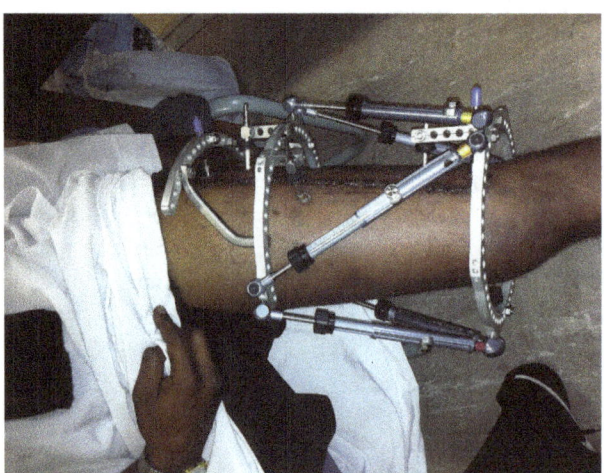

Fig. 2 TL-Hex fixator post correction of femoral deformity

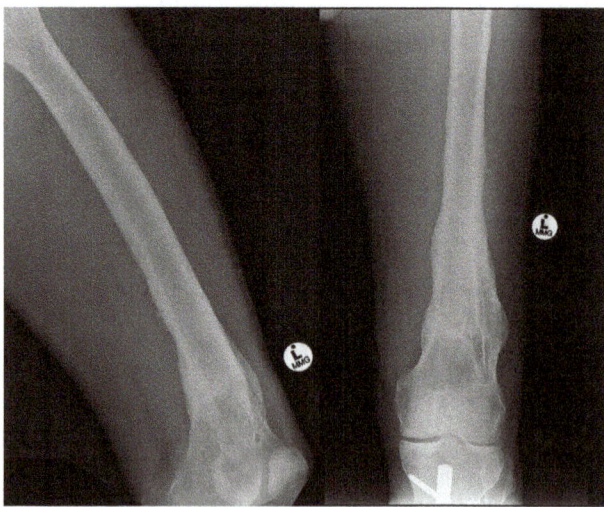

Fig. 3 Anteroposterior and lateral radiographs of united femur after hexapod removal

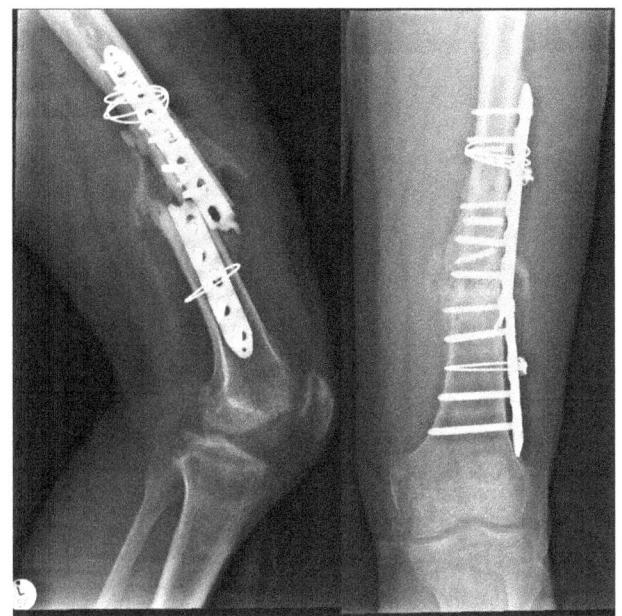

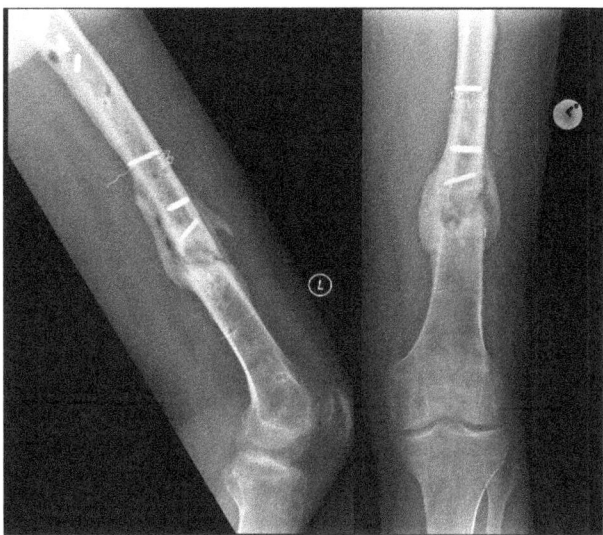

Fig. 5 Anteroposterior and lateral radiographs of united femur after hexapod removal

Fig. 4 Anteroposterior and lateral radiographs of the femur demonstrating angulation, nonunion and failed locking plate at the fracture site

valgus, 18 mm posterior translation and 18° procurvatum deformity. Knee motion was reduced, with a passive range of motion from full extension to 70° flexion. Routine biochemical and subsequent intra-operative sampling confirmed no infection.

Surgery consisted of plate removal and circular external fixator (TL-Hex) application. The plate was exposed along its entire length to facilitate removal of all accessible metalware with several broken screws left in situ and the non-union site left undisturbed. External fixation application followed the same design as described in the first case and with no bone graft used.

After a latency period of 7 days, gradual correction was achieved over 17 days. This included 5 mm of distraction at a rate of 1 mm per day to facilitate reduction. Final anatomical alignment in the coronal and sagittal plane was confirmed on radiographs. After 14 weeks of functional rehabilitation, solid union was confirmed by radiographs and the external fixator removed. No complications were encountered during the treatment process and at last follow-up, 10 months after frame removal, there was no deformity at the union site and knee range of motion had improved from full extension to 110° flexion (Fig. 5).

Discussion

Locking plates are fundamentally different from conventional plates [2, 3, 5]. The biomechanical properties of locking plates are, more appropriately, likened to external fixators than traditional plates and screws [5, 17]. Locking

plates rely on fixed angle screws to provide stability rather than the friction between the plate and bone generated by screw torque [17]. This intrinsic dissimilarity makes conventional plates and locking plates suited for use in different clinical scenarios [3, 18]. Conventional plates are ideal for achieving union through primary bone healing, with precise reduction, interfragmentary compression and rigid fixation [5, 17, 18]. Locking plates on the other hand are better suited for providing elastic fixation that result in secondary fracture healing with callus formation [3, 5, 17, 18].

When the biomechanical principles of locking plates are not adhered to and these plates are applied like conventional plates, a high strain environment may result that exposes the fracture site to potential non-union formation and construct failure [1, 5, 18]. The human body naturally heals fractures by minimising strain across the fracture site. This is achieved by either decreasing the motion across the fracture site, or by increasing the length of the fracture gap [18]. When there is very rigid fixation, resorption at the fracture site attempts to decrease the strain by increasing the gap length [3, 18]. This is seen where short locking plates are applied with a high screw density as normally done in conventional compression plating. In this setting, non-union formation may result, ultimately leading to construct failure [1]. This was evident in both our cases where non-union development was followed by implant failure.

Non-union in the setting of failed internal fixation is challenging to manage [19]. Firstly, infection must be excluded as the management of an infected non-union is fundamentally different from aseptic non-unions. Secondly, classifying these non-unions according to the traditional Weber and Cech system might not be appropriate. This classification relies on the radiographic appearance of the fracture ends to distinguish between avascular and hypervascular non-unions but fail to take account of previous fixation or adequacy of fixation [19–21]. Wu et al. [19] have suggested a revised protocol to classify femoral non-unions following internal fixation. The authors considered non-unions with stable fixation as avascular and non-unions with unstable fixation as hypervascular. Their proposed protocol underlines a need to take the non-union pathogenesis into account when considering the management strategy. In both these case examples, after plate failure, the unstable situation led to hypervascular non-unions.

Femoral non-unions have no clear evidence-based treatment guidelines. A recent systematic review by Somford et al. [22] has suggested a treatment algorithm for femoral non-unions. They specifically provide treatment recommendations for femoral non-unions that occur after initial internal fixation, suggesting reamed nailing after previous plating and plate fixation after previous intramedullary nailing. This underlines the basic reconstructive principle that when one mode of fixation has failed, another mode of fixation should be considered for the revision surgery.

Gershuni [23] outlined the principles for optimal non-union treatment. This included restitution of bony continuity, correction of alignment in all planes, maintenance and recovery of function and limitation of further complications. Hexapod external fixation can fulfil all these requirements. These devices are a modification of the traditional Ilizarov-type fine wire circular external fixator and are able to provide stable fixation and allow early functional rehabilitation [24, 25]. Hexapod fixators consist of two rings connected with six oblique struts in an octahedral configuration. Mathematical algorithms calculate strut length adjustments in order to manipulate the orientations of the two rings to each other [26, 27]. By attaching each of these rings to a bone segment, their position and orientation can be altered, thereby facilitating the reduction of complex multiplanar deformities.

In stiff non-unions, the ability of the hexapod circular external fixator is to provide controlled correction of existing deformities, but, through gradual distraction, the stimulation of new bone formation. This 'tension-stress effect' was initially described by Ilizarov [28–30] and is the biological basis of distraction histogenesis used in limb lengthening and bone transport. It is thus possible, in scenarios involving reduced biological potential, to stimulate natural bone healing without the addition of bone graft or other biologic adjuvants. This was demonstrated in both cases where stiff hypertrophic non-unions healed with exuberant callus formation through gradual distraction without the addition of bone graft.

Conclusion

Locking plate biomechanics are distinctly different from conventional plating. When locking plate principles are not adhered to, non-unions and fixation failure may result. The salvage for these cases can be difficult as broken metalware, bony destruction and deformity is encountered frequently. This treatment strategy using a hexapod circular external fixator provides the option of gradual reduction of deformities together with stable fixation that allows immediate functional rehabilitation.

Informed consent Written consent was obtained from both patients for publication of this report and any accompanying images.

References

1. Leahy M (2010) When locking plates fail. AAOS Now 5(5):9
2. Cronier P, Pietu G, Dujardin C, Bigorre N, Ducellier F, Gerard R (2010) The concept of locking plates. Orthop Traumatol Surg Res. PubMed PMID: 20447888
3. Gardner M, Helfet D, Lorich DG (2004) Has locked plating completely replaced conventional plating? Am J Orthop 33(9):439–446
4. Hak DJ, Toker S, Yi C, Toreson J (2010) The influence of fracture fixation biomechanics on fracture healing. Orthopedics 33(10):752–755
5. Strauss EJ, Schwarzkopf R, Kummer F, Egol KA (2008) The current status of locked plating: the good, the bad, and the ugly. J Orthop Trauma 22(7):479–486
6. Harwood P, Newman J, Michael ALR (2010) An update on fracture healing and non-union. Orthop Trauma 24(1):9–23
7. Abumunaser LA, Al-Sayyad MJ (2011) Evaluation of the calori et Al nonunion scoring system in a retrospective case series. Orthopedics 34(5):359
8. Bhandari M, Schemitsch E (2000) Clinical advances in the treatment of fracture nonunion: the response to mechanical stimulation. Cur Opin Orthop 11:372–377
9. Dimitriou R, Kanakaris N, Soucacos PN, Giannoudis PV (2013) Genetic predisposition to non-union: evidence today. Injury 44(Suppl 1):S50–S53
10. Tzioupis C, Giannoudis PV (2007) Prevalence of long-bone non-unions. Injury 38(Suppl 2):S3–S9
11. Antonova E, Le Kim T, Burge R, Mershon J (2013) Tibia Shaft fracture—costly burden of nonunions.pdf. BMC Musculoskel Disord 14:42
12. Perumal V, Roberts C (2007) (ii) Factors contributing to nonunion of fractures. Curr Orthop. 21(4):258–261
13. Zeckey C, Mommsen P, Andruszkow H, Macke C, Frink M, Stubig T, et al. (2011) The aseptic femoral and tibial shaft nonunion in healthy patients—an analysis of the health-related quality of life and the socioeconomic outcome. Open Orthop J 5:193–7. PubMed PMID: 21686321. Pubmed Central PMCID: 3115668
14. Ferreira N, Marais LC (2012) Osteosarcoma presentation stages at a tumour unit in South Africa. S Afr Med J 102(8):673–676
15. Ferreira N, Marais LC (2012) Prevention and management of external fixator pin track sepsis. Strat Traum Limb Recon 7(2):67–72. PubMed PMID: 22729940. Pubmed Central PMCID: 3535127

16. Checkets RG, Otterburn M, MacEachern G (1993) Pin track infection: definition, incidence and prevention. Int J Orthop Trauma 3(Suppl):16–18

17. Kubiak EN, Fulkerson E, Strauss E, Egol KA (2006) The evolution of locked plates. J Bone Joint Surg [Am]. 88(4):189–200

18. Egol KA, Kubiak EN, Fulkerson E, Kummer FJ, Koval KJ (2004) Biomechanics of locked plates and screws. J Orthop Trauma 18(8):488–493

19. Wu CC, Chen WJ (2000) A revised protocol for more clearly classifying a nonunion. J Orthop Surg 8(1):45–52

20. Judet J, Judet R (1960) L'osteogene et les retards de consolidation et les pseudarthroses des os longs. Huitieme Congress SICOT 15

21. Weber B, Cech O (eds) (1976) Pseudarthrosis. Hans Huber, Bern

22. Somford MP, van den Bekerom MP, Kloen P (2013) Operative treatment for femoral shaft nonunions, a systematic review of the literature. Strat Traum Limb Recon 8(2):77–88. PubMed PMID: 23892497. Pubmed Central PMCID: 3732674

23. Gershuni DH (1989) Fracture nonunion. West J Med 150(6):689–690. PubMed PMID: 2750154. Pubmed Central PMCID: 1026720

24. Fadel M, Hosny G (2005) The Taylor spatial frame for deformity correction in the lower limbs. Int Orthop 29(2):125–129. PubMed PMID: 15703937. Pubmed Central PMCID: 3474509

25. Taylor J. Correction of general deformity with the Taylor Spatial Frame. http://www.jcharlestaylor.com2002

26. Gao XS, Lei D, Liao Q, Zhang GF (2005) Generalized Stewart–Gough platforms and their direct kinematics. IEEE Trans 21(2):141–151

27. Husty ML (1996) An algorithm for solving the direct kinematics of general Stewart–Gough platforms. Mech Mach Theory 31(4):365–379

28. Ilizarov GA (1989) The tension-stress effect on the genesis and growth of tissues: part II. The influence of the rate and frequency of distraction. Clin Orthop Relat Res 239:263–285

29. Ilizarov GA (1989) The tension-stress effect on the genesis and growth of tissues. Part I. The influence of stability of fixation and soft-tissue preservation. Clin Orthop Relat Res 238:249–281

30. Ilizarov GA (1990) Clinical application of the tension-stress effect for limb lengthening. Clin Orthop Relat Res 250:8–26

26

Correction osteotomy of distal radius malunion stabilised with dorsal locking plates without grafting

D. Tiren · D. I. Vos

Abstract The purpose of this study was to evaluate the results of our correction osteotomies of distal radial malunions without a bone graft. Eleven consecutive patients (mean age 52 years, range 18–71) were treated. A dorsal approach was utilised to perform an opening-wedge osteotomy which then was stabilised with two dorsal columnar plates without filling the osteotomy gap. All patients went on to radiographic union with a filling of the osteotomy gap within a mean period of 3 months (range 2–6 months). All patients had satisfactory results in terms of function and pain. Correction osteotomy and stabilisation with bicolumnar locked plate fixation without a bone graft provides sufficient stability to allow the highly vascularised metaphysis to heal. In patients without risk factors predisposing to non-union, this procedure is safe and feasible.

Keywords Correction osteotomy · Corrective osteotomy · Distal radius · Malunion · Bone graft · Locking plates

Introduction

The distal radius fracture is the most common fracture treated in the emergency department. The most common complication of this fracture is malunion which occurs in up to 25 % of conservatively and in 10 % of operatively treated cases [1]. Although a small part of these fractures lead to a symptomatic malunion, correction osteotomy is a frequently performed procedure due to the high incidence of the distal radius fracture [2].

Opening-wedge correction osteotomy of the distal radius is an established but challenging procedure [3]. By this procedure, the foremost complaints such as limited wrist and forearm motion and reduced grip strength are improved and pain diminishes as reported by over 200 papers [3]. The outcome of the procedure is determined by patient selection and adequate restoration of the original anatomy [1, 4, 5].

The procedure consists of correcting the anatomy by performing an osteotomy, filling of the osteotomy gap while maintaining the correction, and stabilising it with plates. Traditionally, the osteotomy gap is filled with an iliac crest corticocancellous bone graft and supported by rigid plate fixation. Although use of other donor sites has been described, the iliac crest remains the golden standard. The harvesting of iliac crest bone can result in donor-site morbidity as high as 20 % [6]. The alternative is to use expensive bone graft substitutes, while the optimal replacement material for the distal radius remains unclear [7].

By leaving the osteotomy gap unfilled, the additional procedure of harvesting the graft is avoided and the surgeon can concentrate on the most important aspect of the procedure that determines the outcome, which is correction of the anatomical deformity.

In this paper, we describe the results of distal radius correction osteotomy in patients with symptomatic malunion with dorsal bicolumnar locked plating, without filling the osteotomy defect.

D. Tiren (✉) · D. I. Vos
Department of General and Trauma Surgery, Amphia Hospital, Postbus 90158, 4800 RK Breda, The Netherlands
e-mail: Davut.Tiren@gmail.com

Patients and methods

Patient selection

Between 2009 and 2011, we treated eleven consecutive patients with a symptomatic dorsal malunion of the distal radius. The medical files, radiographs and outpatient notes were retrospectively analysed.

All patients had undergone an opening-wedge osteotomy through a dorsal approach and dorsal bicolumnar locked plating with 2.4 mm columnar stabilisation plates from Synthes©. The osteotomy gap was left unfilled.

The patient demographics, fracture characteristics and initial treatment method along with the symptoms are summarised in Table 1.

The indication for correction osteotomy of the distal radius was based mainly on clinical findings such as pain and functional impairment in combination with findings on X-ray. A dorsal angulation of more than 15° or a substantial dorsal angulation with a more than 2 mm shortening of the radial height were the accompanying radiological criteria mostly used. The preoperative workup included a CT scan of the malunited fracture. On indication, an MRI and routinely an X-ray of the contralateral wrist to determine the normal anatomical relationship were performed.

Patients with risk factors known to predispose to nonunion of the distal radius, such as morbid obesity, tobacco abuse and diabetes mellitus were treated by other means.

Surgical technique

The dorsal approach to the distal radius was utilised as described by Rikli and Regazzoni [8]. The procedure was carried out under general or regional anaesthesia with a tourniquet and fluoroscopic control. The forearm and hand were disinfected and draped. A 7–10-cm straight incision was performed, over an imaginary line between the base of the second metacarpal, crossing over Listers tubercle towards the border of the muscle belly of the first extensor compartment. For our purpose, the part of the incision distal to the joint crease was not utilised. The subcutaneous tissue was divided, and the extensor retinaculum was incised through the third compartment to identify and free

Table 1 Patient demographics, fracture characteristics, initial treatment and remarks

Patient Nr/sex/age	AO/ Fernandez classification	Delay of osteotomy (weeks)	Fracture side/ dominance	Foremost complaint at presentation	Initial treatment	Additional remarks
1/M/18	C1/III	19	R/R	Pain in rest and movement	Cast immobilisation	–
2/M/63	C1/III	23	L/R	Functional impairment	Cast immobilisation	–
3/M/62	A3/I	14	L/R	Pain in rest and movement	Cast immobilisation	–
4/F/41	C1/III	19	R/R	Pain in rest and movement	Mini AO double plates	Contralateral distal radial fracture
5/F/36	A2/I	13	L/R	Pain in rest and impaired strength	Cast immobilisation	Plates removed at 6 months
6/F/72	A2/I	16	L/R	Pain and functional impairment	Cast immobilisation	CRPS-1
7/F/57	A3/I	26	L/R	Pain and impaired strength	Cast immobilisation	TFCC tear
8/F/49	A2/I	21	R/R	Pain and carpal tunnel compression	Cast immobilisation	CTS
9/M/47	C1/III	15	L/R	Pain and functional impairment	Cast immobilisation	–
10/F/61	A2/I	37	L/R	Carpal tunnel compression and functional impairment	Cast immobilisation	CTS
11/F/66	A2/I	11	L/L	Pain, functional impairment	External fixation	–

M male, *F* female, *L* left, *R* right, *TFCC* triangular fibrocartilaginous complex, *CRPS-1* complex regional pain syndrome type 1, *CTS* carpal tunnel syndrome

the extensor pollicis longus (EPL) tendon. It was held aside with a vessel loop and sometimes behind a Hohmann or a wound retractor. The floor of the third compartment was incised and subperiostally dissected to preserve the second and the fourth compartments. Radially dissection was towards the brachioradialis tendon and ulnarly towards the distal radioulnar joint.

The correction osteotomy was performed as described by Fernandez [4]. Approximately 2 centimetres proximal to the wrist joint the osteotomy site was marked and two K-wires placed; one parallel to the wrist joint and the other tangential to the radius. The osteotomy was performed with an oscillating saw, parallel to the distal K-wire. Using a laminar spreader, the osteotomy was widened until the K-wires were parallel to each other, volar cortical contact being maintained. Using preoperative measurements, additional corrections were performed to correct radial inclination by positioning the laminar spreader more radially while keeping the K-wires parallel. In some cases, an external fixator was placed between the two K-wires to support the reduction with the laminar spreader, while small adjustments were made. When the optimal reduction was achieved under fluoroscopic control, first the dorsoradial plate was positioned underneath the second compartment to support the radial styloid. Then, the radioulnar plate was placed in an angle of approximately 50°–70° to the first plate. After preliminary fixation of the plates, the laminar spreader was removed and the correction verified before definitive fixation of the plates. At least two locked screws were used proximal and distal to the osteotomy site in both plates. The EPL tendon was protected by creating a flap from the extensor tendon retinaculum. The skin was sutured, no wound drains were used, and a compressive bandage was placed over the operated area as far as the elbow.

Postoperative treatment and follow-up

Postoperatively early finger motion and forearm rotation were encouraged. A removable splint was provided for comfort for the first 2 weeks. After splint removal, the wrist was actively and passively mobilised. Powerful and resistive exercises were prohibited until radiographic healing. All other comfortable reasonable daily activities were allowed.

At 2, 6 and 12 weeks and if necessary every 6 weeks after 3 months, patients visited the outpatient clinic where the range of movement of the wrist was assessed and X-rays obtained. Patients were discharged after radiological union and a satisfactory clinical result.

Data collection and statistical analysis

Preoperatively informed consent was obtained, including the disclosure of the possibility of delayed union and non-

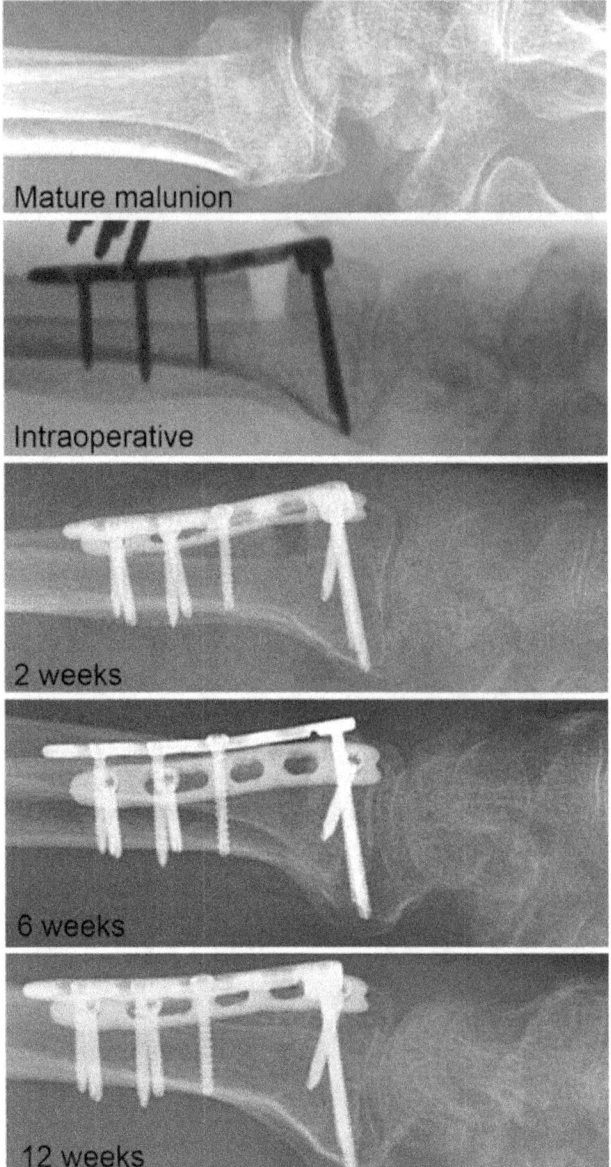

Fig. 1 Correction of the deformity and healing of the osteotomy gap

union which would require a second operation. Range of movement and radiographic changes were documented during each outpatient visit. At the final outpatient visit, the quick-DASH and the Mayo Wrist scores were evaluated. The digitally calibrated radiographs were analysed on high-resolution terminals and measurements performed on preoperative, postoperative and the final radiographs by the first author.

A gradual closing of the osteotomy gap could be observed clearly on the lateral radiographs of the distal radius (Fig. 1). This observation was used to determine union. Closure of the osteotomy gap began at the volar side and followed to the dorsal side until dorsal cortical bridging was complete. The complete dorsal bridging of the osteotomy gap was defined as the moment of union.

Table 2 Summary of radiological and functional results

	Preoperative Mean (±SD)	Postoperative Mean (±SD)	Improvement (±SD)	p value Student's t test
Radiographic measurements				
Volar tilt (°)	−22 (7)	4 (6)	26 (6)	p < 0.0001
Radial inclination (°)	16 (3)	22 (3)	7 (2)	p = 0.0002
Radial height (mm)	7 (3)	14 (2)	6 (5)	p < 0.0001
Range of motion				
Wrist flexion (°)	34 (16)	71 (13)		p < 0.0001
Wrist extension (°)	45 (20)	67 (15)		p = 0.010
Forearm pronation (°)	52 (16)	85 (6)		p < 0.0001
Forearm supination (°)	41 (19)	80 (7)		p < 0.0001
Flexion–extension arc (°)	79 (29)	138 (21)	59 (30)	p < 0.0001
Pronation–supination arc (°)	93 (32)	165 (12)	72 (33)	p < 0.0001
Functional outcome scores				
Mayo wrist score		92 (6)		
q-DASH score		10 (6)		
Time to union		13 (6)		

Pre- and postoperative measurements were compared using dependent sample *t* test for continuous data. *p* values of <0.05 were considered statistically significant.

Results

There were no preoperative or postoperative complications on follow-up evaluation (average of 8 months, range 6–13 months) of our case series. The radiological and functional findings pre- and postoperatively and the results of the outcome scoring postoperatively are summarised in Table 2.

Radiological findings

All osteotomies demonstrated a radiological union of the osteotomy deficit in a mean time of 13 weeks (range 6–24 weeks). There was a correlation between the degree of angular correction and the time to healing of the osteotomy gap (Fig. 2).

The dorsal tilt was corrected by the procedure with a mean of 26°, from a mean dorsal flexion of 22° before the procedure (range 30°–6° dorsal tilt) to a mean palmar flexion of 4° after the procedure (range 2°–15° volar tilt). Radial inclination was improved from a mean of 16 (range 8°–20°) to 22 (range 18°–26°) degrees by the procedure. The radial height was improved from a mean of 7 (range 3–13) mm preoperatively to a mean of 14 (range 12–18) mm postoperatively.

All radiological measurements showed statistically significant improvement postoperatively compared with preoperative measurements.

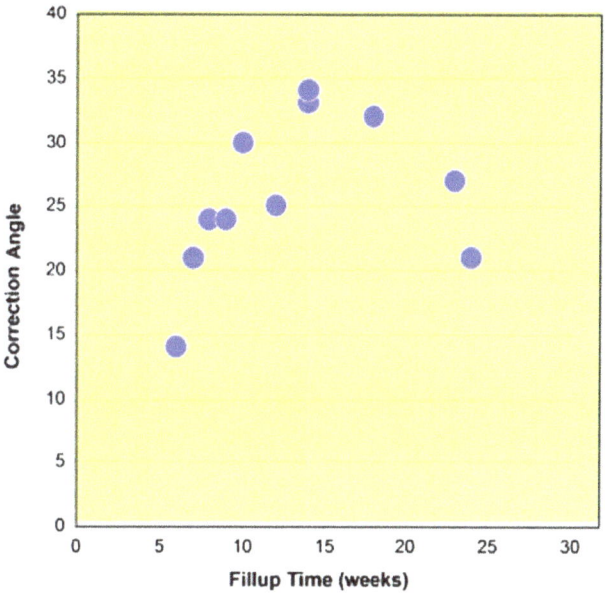

Fig. 2 Correlation between the correction angle and the fill-up time

The follow-up radiographs during the different intervals did not show any loss of reduction or implant failure. Neither were osteoarthritic changes seen during this follow-up.

Clinical outcomes

During the final follow-up visit, a mean wrist and forearm motion was achieved of 71° of flexion (range 40–85), 67° of extension (range 40–90), 85° of pronation (range 70–90) and 80° of supination (range 65–85), when compared with a mean wrist and forearm motion of 34° flexion (range 10–45), 45° of extension, 52° pronation (range 30–70) and 41° of supination (range 10–60) preoperatively. The wrist flexion–extension arc was improved by a mean of 59° (range 20°–110°), and the forearm rotation arc was improved by a mean of 72° (range 10°–135°).

All measurements postoperatively showed a statistically significant improvement.

The modified Mayo Wrist score outcome was excellent in 5 patients, good in 5 patients and satisfactory in one patient. The mean modified Mayo Wrist score was 92 points of 100 (range 80–100).

The q-DASH score was 10 at final follow-up (range 2.3–20.5).

The wrist function gradually improved during the follow-up visits. The pain present in most of the patients and the median nerve compression symptoms in two patients, resolved with the correction.

The TFCC tear of one patient was repaired through a separate incision. After the operation, she had a stable wrist and a good function. All patients were pain-free in rest and could perform their daily activities without pain. One of the patients had some discomfort with forceful forearm rotation during the final visit which did not limit his daily activities.

Only one patient requested removal of the osteosynthesis because of a palpable plate below the scar and a wish for correction of the scar. This procedure was performed 6 months after the correction osteotomy and we could verify the consistency of the new filled up bone which was as solid as the other parts of the distal radius.

We did not encounter complications due to the plate on the dorsal side such as tendon ruptures, tendinitis or adhesions during the follow-up period of this study.

Discussion

We documented good results in our series where we performed a distal radial correction osteotomy for distal radial malunion stabilising it using double-locked plates without filling the osteotomy gap.

The patients had a mean correction of 26° volar tilt and 6 millimetres of radial height resulting in a mean wrist motion of 138° and a forearm rotation of 165°. We had no loss of reduction before healing of the osteotomy gap which occurred after a mean time of 13 weeks. There was no case of infection, implant failure, loss of reduction, delayed union or non-union. However, when the correction of the angle was greater and consequently the osteotomy gap wider, the time for complete union was longer. Even for duration of 24 weeks, the double-dorsal-locked plates construction proved stable enough to maintain the reduction. These results compare with and in some cases are more favourable to other published series [4, 9–11].

As described by Fernandez [4], the traditional correction osteotomy includes correction of the deformity and filling of the opened wedge with a full-thickness iliac crest bone graft. The graft should make a perfect fit with the osteotomy gap to support the reduction. This is held in place with an osteosynthesis. The function of this full-thickness corticocancellous bone graft is twofold: support of the correction and induction of bone healing.

Ring et al. [10] demonstrated that the supportive function of the corticocancellous graft is not necessary when locked plates are used. However, he used cancellous bone graft to induce bone healing in the osteotomy gap. Since cancellous graft harvesting has significant less donor-site morbidity, augmenting the osteotomy gap with cancellous graft has replaced grafting the gap with full-thickness corticocancellous bone graft when used in combination with locked plates in this procedure.

The distal radial metaphysis is a highly vascularised bone with excellent healing capacity [12]. This is why in our opinion there is no reason to induce bone healing by bone grafting, since performing the osteotomy initiates bone healing. Adding cancellous bone or any other biomaterials does not improve fracture healing in distal radial fractures [7, 13], supporting the concept of excellent healing capacity of the distal radial metaphysis.

However, several premorbid conditions seem to predispose to developing a non-union [12]. These conditions include diabetes mellitus, morbid obesity, tobacco abuse and severe peripheral vascular disease. These can be seen as the biological disturbance that affects bone healing.

Even though mechanical support of the correction after osteotomy is achieved well by the double plate construct, this mechanical stability relies on support of the volar cortex. All our osteotomies had volar contact after the procedure. In cases where lengthening is necessary, a circular defect could be created. In our opinion, this would lead to insufficient mechanical support and stability at the osteotomy site. In such cases, we would advise harvesting a full-thickness corticocancellous graft for mechanical support of the defect.

Another area, similar to the distal radius in terms of healing capacity and in being a donor site for cancellous bone, is the proximal tibia. High tibial osteotomies are performed in the proximal tibia. Since the advent of locked plates for high tibial osteotomy, the osteotomy defect is not filled. In a study [14] published on this subject, the authors reported good results. The osteotomy gap healed in 91 of the 92 included patients in this study without augmentation of the osteotomy defect.

One questions why hand and wrist surgeons still use bone graft or bone substitutes for correction osteotomies in the distal radius while surgeons performing correction osteotomy on the proximal end of the tibia find them unnecessary.

In 2005, Wieland et al. [11] described a series of 47 patients where they performed correction osteotomy in the distal radius without filling of the osteotomy gap. They observed that all osteotomy gaps healed within 3 months. Furthermore, they found that leaving the gap empty, simplified the procedure substantially. However, their group was heterogeneous with inclusion of volar and dorsal displaced fractures and stabilisation was with dorsal or volar plates. Notably, they stabilised the osteotomy with conventional plates. Distal radius osteotomy and stabilisation with conventional plates leads to non-union occasionally, probably due to the poorer stability these plates provide [12].

Ozer et al. [9] described a case–control study of 14 distal radius osteotomies stabilised by a locked volar plate, without filling of the osteotomy gap, and found no delay in healing compared with the control group.

Our study is the first to describe correction osteotomies of the distal radius for dorsal malunion, with double dorsal plating, without filling of the osteotomy defect. With the latter, surgical—and tourniquet time was reduced. The patient did not have to undergo a bone-grafting procedure. Nor were bone substitutes or bioactive materials, which increase the costs for this procedure substantially, used. Despite this, our functional and radiological results were similar if not better than comparable series where bone grafting or bone substitutes were used.

The limitations of this study include factors relating to the retrospective nature of this study. Preoperative functional outcome scores were not measured, and there was no control group.

Another important limitation is the small number of patients included in this study. Even though the numbers are small, these eleven patients show that it is possible to promote union in the osteotomy gap of the distal radius without filling of the gap when locked dorsal plates are used.

Furthermore, since our primary endpoint was union, our follow-up time was relatively short to report reliably on complications related to this procedure such as osteoarthritic changes, tendon irritation or tendon ruptures. To measure the time saved and the effect limiting the surgery has on the adequate correction of the anatomy, a prospective study would be necessary.

In conclusion, performing distal radial correction osteotomy for dorsally displaced distal radius malunion, stabilised by dorsal bicolumnar locked plates can be performed safely in most patients with symptomatic malunion of the distal radius without filling of the osteotomy gap. The latter reduces surgical trauma and the operating time and simplifies the procedure. The surgeon can then concentrate on the most important part of the procedure: adequate correction of the deformity.

Acknowledgments We would like to express our sincere gratitude to Dr. Frank X. O' Connor, our valued colleague from the department of anesthesiology of our hospital, for editing the manuscript for style and language.

References

1. Fernandez DL (2008) Osteotomy for extra-articular malunion of the distal radius. In: Slutsky DJ, Osterman L (eds) Fractures and injuries of the distal radius and carpus: the cutting edge. Saunders, Philadelphia, pp 529–541
2. Vroemen JC, Strackee SD (2012) Three-dimensional computer-assisted corrective osteotomy techniques for the malunited distal radius. In: Waddell JP (ed) The role of osteotomy in the correction of congenital and acquired disorders of the skeleton, pp 115–128. www.Intechopen.com
3. Prommersberger KJ, Pillukat T, Mühldorfer M, van Schoonhoven J (2012) Malunion of the distal radius. Arch Orthop Trauma Surg 132(5):693–702
4. Fernandez DL (1982) Correction of post-traumatic wrist deformity in adults by osteotomy, bone-grafting, and internal fixation. J Bone Joint Surg 64(8):1164–1178
5. Jupiter JB, Fernandez DL (2001) Complications following distal radial fracture. J Bone Joint Surg 83(8):1244–1265
6. Dimitriou R, Mataliotakis GI, Angoules AG, Kanakaris NK, Giannoudis PV (2011) Complications following autologous bone graft harvesting from the iliac crest and using the RIA: a systematic review. Injury 42(Suppl 2):S3–S15
7. Hartigan BJ, Makowiec RL (2008) Use of bone graft substitutes and bioactive materials in treatment of distal radius fractures. In: Slutsky DJ, Osterman L (eds) Fractures and injuries of the distal radius and carpus: the cutting edge. Saunders, Philadelphia, pp 241–245
8. Rikli DA, Regazzoni P (2000) The double plating technique for distal radius fractures. Tech Hand Upper Extrem Surg 4–2:107–114
9. Ozer K, Kilic A, Sabel A, Ipaktchi K (2011) The role of bone allografts in the treatment of angular malunions of the distal radius. J Hand Surg 36–11:1804–1809
10. Ring D, Roberge C, Morgan T, Jupiter JB (2002) Osteotomy for malunited fractures of the distal radius: a comparison of structural and nonstructural autogenous bone grafts. J Hand Surg 27–2:216–222
11. Wieland AWJ, Dekkers GHG, Brink PRG (2005) Open wedge osteotomy for malunited extraarticular distal radius fractures with plate osteosynthesis without bone grafting. Eur J Trauma 31:148–153
12. Prommersberger KJ, Fernandez DL (2004) Nonunion of distal radius fractures. Clin Orthop Relat Res 419:51–56
13. Handoll HH, Watts AC (2008) Bone grafts and bone substitutes for treating distal radial fractures in adults. Cochrane Database Syst Rev 2:CD006836
14. Staubli AE, De Simoni C, Babst R, Lobenhoffer P (2003) TomoFix: a new LCP-concept for open wedge osteotomy of the medial proximal tibia–early results in 92 cases. Injury 34(Suppl 2):B55–B62

27

An accurate method of determining a single-plane osteotomy to correct a combined rotational and angular deformity

James Youngman[1] · Dimitri Raptis[2] · Khalid Al-Dadah[1,3] · Fergal Monsell[4]

Abstract   Conventional osteotomy used for the correction of deformity is performed out of the plane of deformity creating a wedge either opening or closing when the deformity is corrected. Deformity that is a combination of rotation and angulation exists in a single plane that is oblique to the coronal, sagittal and axial planes depending on the magnitude of deformity measured in each plane. Accurate planning and a simple method of finding this oblique plane operatively is presented. This method starts by finding the bisector of angulation. This is marked by a wire that lies in the plane of angulation and along the bisector of angulation. The saw blade is rotated about this bisector axis according to the proportion of angulation and rotation. There is no second reorientation of the saw blade required making the final plane much easier to define. This single-plane oblique osteotomy allows accurate realignment of the limb.

Keywords   Osteotomy · Correction · Deformity · Realignment · Single cut

Introduction

Bone deformity is a combination of angulation and rotation commonly. Coronal plane angular deformity (varus and valgus) is seen on AP radiographs, and sagittal plane angular deformity (procurvatum and recurvatum) is seen on lateral radiographs. Deformity measured on both AP and lateral radiographs can be resolved into a single oblique plane. Imaging at right angles to this oblique plane of deformity shows the maximum deformity (as seen in profile), whereas imaging into the plane of deformity shows no deformity.

The plane of a pure angular deformity lies in the long axis of the bone. Rotational deformity is angulation in the axial plane. Rotational deformity is not seen on coronal or sagittal plane imaging directly and can only be measured directly on axial imaging. The plane of rotational deformity is transverse to the long axis. Osteotomy in this plane is used to correct pure rotational deformity allows full bone contact after correction.

A transverse or axial plane osteotomy used for correction of angulation creates an opening wedge requiring bone graft (or not if performed by distraction osteogenesis) or requires removal of a wedge of bone (closing wedge). If an osteotomy is carried out in the plane of deformity, it allows correction of the deformity by rotating the opposing bone surfaces while maintaining maximum bone contact. Where the deformity is both angulation and rotation, the true plane of deformity is oblique to both the long axis and the transverse plane. Osteotomy in this plane allows rotation of opposing flat surfaces that correct angular and rotational deformity simultaneously and maintain full bone contact. We present a simple graphical method for determining this total plane of deformity and the plane of osteotomy about which the total deformity can be corrected.

✉ Khalid Al-Dadah
khalidaldadah@gmail.com

James Youngman
james.youngman@uclh.nhs.uk

[1]   Department of Trauma and Orthopaedic Surgery, University College London Hospital, 235 Euston Road, London NW1 2BU, UK

[2]   University Hospital Zurich, Zurich, Switzerland

[3]   Imperial College London, London, UK

[4]   Bristol Royal Hospital for Children, Bristol, UK

Method

The following is the description of the full planning method.

Measurement of deformity

The angular deformity is measured in degrees on the AP radiograph (coronal angle C) and lateral radiograph (Sagittal angle S) using standard methods (Fig. 1). A CT scan of both the affected and normal limb is used to measure the rotational deformity (rotational angle R). The rotational angle can also be measured using clinical measurement. This method combines deformity measured on coronal, sagittal and axial images and resolves them into a single oblique plane. The coronal and sagittal planes are first resolved into the true angular deformity in the oblique plane (of the longitudinal axis), and this is combined with axial angulation (the rotational deformity, which is in effect an angular deformity in the axial plane) to determine the total deformity in a different plane.

Part one calculates the plane and magnitude of angular deformity from the AP and lateral radiographs giving the total deformity in the longitudinal plane. Part two calculates the total deformity by combining rotational and angular deformity.

The method is described using a worked example; the AP radiograph (Fig. 1) shows a valgus angulation (C) of 21° for a right tibia, the lateral radiograph shows an anterior angulation (S) of 6° and the axial imaging shows a 31° external rotation deformity (Fig. 2 which shows rotation markers when looking down onto a right tibia).

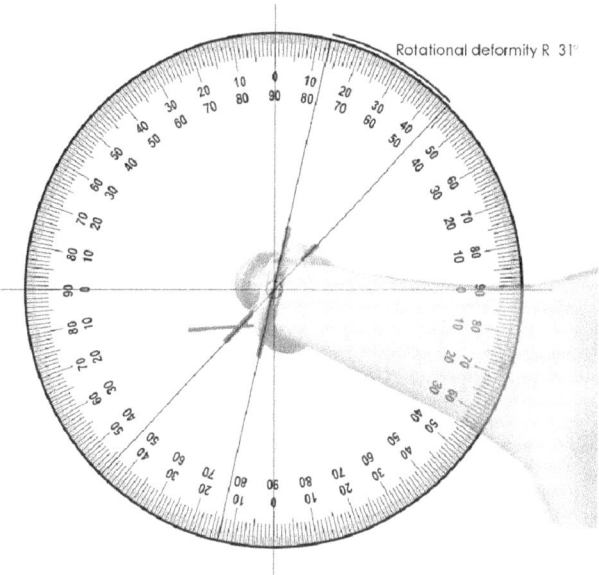

Fig. 2 Rotational deformity in axial plane

Part one

The simplest method of measuring the true magnitude of angular deformity is to image the deformity across the plane of maximal angulation and measure it directly. Alternatively, the magnitude and plane of deformity can be calculated from measurements taken from true AP and lateral radiographs. This can be done graphically:

> The coronal plane deformity is drawn as a vertical line (Line C) Fig. 1. This vertical line intersects the circumference of the protractor at the measured angle C (21°) subtended from the central point starting at the AP axis (0°). For a small angular deformity, line C lies close to the AP axis. For a bigger angular deformity, line C is deflected further from the AP axis. For a valgus deformity, Line C is drawn towards the lateral side and varus is drawn on the medial side.

> The process is repeated for the sagittal plane deformity. The sagittal plane deformity is drawn as a horizontal line (Line S) Fig. 1. This horizontal line intersects the circumference of the protractor at the measured angle S (6°) subtended from the central point starting at the horizontal axis (0°). For a small angular deformity, line S lies close to the horizontal axis. For a bigger angular deformity, line S is deflected further from the horizontal axis. For a recurvatum (anterior angulation), deformity line S is drawn towards the anterior side and if procurvatum (posterior angulation) it is drawn on the posterior side.

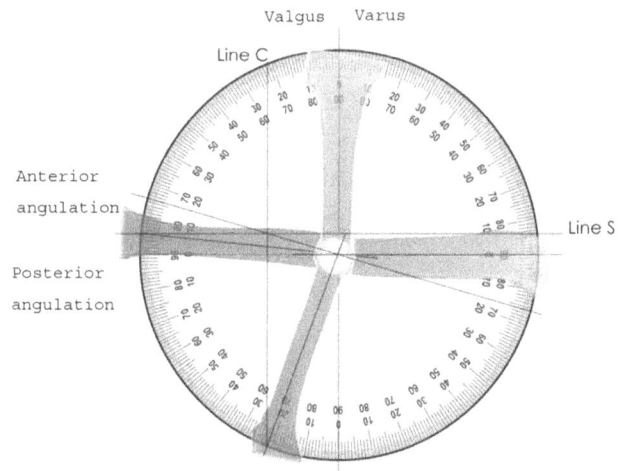

Fig. 1 Angular deformity in anterior–posterior and lateral planes

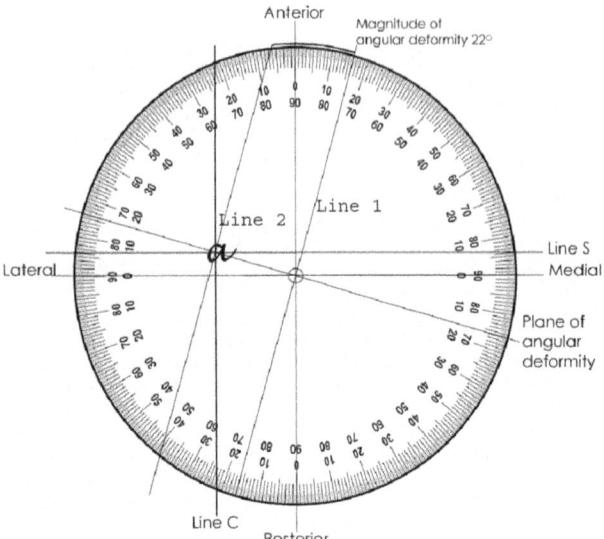

Fig. 3 Plane and magnitude of angular deformity

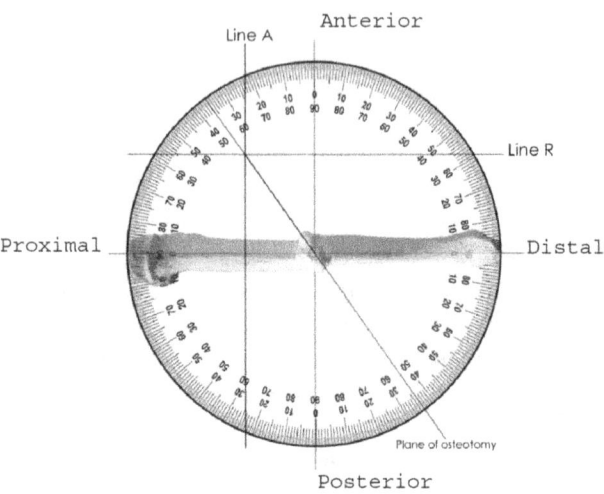

Fig. 4 Plane of osteotomy

A line is drawn from the central point through the intersection of Line C and Line S. This represents the resolved plane of angular deformity. Line C and Line S intersect at point *a* (Fig. 3). In this example the plane of angular deformity is 16° to the coronal plane.

To measure the magnitude of deformity, two lines are drawn at right angles to the plane of angular deformity (Fig. 3). Line 1 is drawn through the central point and Line 2 is drawn through the intersection. The magnitude of angular deformity is the separation of these lines measured in degrees at the circumference.

The plane of angulation is 16° anterior to the coronal plane or 74° external to the sagittal plane. The magnitude of angular deformity is measured as 22° (A). An AP radiograph taken with the leg 16° externally rotated would demonstrate the full angular deformity (A) of 22°.

Part two

The angular and rotational deformities are now resolved into a final single plane. The starting position for this is the bisector of the angulation in the plane of the first resolved angular deformity.

Step one is to define the bisector of the angular deformity. This is calculated [90 + (A/2)] for the convexity and [90 − (A/2)] for the concavity of the deformity. In this example it is 101° to both proximal and distal segments in the plane of the angular deformity when viewed from the apex of the convexity.

The bisector is marked by a K-wire in the plane of angular deformity. *A simple line diagram will help understand this part.*

A photocopy of a standard circular protractor is marked proximal, distal, anterior and posterior with axes intersecting at the central point (Fig. 4). The horizontal axis is marked proximal and distal matching the operative view of the bone. In this example proximal is marked on the left and distal on the right.

The horizontal axis on the protractor lies in the plane of angular deformity; this means that when viewing the bone as in the example on Fig. 4, the bone has been rotated such that the true plane of angular deformity faces the viewer. In this example, the bone has been rotated 16° externally. The AP axis now lies at right angles to the bisector of the angular deformity. The central point is looking down the axis of the bisector of angular deformity.

The resolved angular deformity of 22° in the oblique plane (A) is represented by (line A) in Fig. 4. A vertical line is drawn that intersects the circumference of the protractor at the measured angle (22°) from the central point starting at the AP axis. For a deformity approached from the convexity, as in this example, this is marked to the proximal side but if seen from the concavity it is marked to the distal. In this example line A is drawn proximal from the AP axis.

The process is repeated for the rotational deformity which is drawn as a horizontal line (line R) in Fig. 4. This horizontal line intersects the circumference of the protractor at the measured angle R (31°)

subtended from the central point starting at the horizontal axis (0°). For a small rotational deformity, line R lies close to the horizontal axis. For a bigger angular deformity, line R is deflected further from the horizontal axis. External rotation is drawn anterior to the horizontal axis and internal rotation is drawn posterior to the horizontal axis. In this example line R is anterior.

A straight line is drawn from the central point to the intersection of line A and line R and continued to the circumference. This defines the plane of osteotomy. In this example it is measured as 54° from the horizontal axis or plane of angular deformity and 36° from the transverse plane rotated about the bisector of angulation.

For a deformity that is mainly angular, the final plane is close to the plane of angular deformity (horizontal axis). For deformity that is mainly rotational, the plane is closer to the transverse or axial plane (vertical axis).

If this convention is not followed correctly, it is possible to plan an osteotomy that achieves a mirror image of the desired correction, creating, for example, external rotation with varus rather than internal rotation with varus. The osteotomy rule that confirms the correct orientation is: the apex (acute angle) of the distal fragment rotates towards the concavity of the angulation. If this rotation corrects the rotational deformity, the osteotomy is correctly orientated.

Surgical technique

The starting point for the osteotomy is the bisector of the angular deformity in the plane of the angular deformity (the resolved oblique plane performed in part one). The deformity is imaged in the plane of maximum deformity by rotating the limb until the maximum angular deformity is seen. A Kirschner wire (K-wire) is then placed along the bisector in the plane of angular deformity.

The saw blade is rotated from longitudinal to transverse around this bisector axis depending on the combination of rotation and angulation. The more rotation the more transverse the cut, the more angulation the more longitudinal the cut. The calculation of the combination of rotation and angulation to provide the final plane uses the circular protractor method (part two).

The osteotomy rule to correctly orient the cut is: the apex (acute angle) of the distal fragment rotates towards the concavity of the angulation. This osteotomy rule is critical as it is easy to rotate the saw blade to produce a mirror image of the desired cut that increases the rotation deformity with correction of angulation.

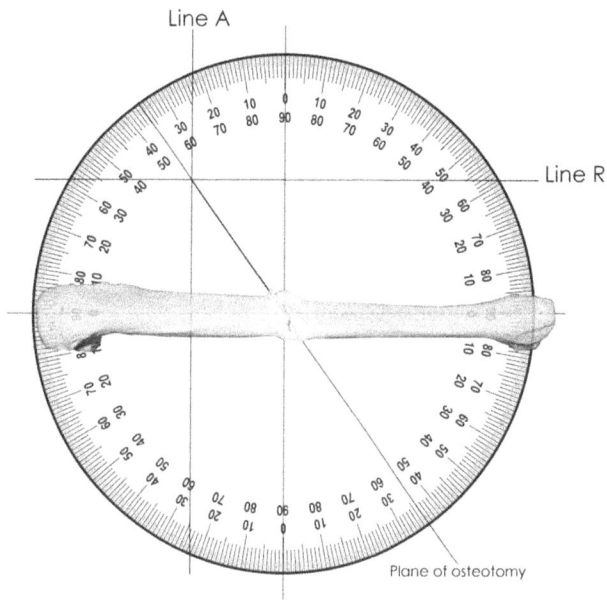

Fig. 5 Full correction of angular and rotational deformity following rotation around the osteotomy plane

Figure 5 shows the full correction of angular and rotational deformity following rotation around the osteotomy plane.

Discussion

Oblique plane osteotomy has been described for the correction of Blount's disease, proximal femoral deformity, metatarsal deformity and the correction of tibial malunion [1, 2].

A single-plane osteotomy has a number of advantages over a wedge osteotomy: the second cut of a wedge osteotomy is difficult to make accurately once the bone is divided, making it easy to create a new deformity; it is possible to under-correct the original deformity; and an incorrectly created wedge can produce a bone gap. Resection of a bone wedge creates shortening that can be avoided by the use of a single-plane osteotomy. Obliquity of this single-plane osteotomy often allows stable interfragmentary screw fixation with compression and a large area of bone contact that is not possible with a transverse osteotomy. Translation along the plane of osteotomy allows correction of translational deformity with restoration of length. Where the surgical anatomy dictates the need for an approach to the concavity of angulation, a closing wedge may be technically challenging, whereas a single cut and rotation about a single oblique plane provides an elegant solution.

When a hexapod external fixator is used to simultaneously correct angular and rotational deformity, the segments are rotated about this single plane. If an osteotomy can be performed in this plane, the cut bone surfaces rotate about each other without creating a bone gap [3].

The starting points for describing this plane of osteotomy are the plane of angular deformity and the bisector of the angular deformity. These are both relatively easy to define and identify using the image intensifier in theatre. Rotation of the saw blade is made around the axis that is the bisector of the angular deformity. This method of planning can also be used to identify the correct plane for a focal dome osteotomy, the axis of which lies at right angles to the final osteotomy plane described. A deformity that is predominantly angular with little rotation exists predominantly in the long axis of the bone, and therefore, a focal dome osteotomy may be preferred.

When rotating about the final plane, assuming the proximal segment remains static, the movement of the distal segment is through the arc of a cone, the central axis of which is at 90° to the plane of osteotomy. The correction of angulation therefore occurs in a circular movement and not in a straight line. The use of the bisector of angulation as the initial reference corrects for this circular movement to produce the desired correction. If the chosen plane is parallel to the bisector but not accurately rotated, the angular correction is achieved with either excessive or insufficient rotation. If the chosen plane is not parallel to the bisector, rotational correction is accompanied by angulation in a different plane.

Other methods of describing this plane of osteotomy reference from the plane of the proximal or distal segment as the starting point and require two re-orientations of the blade to find the plane of osteotomy with the second reorientation towards the direction of rotation by half the rotational deformity. Any inaccuracy with this reorientation may cause significant angular deformity.

The graphical method of combining angulation on AP and lateral radiographs using a circular protractor has been shown to produce results to within 1.5° of the correct mathematical results. This graphical method of calculating the plane of osteotomy is accurate for deformities up to 90°, whereas the vector method of planning is less accurate when the total deformity exceeds 30°. This method may be applied to deformity correction in any bone where rotational and angular deformities are combined and considerably simplifies the planning of single-plane osteotomy for the correction of complex deformity.

Acknowledgments No grants or funds were received for this study.

Informed consent Written informed consent from the donors was obtained prior to their inclusion in this study.

References

1. Nyska M, Trnka HJ, Parks GB, Myerson MS (2003) The Ludloff metatarsal osteotomy: guidelines for optimal correction based on geometric analysis conducted on a saw bone model. Foot Ankle Int 24:34–39
2. Paley D (2002) Principles of deformity correction. Ch 9. Springer, Berlin, pp 235–268
3. Waanders NA, Herzenberg JE (1992) The theoretical application of inclined hinges with the Ilizarov external fixator for simultaneous angulation and rotation correction. Bull Hosp Jt Dis 52:27–35

28

Efficacy of 1 % silver sulphadiazine dressings in preventing infection of external fixation pin-tracks

Alfred O. Ogbemudia[1] · **Anirejuoritse Bafor**[1] · **Ehimwenma J. Ogbemudia**[2] ·
Edwin Edomwonyi[3]

Abstract Pin-track infection (PTI) is a common complication of external fixation. Antimicrobial dressings of the pin-site interface should reduce the severity and incidence of PTI. This study is aimed at determining the efficacy of 1 % silver sulphadiazine dressings in preventing PTI in external fixation. We compared the incidence of PTI between group A (dry sterile gauze dressing) and group B (1 % silver sulphadiazine impregnated gauze dressing). PTI was diagnosed when there was: (1) redness around any pin-site, (2) tenderness near a pin-site and (3) serous or purulent discharge from the pin-skin interface. With infection, swab was obtained for microscopy, culture and sensitivity. Pin-track infections were diagnosed in 22.5 and 4.1 % of patients in groups A and B, respectively. This difference was statistically significant. The commonest organism isolated from swabs was *Staphyloccus aureus*. In patients with external fixation, 1 % silver sulphadiazine lowered PTI. This further underlines the need for antimicrobial dressings of pin-sites. We recommend the use of 1 % silver sulphadiazine impregnated ribbon gauze for pin-site dressings.
Level of evidence II.

✉ Alfred O. Ogbemudia
alfredoghogho@yahoo.com

[1] Department of Orthopaedics and Trauma, University of Benin Teaching Hospital, PMB 1111, Benin City, Edo State, Nigeria

[2] Department of Medicine, University of Benin, Benin City, Edo State, Nigeria

[3] Department of Orthopaedics and Trauma, Irrua Specialist Teaching Hospital, Irrua, Edo State, Nigeria

Keywords 1 % silver sulphadiazine · Pin-skin interface · External fixation · Infection

Introduction

External fixation is integral to trauma and orthopaedic surgery. In addition to its use in stabilizing open fractures, the device is used in limb lengthening, bone transport and stabilization of the limb after corrective osteotomy and arthrodesis.

The pins used in external fixation maintain an open wound for bacterial invasion of tissues, making infection along the pin-track the most frequent complication of external fixation. The incidence of infection ranges between 11 and 96.6 % [1–6]. The first point of infection is the interface between the skin and pin. The infection then extends along the pin-track and, if allowed to continue, may lead to osteomyelitis, cellulitis and loosening of the pins. Even an infection as rare as myiasis has been reported [7].

Prevention of pin-track infection is, therefore, wise. Several studies describe varying methods for the control or prevention of infection. These methods include: technique of insertion such as prevention of thermal injury [8]; use of antimicrobial coated pins [9–11]; silver-coated pins [12]; and the use of antimicrobial impregnated patches [13].

In a related study, a combination of chlorhexidine and silver sulphadiazine in dressings was found very effective in reducing the incidence of pin-track infection [14].

Silver sulphadiazine is a very highly effective topical antimicrobial agent used in the dressing of burn wounds with the capacity to reduce bacterial colonization [15–17]. Silver sulphadiazine cream causes a slow and sustained release of silver ions which bind to bacterial deoxyribonucleic acid, inhibiting growth and multiplication of bacterial cells. It penetrates into exudates and necrotic tissue and is effective against *Staphylococcus aureus*, *Escherichia coli*, *Pseudomonas aeruginosa*, and strains of Proteus, Klebsiella, and *Candida albicans* [17]. The use of silver sulphadiazine in the management of extensive burns has not been found to be associated with systemic complications [18].

This longstanding safety and efficacy of silver sulphadiazine in the treatment of burns led to its choice as the agent for dressing of external fixator pins. A sterile ribbon gauze enmeshed in the creamy preparation of silver sulphadiazine and rolled around the skin-pin interface prolongs the antimicrobial activity of 1 % silver sulphadiazine at the pin-site and prevents bacterial colonization and subsequent infection. The potential here is to prevent infection to an extent similar to that from use of long-acting antimicrobial coated pins which are not available readily in the average clinical setting in most developing countries and are costlier than noncoated pins.

This study was designed to assess the efficacy of silver sulphadiazine dressings in the prevention of PTI by comparing the incidence of infection in a group dressed with 1 % silver sulphadiazine to another dressed with dry sterile gauze.

Patients and methods

This study was conducted from January 2003 to December 2012 in a teaching hospital and two other hospitals in the same city. Institutional approval was obtained from the teaching hospital's ethics and research committee.

All patients who gave consent (or had their guardians' consent in the case of minors) to participate in the study were allocated to group A or B with the aid of a continuously updated register. Each nonconsenting patient received care with established treatment protocols. We excluded patients with chronic osteomyelitis or limb ischaemia lasting more than 8 h or established wound sepsis.

Ninety-eight patients were recruited consecutively into either group A or B. We recorded their clinical and demographic data. In determining the sample size, we planned to detect a double-fold reduction in the rate of pin-track infection amongst patients treated using silver sulphadiazine with a 90 % power of achieving 5 % significance. A sample size of 43 was determined per group. We made adjustment for a 12 % loss to follow-up. As a result, the final sample per group came to 49 patients. The resulting data were evaluated for statistical significance of the rate of infection using Chi-square test.

Technique of application of pins

Each pin (a 4.5-mm Schanz screw) was applied through a 5-mm stab wound in the skin with a size 10 blade. The holes in the near cortex were pre-drilled with a hand drill using a 2.7-mm drill bit through a drill guide and the pins inserted until the far cortex was engaged. There was no pre-drilling for the insertion of 1.8 mm Kirschner wires for the Ilizarov circular external fixator. Each AO unilateral external fixators had four 4.5 mm Schanz screw pin-sites per limb; each unilateral rail had six 5 mm pin-sites, and each Ilizarov device had sixteen 1.8 mm pin-sites.

Dressing protocol

Group A patients (the control group) had daily pin-site dressings with dry sterile strip of gauze after cleaning the pin-site with methylated spirit, while group B patients (the study group) had once-weekly pin-site dressing with a sterile strip of gauze that was impregnated with 1 % silver sulphadiazine cream (Dermazin®, Lek Pharmaceutical and Chemical Company, Ljubljana, Slovenia) and wound round the pin or wire after cleaning with methylated spirit. The immediate post-surgical dressings were removed 72 h, and fresh dressings were applied accordingly.

Antibiotic prophylaxis

All the patients had intravenous ceftriazone 1 g daily for 48 h and metronidazole 500 mg 8-hourly for 24 h. Children were given 20 mg per kg of a single daily dose of ceftriazone and 7.5 mg/kg per dose of metronidazole. Our choice of post-operative antibiotics is based on the need for prophylaxis [19].

Duration of hospital stay

All the cases were managed as inpatients for a minimum of 5 weeks and followed up for at least 16 weeks after removal of pins.

Assessment of pin-sites

The presence or absence of pin-track infection was determined during dressing change at the ward round. Redness or tenderness near a pin (stage 1) or serous discharge (stage 2) or seropurulent or purulent discharge (stage 3) was taken as evidence of infection. The above classification set aside grades 4 and 5 of the Dahl classification [20] (4 = osteolysis requiring pin removal and 5 = ring sequestrum requiring debridement) which we presume are representative of a complicated infection. Swabs were taken from any pin-site with serous, seropurulent and purulent discharge for microscopy, culture and sensitivity. Antibiotic therapy was recommended in those patients with pin-track infection.

Results

There were 49 patients (49 fixators across forty-nine bones) in group A and 49 patients (51 fixators across fifty-one bones) in group B. The entire study group was made up of sixty-four males and thirty-four females with an average age of 37.2 ± 15.8 years (range 4–75 years). There were 33 males and 16 females in group A with an average age of 36.7 ± 16.8 years (a range of 7–75 years) as well as 31 males and 18 females in group B with an average age 37.7 ± 15.2 years (a range of 4–75 years). There was no loss to follow-up within 16 weeks after removal of pins.

Tables 1 and 2 show the details of demographic and clinical data of the study groups. The external fixators remained in place for an average of 9.8 weeks in group A and 13.2 weeks in group B. Eleven patients (22.5 %) in group A and two (4.1 %) in group B had pin-track infections, respectively $(p = 0.01)$. Thirty-eight pin-tracks (14.2 %) were infected in group A, while seven pin-tracks (1.9 %) were infected in group B $(p < 0.01)$. The types of fixation, number of pin-sites and infection rates are shown in Table 3.

All infections were superficial in both groups. There was no difference in the two groups in terms of pin complications post-removal.

Discussion

The incidence of infection amongst patients who had dry dressings (22.5 %) against those who had silver sulphadiazine dressings (4.1 %) indicates that the antimicrobial effect of silver dressing is efficacious. This significantly lower incidence of infection inpatients who had silver sulphadiazine dressings is attributable to the antimicrobial qualities of 1 % silver sulphadiazine in controlling microbial invasion of the pin-site since both control and study groups were given the same dose of antibiotics for the same duration and had cleaning with methylated spirit before

Table 1 The demographic characteristics of the study groups

Feature	Control group (A)	Study group (B)
No of patients	49	49
Age in years (range)[a]	36.7 ± 16.8 (7–75)	37.7 ± 15.2 (4–75)
Male/female	33:16	31:18

[a] Mean ± standard deviation and (range)

Table 2 Site of fixation and indication for external fixation

Feature	Control group (A)	Study group (B)
Site of external fixation		
Humerus	7	6
Radius	2	2
Ulna	2	1
Hand	1	0
Femur	5	11
Tibia	29	31
Foot	2	0
Ankle	1	0
Total	49	51
Indication (diagnosis)		
Gunshot Injury	14	17
Road traffic accident	32	28
Achondroplasia	1	1
Blount disease	2	3

Table 3 Types of fixation, number of pin-sites and infection rates

Feature	Control group (A)	Study group (B)
Number of pin-sites	268	368
AO tubular external fixation	43	41
Unilateral rail	0	2
Ilizarov device	6	8
Pin tract infection (patients)[a]	11 (22.5 %)	2 (4.1 %)
Pin tract infection (pin-sites)[a]	38 (14.2 %)	7 (1.9 %)

[a] Number and (percentage)

application of dressings. The inpatient care offered to the patients eliminated the confounding influence of environmental and related caregivers' factors on the results.

Infection at the pin-site from external fixation may lead to loosening, early discontinuation of external fixation and systemic sepsis in some cases. Loosening and early discontinuation of external fixation would mar any procedure despite being well done.

The results of this study support several others which have found antimicrobial preparations effective in preventing pin-track infection [9–12, 14]. The value of antimicrobial preparations has been demonstrated by use of chlorhexidine coating in controlling microbial colonization of epidural and central venous catheters [21–23]. Similarly, the reduction in incidence of PTI in this study is attributed to the antimicrobial activity provided by the 1 % silver sulphadiazine and is consistent with the efficacy of silver-coated pins in reducing pin-track infection.

The choice of once-weekly dressings was determined by a need to have a dressing routine that would be feasible in a busy unit that has to maintain time for other aspects of patient care. This choice is supported by an earlier study showing no difference in outcome between daily and weekly dressing changes in the incidence of pin-track infection [24]. Use of an effective antimicrobial dressing has been described previously to be as effective as systemic antibiotic administration in preventing pin-track infections [25].

Whilst self-applied nonantimicrobial based dressings are feasible, it is associated with a high incidence of pin-track infection [26]. The possibility of adding 1 % silver sulphadiazine cream once or twice daily to the pin-site interface (PSI) at home by a patient has potential to be an effective solution in cases where home dressings are associated with increased incidence of infection. The outcome of this study parallels the established efficacy of silver sulphadiazine in burn wound management [17, 18].

There are limitations to this study. We were unable to blind patients and caregivers to the type of dressing used, and the prolonged admission in hospital in order to eliminate environmental factors may influence pin-site contamination. This absence of blinding did not seem to have had a significant influence on the results because the diagnosis of infection was determined during dressing changes on ward rounds using the outlined criteria.

Conclusion

The incidence of pin-track infection was significantly reduced by the use of 1 % silver sulphadiazine cream impregnated gauze dressings at the pin-site. There was no significant difference in complications after pin or wire removal. On the basis of our findings, we recommend the use of 1 % silver sulphadiazine dressings for external fixator pins.

Acknowledgments The authors declare that no funding or financial support was received from any individual or group.

Research involving Human Participants and/or Animals This study had been approved by the Research and Ethics Committee of the institution where it was conducted. This study was conducted in conformity to ethical standards comparable to those espoused in the 1964 Helsinki Declaration.

Informed consent We obtained informed consent from each patient or guardian of minors and accorded all patients their full rights to treatment and continuity of care.

References

1. Thakur AJ, Patankar J (1991) Open tibial fractures. Treatment by uniplanar external fixation and early bone grafting. J Bone Jt Surg Br 73:448–451
2. Ahlborg HG, Josefsson PO (1999) Pin tract complications in external fixation of fractures of the distal radius. Acta Orthop Scand 70:116–118
3. Parameswaran AD, Roberts CS, Seligson D, Voor M (2003) Pin tract Infection with contemporary external fixation: how much of a problem. J Orthop Trauma 17:503–507
4. Mostafavi HR, Tornetta P (1997) Open fractures of the humerus treated with external fixation. Clin Orthop Rel Res 337:187–197
5. Schalamon J, Petnehazy T, Ainoedhofer H, Zwick EB, Singer G, Hoellwarth ME (2007) Pin tract infection with external fixation of pediatric fractures. J Pediatr Surg 42(9):1584–1587
6. Antoci V, Ono CM, Antoci V, Raney EM (2008) Pin-track infection during limb lengthening using external fixation. Am J Orthop 37(9):E150–E154
7. Paris LA, Viscarret M, Uban C, Vargas J, Rodriguez-Morales AJ (2008) Pin-site myiasis: a rare complication of a treated open fracture of tibia. Surg Infect 9(3):403–406
8. Nayagam S (2010) Femoral lengthening with a rail external fixator: tips and tricks. Strat Trauma Limb Reconstr 5(3):137–144
9. DeJong ES, DeBerardino TM, Brooks DE, Nelson BJ, Campbell AA, Bottoni CR, Pusateri AE, Walton RS, Guymon CH, McManus AT (2001) Antimicrobial efficacy of external fixator pins coated with a lipid stabilized hydroxyapatite/chlorhexidine complex to prevent pin tract infection in a goat model. J Trauma 50(6):1008–1014
10. Voos K, Rosenberg B, Fagrhi M, Seligson D (1999) Use of a tobramycin-impregnated polymethyl methacrylate pin sleeve for the prevention of pin tract infection in goats. J Orthop Trauma 13:98–101
11. Massè A, Bruno A, Bosetti M, Biasibetti A, Cannas M, Gallinaro P (2000) Prevention of pin track infection in external fixation with silver coated pins: clinical and microbiological results. J Biomed Mater Res (Appl Biomater) 53:600–604
12. Davies R, Holt N, Nayagam S (2005) The care of pin sites with external fixation. J Bone Jt Surg Br 87(5):716–719
13. Wu SC, Crews RT, Zelen C, Wrobel JS, Armstrong DG (2008) Use of chlorhexidine-impregnated patch at pin site to reduce local morbidity: the ChIPPS pilot trial. Int Wound J 5(3):416–422
14. Ogbemudia AO, Bafor A, Edomwonyi E, Enemudo R (2010) Prevalence of pin tract infection: the role of combined silver sulphadiazine and chlorhexidine dressing. Niger J Clin Pract 13:268–271
15. Margaret I, Lui SL, Poon VKM, Lung I, Burd A (2006) Antimicrobial activities of silver dressings: an in vitro comparison. J Med Microbiol 55:59–63
16. Robb EC, Nathan P (1981) Control of experimental burn wound infections: comparative delivery of the antimicrobial agent (silver sulphadiazine) either from a cream base or from a solid synthetic dressing. J Trauma 21:889–893
17. Silver S, Phung LT, Silver G (2006) Silver as biocides in burn and wound dressings and bacterial resistance to silver compounds. J Ind Microbiol Biotechnol 33:627–634
18. Boosalis MG, McCall JT, Ahrenholz DH, Solem LD, McClain CJ (1987) Serum and urinary silver levels in thermal injury patients. Surgery 101:40–43
19. Zimmerli W (2001) Antibiotic prophylaxis. In: AO principles of fracture management. Stuttgart. Thieme, pp.703–708
20. Al-Sayyad MJ (2008) Taylor spatial frame in the treatment of open tibial shaft fractures. Indian J Orthop 42(4):431–438

21. Shapiro JM, Bond EL, Garman JK (1990) Use of chlorhexidine dressing to reduce microbial colonization of epidural catheters. Anaesthesiology 73:625–631
22. Hanazaki K, Shingu K, Adachi W, Miyazaki T, Amano J (1999) Chlorhexidine dressing for reduction in microbial colonization of the skin with central venous catheters: a prospective randomized controlled trial. J Hosp Infect 42:165–168
23. Hannan M, Juste RN, Umasanker S, Glendenning A, Nightingale C, Azadian B, Soni N (1999) Antiseptic-bonded central venous catheters and bacterial colonization. Anaesthesia 54:868–872
24. Dahl AW, Toksvig Larsen S, Lindstrand A (2003) No difference between daily and weekly pin site care: randomized study of 50 patients with external fixation. Acta Orthop Scand 74:704–708
25. Bhattacharyya M, Bradley H (2006) Antibiotics vs an antimicrobial dressing for pin tract infection. Wounds 2(2):26–33
26. Saw A, Chan CK, Penafort R, Sengupta S (2006) A simple practical protocol for care of metal-skin interface of external fixation. Med J Malays 61(Suppl A):62–65

29

Distal humerus prosthetic hemiarthroplasty: midterm results

Andras Heijink[1,4] · Marc L. Wagener[2] · Maarten J. de Vos[3] · Denise Eygendaal[4]

Abstract Treatment of comminuted distal humeral fractures remains challenging. Open reduction–internal fixation remains the preferred treatment, but is not always feasible. In selected cases with non-reconstructable or highly comminuted fractures, total elbow arthroplasty has been used, however, also with relatively high complication and failure rates. Distal humerus prosthetic hemiarthroplasty (DHA) may be an alternative in these cases. The purpose of this study was to report the midterm results of six patients that were treated by DHA for acute and salvage treatment of non-reconstructable fractures of the distal humerus. All six patients were treated by DHA for acute and salvage treatment of non-reconstructable fractures of the distal humerus. Medical records were reviewed, and each patient was seen in the office. Mean follow-up was 54 months (range 21–76 months). Implant survival was 100 %. Three were pain free and three had mild or moderate residual pain. Average flexion–extension arc was 95.8° (range 70°–115°) and average pronation–supination arc was 165° (range 150°–180°). In three, there was some degree of instability, which was symptomatic in one. One had motoric and sensory sequelae of a partially recovered traumatic ulnar nerve lesion. According to the Mayo Elbow Performance Score, there were three excellent, one good and two poor results. Four were satisfied with the final result, and two were not. In this case series of six patients with DHA for non-reconstructable distal humerus fractures, favorable midterm follow-up results were seen; however, complications were also observed.

Keywords Arthroplasty · Elbow · Posttraumatic · Trauma · Replacement · Upper extremity

Introduction

Treating comminuted distal humerus fractures remains challenging. Open reduction–internal fixation by means of double plating remains the gold standard, certainly in the young patient. However, the incidence of complications has been high, including reoperations and disappointing functional outcomes [1]. Also, in the elderly, results have been somewhat less predictable [1]. Some fractures are not amendable to open reduction–internal fixation (ORIF) due to the severity of comminution or poor bone quality. Total elbow arthroplasty (TEA) has been used as alternative treatment for non-reconstructable or severely comminuted fractures in the elderly [1]. Unfortunately, the incidence of complications after TEA has been relatively high [2]. This is even more so for posttraumatic indications [2]. Distal humerus prosthetic hemiarthroplasty (DHA) may be an alternative. DHA involves replacement of the distal humerus by a humeral component of a convertible total elbow system, mounted with an anatomical spool. Avoiding the ulnar component, loosening of which is responsible for large part of TEA failures, may reduce the complication rate as compared to TEA. Late conversion to total elbow

✉ Andras Heijink
aheijink@yahoo.com

1 Department of Orthopaedic Surgery, Academic Medical Center (AMC), Meibergdreef 9, 1105 AZ Amsterdam, The Netherlands

2 Department of Orthopaedic Surgery, St. Radboud University Hospital, Nijmegen, The Netherlands

3 Department of Orthopaedic Surgery, Tergooi Hospitals, Hilversum, The Netherlands

4 Department of Orthopaedic Surgery, Amphia Hospital, Breda, The Netherlands

arthroplasty is possible. First reported on in 1947, the earlier seven reports involving 28 cases with various indications date back to a time in which prosthetic material and design, understanding of elbow biomechanics, and surgical technique were less developed than they are today [3–9]. More recently, with advancement of understanding of elbow anatomy and biomechanics and the development of new prostheses, DHA has regained interest. Current expert opinion is that DHA may be considered for acute non-reconstructable fractures of the distal humerus or failed open reduction–internal fixation and/or posttraumatic sequelae of such fractures without realistic reconstruction options (e.g., nonunion, avascular necrosis). Some include fracture types that are generally associated with complete disruption of the vascularization of the distal fragments (e.g., coronal shear fracture of the capitellum and lateral trochlea combined with low transverse bicondylar extension). The decision as to when a fracture is considered non-reconstructable depends on fracture characteristics, bone quality and surgeon experience. To date, clinical data related to DHA using modern era prostheses and surgical principles are limited to eight peer-reviewed publications reporting on six series including 60 cases (Table 1) [10–17]. Forty-nine of those cases involved treatment of acute fractures, and 11 were salvage procedures (i.e., reconstruction after failed open reduction–internal fixation). Three commercial implant systems were used: the Sorbie-Questor total elbow prosthesis (Wright Medical, Arlington, TN, USA), the Kudo total elbow prosthesis (Biomet, Warsaw, IN, USA) and the Latitude Total Elbow Prosthesis (Tornier, Montbonnot, France).

The midterm follow-up results of six patients that were treated by distal humerus prosthetic hemiarthroplasty for non-reconstructable fracture of the distal humerus or failure of ORIF of such fractures are reported.

Materials and methods

Approval for this study was waived from our institutions' Medical Ethical Committee, and each patient was informed that data concerning their case would be submitted for publication.

Six patients were treated in our institution by distal humerus prosthetic hemiarthroplasty (DHA) between April 2006 and November 2009: One was treated for a closed non-reconstructable fracture of the distal humerus, while five were treated for failed earlier treatment and/or sequelae of such a fracture without realistic reconstruction options.

During surgery, the patient was in the lateral decubitus position with the arm in a support and flexed to 90°, the humerus parallel and forearm perpendicular to the floor.

Prophylactic antibiotic coverage consisted of 2 g cefazolin intravenously. A tourniquet was used. An (extensile) posterior approach was carried out, during which both epicondyles were exposed and the ulnar nerve was identified and mobilized, but not anteriorly transposed. In three patients (cases 3, 4 and 5), an apex-distal chevron olecranon osteotomy was performed at the bare area of the sigmoid fossa and the triceps mechanism was reflected sufficiently proximally to expose the distal humerus. In three others (cases 1, 2 and 6), the ulnohumeral joint was dislocated after subperiosteal release of the lateral collateral ligament complex. The comminuted articular segments were then removed, taking care to preserve the medial and lateral epicondyles and to protect the origin of the collateral ligament. The distal humeral articular segments, the radial head and coronoid were used as templates for choosing the correct implant size. The superior aspect of the olecranon fossa was resected, and the humeral canal was broached and reamed. A trial component was then placed, using local landmarks such as the insertion of the collateral ligaments and the condyles to determine adequate depth. With the trial prosthesis in situ, the elbow was reduced and range of motion and stability were tested. Subsequently, the final prosthesis was cemented in place. The olecranon osteotomy was repaired using a tension band technique consisting of a large screw 6.0 mm in diameter and an Orthocord® (Biomet, Warsaw, IN, USA) tension band. Alternatively, the lateral collateral ligament was reconstructed using transosseous sutures. A removable splint for the night was provided for 6 weeks to allow proper soft tissue healing. Passive range of motion started on the first postoperative day, and active range of motion was resumed after 6 weeks, both under the supervision of a physical therapist. All procedures were performed by two senior shoulder and elbow surgeons (D.E. and M.V.).

Medical records were reviewed, and each patient was seen in the office for a clinical assessment and radiographic evaluation. At the office, range of motion was measured using a goniometer and instability was tested for in extension and 30° of flexion by the moving valgus stress test. Instability was graded none (grade 0), medial tenderness with valgus stress (grade 1), mild instability (grade 2) or subluxation (grade 3). Elbow function was further assessed using the Mayo Elbow Performance Score [18, 19] and Oxford Elbow Score (OES). In addition, the Disabilities of Arm, Shoulder and Hand (DASH) questionnaire and Short Form (SF)-36 questionnaire were administered. For one patient that had died of natural causes (case 5), documentation from the last clinic visit was used. Radiographs of the elbow were reviewed for signs of implant loosening, degenerative changes of the ulnar trochlea and periarticular heterotopic ossifications. Periarticular heterotopic ossifications were graded as previously described by Brooker et al. [20].

Table 1 Summary of recent literature

References	Study design	N	Average follow-up	Prosthesis type	Data	Implant failure (%)	Average postoperative flexion–extension arc (°)	MEPS	Degeneration proximal ulna leading to (planned) conversion
Parsons et al. [15]	Case series	8 (4 acute, 4 salvage)	Not provided, short-term	Sorbie-Questor	Pooled	100	Not provided	Not provided	1
Burkhart et al. [13, 14]	Case series	10 (8 acute, 2 salvage)	12.1 (6–23) months	Latitude	Individualized	100	107 (range 75–135)	8 excellent, 1 good, 1 fair	1
Adolfsson et al. [10, 11]	Case series	8 (all acute)	4.1 (range 2.5–6) years	Kudo	Individualized	100	96.3 (range 60–120)	5 excellent, 3 good	None
Argintar et al. [12]	Case series	10 (9 acute, 1 salvage)	12 months (range not provided)	Latitude	Individualized	100	102 (range 110–140)	3 excellent, 2 good, 3 fair, 1 poor, 1 n/a	None
Smith et al. [17]	Case series	17 (15 acute, 2 salvage)[a]	80 (range 25–133) months	5 Sorbie-Questor, 12 Latitude	Individualized	15 %[b]	116 (range 70–133)	4 excellent, 4 good, 1 fair, 1 poor	None
Hohman et al. [16]	Case series	7 (5 acute, 2 salvage)[c]	36 months (range not provided)	Latitude	Individualized	100	96 (range 70–130)	1 excellent, 3 good, 2 fair, 1 poor	None

[a] Four revised prostheses were not included in the review, and four patients had died. One was lost to follow-up for reasons not discussed

[b] Implant failure was calculated based on four failures/revisions of a total of 26 placed prostheses, assuming the nine prosthesis that were lost to follow-up have not failed

[c] One patient was lost to follow-up

179

All six patients were females. There were four right and two left and four dominant elbows involved. Mean age at surgery was 69 (range 55–77 years). In one patient,

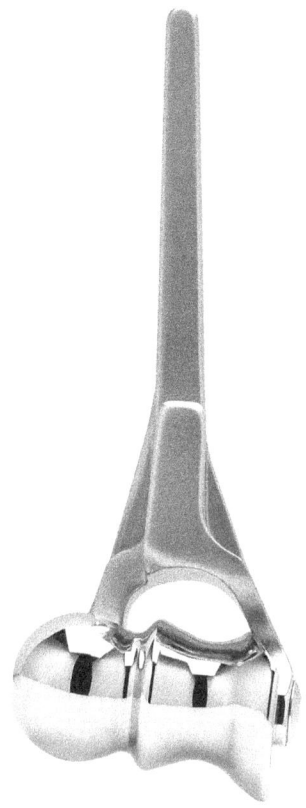

Fig. 1 Humeral component with anatomical spool (i.e., distal humerus prosthesis) of the Lattitude® Total Elbow

treatment was for acute fracture (case 5), in one for avascular necrosis of the capitellum (case 2) and in four for symptomatic nonunion. None had open wounds or impaired skin or soft tissues. None had degenerative changes of the proximal ulna on the preoperative imaging studies. In all patients, the humeral component of the Latitude® Total Elbow Prosthesis (Tornier, Montbonnot, France) was used with an anatomical spool (Fig. 1). All were cemented in place and inserted according to the manufacturer's recommendations. Mean follow-up was 54 months (range 21–76 months).

Results

Demographic data, overall clinical outcome data and patient-derived outcome data of this patient sample are presented (Tables 2, 3, 4, respectively). Three patients had no pain, two had mild, and one had moderate pain. Four were satisfied and two were dissatisfied with the final result. Average flexion was 122.5° (range 110°–130°), average extension deficit was 26.7° (range 20°–40°), and the average flexion–extension arc was 95.8° (range 70°–115°). Average pronation was 84.2° (range 75°–90°), average supination was 80.1° (range 75°–90°), and the average pronation–supination arc was 165° (range 150°–180°). One patient had grade 1 (case 1), one patient had grade 2 (case 3), and one patient had grade 3 (case 2) valgus instability with testing. The patient with grade 3 instability also complained of subjective instability during activities of daily living. Interestingly, two of those three patients with valgus instability (cases 1 and 2) had had a subperiosteal

Table 2 Demographic data for the individual patients

Case	Sex	Injured side	Dominant side	Age at surgery	AO classification initial fracture	Indication	Surgical procedures prior to distal humerus hemiarthroplasty	Time from initial fracture treatment (months)
1	Female	Right	Right	62	13 type b2	Nonunion capitellum w/secondary avascular necrosis	ORIF	29
2	Female	Right	Right	55	13 type c3	Severe avascular necrosis capitellum	ORIF	10
3	Female	Right	Right	77	13 type b3	Nonunion capitellum w/secondary avascular necrosis	ORIF	1
4	Female	Left	Right	65	13 type b3	Nonunion capitellum w/secondary avascular necrosis	ORIF	4
5	Female	Right	Right	76	13 type c3	Acute non-reconstructable distal humerus fracture	None	0
6	Female	Left	Right	68	13 type b3	Nonunion capitellum w/secondary avascular necrosis capitellum	ORIF	7

ORIF open reduction–internal fixation

Table 3 Clinical outcome data for the individual patients

Case	F/U (mos)	Pain[a]	Instability[b]	Flexion–extension (arc) (zero method, °)	Pronation–supination (arc) (zero method, °)	Mayo Elbow Performance Score[c]	Neurovascular or infectious complications	Additional comments	Patient satisfaction
1	76	Mild	Grade 1 valgus	110–40–0 (70)	75–0–75 (150)	55/poor	Fully recovered lesion ulnar nerve not neurophysiologically investigated	None	Unsatisfied
2	61	Moderate	Grade 3 valgus	115–30–0 (85)	90–0–80 (170)	40/poor	Partially recovered EMG-proven axonotmesis ulnar nerve	Persistent subluxation	Unsatisfied
3	57	Mild	Grade 2 valgus	130–30–0 (100)	90–0–90 (180)	80/good	None	None	Satisfied
4	66	None	None	135–20–0 (115)	80–0–80 (160)	100/excellent	None	None	Satisfied
5[d]	21	None	None	115–20–0 (95)	80–0–70 (150)	95/excellent	None	None	Satisfied
6	43	None	None	130–20–0 (110)	90–0–90 (180)	100/excellent	None	None	Satisfied

[a] Pain is graded as none, mild, moderate or severe

[b] Instability is graded as none (i.e., stable), mild, moderate or gross

[c] The Mayo Elbow Performance Score total score is graded as excellent (95–100), good (80–94), fair (60–79) and poor (<59). All revisions are considered a poor result, regardless of total score

[d] Patient deceased due to old age. Documentation from last office visit was used

Table 4 Patient-derived outcome scores

Case	DASH	Oxford Elbow Score			SF-36	
		Pain domain	Elbow function	Socio-psychological	Physical component summary	Mental component summary
1	20	100	68.8	50	43.6	49.1
2	57.5	43.8	25	31.3	37.5	51.5
3	7.4	100	100	87.5	47.8	56.4
4	5.0	87.5	87.5	93.8	54.3	39.4
5	n/a	n/a	n/a	n/a	n/a	n/a
6	2.5	87.5	100	87.5	53.9	59.5

release and subsequent reattachment of the lateral collateral ligament complex, and both were also the patients that were unsatisfied with the final outcome. According to the Mayo Elbow Performance Score, there were three excellent, one good and two poor results. There were two neurovascular complications. One patient had motoric and sensory sequelae of an EMG-proven axonotmesis of the ulnar nerve that has only partially recovered to date. Another had decreased sensation in the ulnar nerve distribution preoperatively that had fully recovered at end follow-up. There were no infections and no systemic complications.

At end follow-up, implant survival was 100 % with no radiographic signs of loosening in any case (case 6, Fig. 2a–d). In one patient (case 2), there was subluxation of the ulnohumeral joint with slight radiographic attrition of the proximal ulna (case 2, Fig. 3a–d). This was the same patient with grade 3 valgus instability. Heterotopic ossifications (Brooker II) had developed in one patient (case 5). Two patients had developed calcifications related to reconstruction of the lateral collateral ligament (cases 1 and 2). None of the others showed erosion of the proximal ulna.

Discussion

Distal humerus hemiarthroplasty (DHA) involves replacement of the distal humerus by a humeral component of a convertible total elbow system, mounted with an

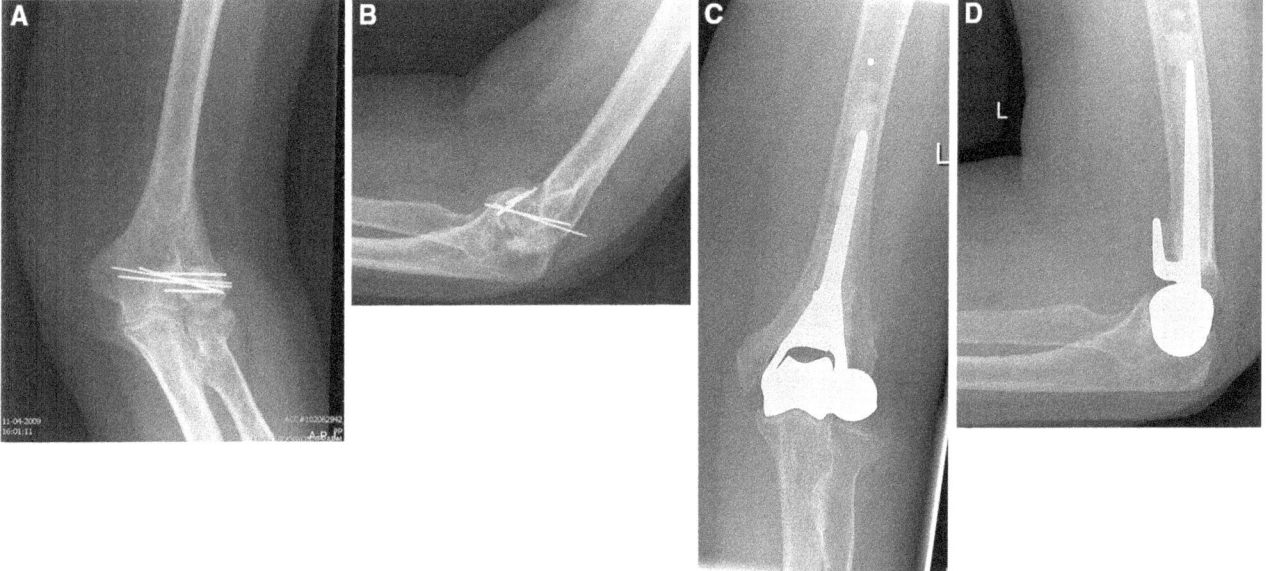

Fig. 2 a–d Antero-posterior and lateral radiographic images of the elbow before (**a, b**) and at end follow-up (**c, d**) 43 months after distal humerus prosthetic hemiarthroplasty (humeral component of Latitude® Total Elbow with anatomical spool) at end follow-up of case 6. The prosthesis is well positioned, without signs of loosening

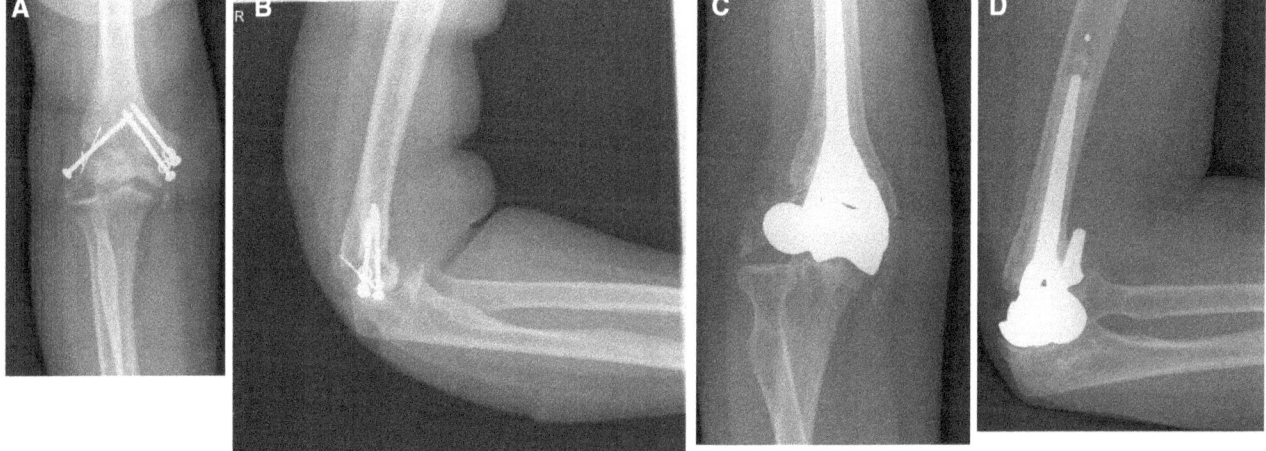

Fig. 3 a–d Antero-posterior and lateral radiographic image of the elbow before (**a, b**) and at end follow-up (**c, d**) 61 months after distal humerus prosthetic hemiarthroplasty (humeral component of Latitude® Total Elbow with anatomical spool) of case 2. Subluxations of the ulnohumeral joint and discrete irregularity of the articulating surface of the proximal ulna are noted

anatomical spool. The midterm follow-up results of six consecutive cases were reported.

Terminology has been variable and mostly not discerning well-enough isolated distal humerus replacement from total elbow replacement. We suggest using the term *distal humerus prosthetic hemiarthroplasty* in future when describing this procedure, as it is (1) descriptive of the procedure, (2) avoids confusion with radiocapitellar prosthetic arthroplasty, which has also been referred to as a hemiarthroplasty and (3) avoids confusion with other types of arthroplasties, such as resection arthroplasty, interposition arthroplasty.

Anatomical prerequisites for DHA are (1) an intact or stable radial head, (2) an intact or reconstructable coronoid process, (3) intact or reconstructable columns, (4) a presumably stable (i.e., ligamentous intact) elbow or reconstructable collateral ligaments and (5) absence of ulnohumeral degenerative changes. Patients should also be too young for TEA. DHA is considered an *'unlinked'* construction and therefore must mimic the native distal humerus anatomy in order to provide optimal stability and transmission of forces. The implant must be inserted at the correct level and orientation to restore the axis of flexion in relation to the insertions of the medial and lateral collateral ligaments.

Our observations made in and conclusions drawn from this study are obviously only as strong and valid as can be with a case series. However, cases series are still the only and therefore *best available* evidence to date on this topic and will probably remain so for quite some time.

Over all, our results compare well with the current literature [10–17]. Smith et al. reported 4 failures of 26 placed prostheses (15 %, assuming the nine prostheses that were lost to follow-up have not failed) due to periprosthetic fracture and loosening. All other authors reported 100 % implant survival, although both Parsons and Burkhart had scheduled a conversion to total elbow arthroplasty (TEA) for symptomatic ulnar wear. In the current series, no implants failed. None of the authors reports an objective measurement of residual pain, and only Hohman et al. comment on patient satisfaction by reporting a mean Likert satisfaction scale of 7 of 10. Comparison with the current series, in which two out of six patients (33 %) were unsatisfied with the final outcome, is therefore not possible. Our results expressed in terms of Mayo Elbow Performance Score (MEPS) are with 67 % combined excellent or good results mid-range when compared to the current literature (range 50–100 %), as is the range of ulnohumeral motion. Complications are not all that uncommon, some minor, but some more serious. Hohman et al. reported one peroperative diaphyseal humerus fracture and Argintar et al. one peroperative olecranon fracture, both successfully treated by plate fixation. As stated, Smith et al. reported two periprosthetic fractures for which conversion to total elbow arthroplasty was performed, respectively, 54 and 140 months after placement of the prosthesis. Adolfsson et al. observed one periprosthetic fracture 3 years after placement of the prosthesis, which was successfully treated by plate fixation. Smith et al. also revised 2 of 26 placed prostheses (8 %, assuming the nine prostheses that were lost to follow-up have not failed) for loosening. All but one author reported ulnar nerve neuropathy, either transient or persistent, requiring transposition, mostly in around 10 % of the cases, but for Smith et al. even in up to 4 of 17 (24 %). In the current series, two of six patients (33 %) had ulnar nerve problems, one a transient neuropathy, the second a not recovered axonotmesis, which was sustained during the trauma. We appear to be first to encounter valgus instability, which will be discussed in the next paragraph. Wound problems or infection were uncommon, as were nonunion of the olecranon osteotomy. Frequently, Smith et al. reported in up to 59 % of reviewed patients, symptomatic hardware, used to fix the olecranon

osteotomy, had to be removed. Smith et al. reported one case of elbow stiffness, requiring arthrolysis. Radiographically, all but one author reported wear of the proximal ulna to some extent. Parsons et al. had scheduled one of eight (12.5 %) patients for conversion for the same reason at not specified short-term follow-up for symptomatic ulnar wear and Burkhart one of 10 (10 %) after 13-month follow-up. Further, Adolfsson et al. observed attrition of the proximal ulna in three of eight (37.5 %) that was only mildly symptomatic at most, which could already be noticed at 2 years in two patients and after 6 years in three. Smith et al. reported ulnar wear in 13 of 17 (76 %) reviewed patients: grade 1 (partial-thickness cartilage loss) in 7, grade 2 (full-thickness cartilage loss) in 4 and grade 3 (bone loss) in 2. Hohman et al. report ulnar wear in all seven patients: mild (preserved joint space) in three, moderate (loss of joint space, but no bone loss) in two and severe (significant bone loss) in two. In the current series, the one patient with the subluxed ulnohumeral joint had attrition of the proximal ulna, but the other did not at midterm follow-up.

From the current series, an important observation can be made. Two out of three patients in whom the lateral collateral ligament was released to dislocate the joint without olecranon osteotomy (cases 1 and 2) were unsatisfied with the final outcome. The first patient has mild residual pain and mild (grade 1) valgus instability. The second (case 2) has moderate residual pain gross (grade 3) valgus instability and a radiographically subluxed prosthesis. In the first case (case 1), possibly the stress on the medial ulnar collateral ligament (MUCL) during the period of dislocation was too great that it resulted in persistent insufficiency of the ligament. In the second case (case 2), it seems the reattachment of the lateral ligament complex has failed. Although being unsatisfied with the final outcome, this patient refused further surgery. We therefore feel very strongly that release of the lateral collateral ligament should not routinely be performed, and we prefer an olecranon osteotomy for exposure and dislocation of the joint without ligamentous release.

Another observation is that salvage procedures, as is the case for five of six cases in the current series, show comparable results and complication ratios as acute cases, of which the majority (82 %) of data of the current literature are derived from [10–17].

In this case series of six patients with DHA for non-reconstructable distal humerus fracture, favorable midterm follow-up results were seen, albeit fair to say that two patients are not satisfied with the final outcome. We feel very strongly that release of the lateral collateral ligament should not routinely be performed and would advise an olecranon osteotomy without ligamentous release to be performed for exposure and dislocation of the joint. The role of DHA in acute fracture care is not well defined to date, but the technique may increasingly need to be considered with the increasing incidence of complex, osteopenic fractures in the elderly.

References

1. McKee MD, Veillette CJ, Hall JA, Schemitsch EH, Wild LM, McCormack R, Perey B, Goetz T, Zomar M, Moon K, Mandel S, Petit S, Guy P, Leung I (2009) A multicenter, prospective, randomized, controlled trial of open reduction—internal fixation versus total elbow arthroplasty for displaced intra-articular distal humeral fractures in elderly patients. J Shoulder Elbow Surg 18:3–12. doi:10.1016/j.jse.2008.06.005

2. Voloshin I, Schippert DW, Kakar S, Kaye EK, Morrey BF (2011) Complications of total elbow replacement: a systematic review. J Shoulder Elbow Surg 20:158–168. doi:10.1016/j.jse.2010.08.026

3. Barr JS, Eaton RG (1965) Elbow reconstruction with a new prosthesis to replace the distal end of the humerus. A case report. J Bone Joint Surg Am 47:1408–1413

4. Macausland WR (1947) Arthroplasty of the elbow. N Engl J Med 236:97–99. doi:10.1056/NEJM194701162360303

5. Mellen RH, Phalen GS (1947) Arthroplasty of the elbow by replacement of the distal portion of the humerus with an acrylic prosthesis. J Bone Joint Surg Am 29:348–353

6. Shifrin PG, Johnson DP (1990) Elbow hemiarthroplasty with 20-year follow-up study. A case report and literature review. Clin Orthop Relat Res 254:128–133

7. Street DM, Stevens PS (1974) A humeral replacement prosthesis for the elbow: results in ten elbows. J Bone Joint Surg Am 56:1147–1158

8. Swoboda B, Scott RD (1999) Humeral hemiarthroplasty of the elbow joint in young patients with rheumatoid arthritis: a report on 7 arthroplasties. J Arthroplasty 14:553–559

9. Venable CS (1952) An elbow and an elbow prosthesis; case of complete loss of the lower third of the humerus. Am J Surg 83:271–275

10. Adolfsson L, Hammer R (2006) Elbow hemiarthroplasty for acute reconstruction of intraarticular distal humerus fractures: a pre-liminary report involving 4 patients. Acta Orthop 77:785–787. doi:10.1080/17453670610012999

11. Adolfsson L, Nestorson J (2012) The Kudo humeral component as primary hemiarthroplasty in distal humeral fractures. J Shoulder Elbow Surg 21:451–455. doi:10.1016/j.jse.2011.07.011

12. Argintar E, Berry M, Narvy SJ, Kramer J, Omid R, Itamura JM (2012) Hemiarthroplasty for the treatment of distal humerus fractures: short-term clinical results. Orthopedics 35:1042–1045. doi:10.3928/01477447-20121120-06

13. Burkhart KJ, Muller LP, Schwarz C, Mattyasovszky SG, Rommens PM (2010) Treatment of the complex intraarticular fracture of the distal humerus with the latitude elbow prosthesis. Oper Orthop Traumatol 22:279–298. doi:10.1007/s00064-010-8031-z

14. Burkhart KJ, Nijs S, Mattyasovszky SG, Wouters R, Gruszka D, Nowak TE, Rommens PM, Muller LP (2011) Distal humerus hemiarthroplasty of the elbow for comminuted distal humeral fractures in the elderly patient. J Trauma 71:635–642. doi:10.1097/TA.0b013e318216936e

15. Parsons M, O'Brien RJ, Hughes JS (2005) Elbow hemiarthroplasty for acute and salvage reconstruction of intra-articular distal humerus fractures. Tech Shoulder Elbow Surg 6:87–97

16. Hohman DW, Nodzo SR, Qvick LM, Duquin TR, Paterson PP (2014) Hemiarthroplasty of the distal humerus for acute and chronic complex intra-articular injuries. J Shoulder Elbow Surg 23:265–272. doi:10.1016/j.jse.2013.05.007

17. Smith GC, Hughes JS (2013) Unreconstructable acute distal humeral fractures and their sequelae treated with distal humeral hemiarthroplasty: a two-year to eleven-year follow-up. J Shoulder Elbow Surg 22:1710–1723. doi:10.1016/j.jse.2013.06.012

18. Morrey BF, Chao EY, Hui FC (1979) Biomechanical study of the elbow following excision of the radial head. J Bone Joint Surg Am 61:63–68

19. Turchin DC, Beaton DE, Richards RR (1998) Validity of observer-based aggregate scoring systems as descriptors of elbow pain, function, and disability. J Bone Joint Surg Am 80:154–162

20. Brooker AF, Bowerman JW, Robinson RA, Riley LH Jr (1973) Ectopic ossification following total hip replacement. Incidence and a method of classification. J Bone Joint Surg Am 55:1629–1632

30

Computer-assisted 3D planned corrective osteotomies in eight malunited radius fractures

M. M. J. Walenkamp[1] · R. J. O. de Muinck Keizer[1] ⓘ · J. G. G. Dobbe[2] ·
G. J. Streekstra[2,3] · J. C. Goslings[1] · P. Kloen[4] · S. D. Strackee[5] · N. W. L. Schep[6]

Abstract In corrective osteotomy of the radius, detailed preoperative planning is essential to optimising functional outcome. However, complex malunions are not completely addressed with conventional preoperative planning. Computer-assisted preoperative planning may optimise the results of corrective osteotomy of the radius. We analysed the pre- and postoperative radiological result of computer-assisted 3D planned corrective osteotomy in a series of patients with a malunited radius and assessed postoperative function. We included eight patients aged 13–64 who underwent a computer-assisted 3D planned corrective osteotomy of the radius for the treatment of a symptomatic radius malunion. We evaluated pre- and postoperative residual malpositioning on 3D reconstructions as expressed in six positioning parameters (three displacements along and three rotations about the axes of a 3D anatomical coordinate system) and assessed postoperative wrist range of motion. In this small case series, dorsopalmar tilt was significantly improved ($p = 0.05$). Ulnoradial shift, however, increased by the correction osteotomy (6 of 8 cases, 75 %). Postoperative 3D evaluation revealed improved positioning parameters for patients in axial rotational alignment (62.5 %), radial inclination (75 %), proximodistal shift (83 %) and volodorsal shift (88 %), although the cohort was not large enough to confirm this by statistical significance. All but one patient experienced improved range of motion (88 %). Computer-assisted 3D planning ameliorates alignment of radial malunions and improves functional results in patients with a symptomatic malunion of the radius. Further development is required to improve transfer of the planned position to the intra-operative bone.
Level of evidence IV.

M. M. J. Walenkamp and R. J. O. de Muinck Keizer have contributed equally to this work.

✉ R. J. O. de Muinck Keizer
rjodemuinckkeizer@amc.nl

[1] Trauma Unit, Department of Surgery, Academic Medical Centre, University of Amsterdam, room G4-137, P.O. Box 22660, 1100 DD Amsterdam, The Netherlands

[2] Biomedical Engineering and Physics, Academic Medical Centre, University of Amsterdam, Amsterdam, The Netherlands

[3] Department of Radiology, Academic Medical Centre, University of Amsterdam, Amsterdam, The Netherlands

[4] Department of Orthopaedic Surgery, Academic Medical Centre, University of Amsterdam, Amsterdam, The Netherlands

[5] Department of Plastic, Reconstructive and Hand Surgery, Academic Medical Centre, University of Amsterdam, Amsterdam, The Netherlands

[6] Department of Surgery, Maasstad Hospital, Rotterdam, The Netherlands

Keywords Malunion · Radius · Corrective osteotomy · 3D

Introduction

Malunion of a radial fracture may result in chronic pain and loss of function and occurs in around 5 % of the cases [1–3]. A corrective osteotomy for patients with a malunited radius fracture can improve wrist function and reduce stiffness and pain [4]. Previous studies showed that accuracy of the anatomical reconstruction is essential to achieving an optimal outcome [5–7]. Therefore, conscientious preoperative planning of the procedure and accurate surgical repositioning is required [1, 5]. Conventionally, planning is based on two orthogonal radiographs depicting lateral and posteroanterior views of the radius.

However, malunion of the radius commonly involves complex three-dimensional (3D) deformations in different planes, which may not be acknowledged on conventional preoperative 2D radiographs [8–12]. Two-dimensional radiographic planning does not always result in adequate restoration of alignment, as was demonstrated by a recent study performed by members of our study group [7].

A potential solution of the challenge presented by the complex deformity of radius malunions is the use of computer-assisted 3D planning techniques. With these techniques, both physical and virtual models of the deformed radius and the mirrored contralateral radius can be created. The models are used preoperatively to conceptualise the multiple planes of deformity and to preoperatively plan the osteotomy [4, 13]. Preoperative 3D planning also provides the possibility to create patient-specific cutting guides to transfer the planned osteotomy plane to the patient's bony anatomy during surgery. Patient-specific guides for cutting or drilling have been successfully introduced before [14–16]. They have proven to enable accurate positioning of surgical instruments or implants with respect to bony anatomy. However, these studies mostly focus on functional results without properly evaluating residual postoperative malpositioning using 3D imaging techniques.

Therefore, the aim of this study was to assess whether computer-assisted 3D planning and the intra-operative use of personalised cutting guides improve the accuracy of bone alignment.

Materials and methods

All patients who underwent a computer-assisted 3D planned corrective osteotomy of the radius for the treatment of symptomatic radius malunion between January 2009 and March 2014 were eligible for inclusion. Only patients who underwent a postoperative CT scan of both (full length) radii were included. Patients with a previous fracture of the contralateral radius were excluded.

Preoperative planning

Preoperative planning was based on computed tomography (CT) scans of both the affected and the contralateral radius. The unaffected contralateral bone served as reference for determining malalignment. All CT scans were obtained using a Brilliance 64-channel CT scanner (Phillips Healthcare, Best, The Netherlands) reconstructed to a 3D volume with a voxel spacing of $0.45 \times 0.45 \times 0.45$ mm. Data were imported by a dedicated application program

which helps quantifying pre- and postoperative malalignment [17]. In short, the program enables segmenting the affected bone using a threshold-connected region growing algorithm that collects voxels that belong to the affected bone, followed by a binary closing algorithm to close residual gaps. A Laplacian level-set segmentation growth algorithm advances the outline towards the boundary of the bone. A polygonal mesh is finally extracted, which is used for visualisation of the bone deformity. It also serves to create a double-contour polygon by sampling the grey-level image 0.3 mm towards the inside (bright) and outside (dark) for each point of the polygonal bone model. This double-contour polygon with image grey levels assigned to each point enables efficient and accurate point-to-image registration.

Next, distal and proximal segments are clipped to exclude the malunited fracture region. The clipped segments are aligned with the mirrored image of the healthy contralateral bone, by point-to-image registration. This procedure provides a position matrix that brings the distal bone segment in a position that agrees with that of the mirrored contralateral bone. The matrix is used to quantify malpositioning in terms of three displacements along and three rotations about the axes of a 3D anatomical coordinate system (Fig. 4) [7]. The centroid of the clipped bone segment polygons is used as centre of rotation. Translations are determined in the ulnoradial, volodorsal and proximodistal directions. Rotations are expressed in terms of dorsopalmar tilt, radial inclination and axial rotation (pronation and supination). In case of an oblique single-cut rotation osteotomy [14], the matrix is used to determine the orientation of the osteotomy and the rotation angle for aligning the distal and proximal bone segments. The software further enables to create (1) both virtual and physical models of both radii on which the osteotomy planning was simulated (Fig. 1), and (2) patient-specific cutting guides and jigs for intra-operative guidance of the osteotomy (Fig. 2).

Patient-specific bone models and cutting guides

During the preoperative planning, the surgeon was able to interactively set the position and orientation of the cutting plane in the virtual radius (Fig. 1). Synthetic acrylonitrile butadiene styrene (ABS) bone models were created using additive manufacturing technology (SST1200es 3D printer, Dimension Inc, Eden Prairie, MN, USA) with a resolution of 254 µm.

In four patients, a patient-specific cutting guide was used which snugly fitted to the bone geometry (see Fig. 2b). Polyamide cutting guides were manufactured (Materialise, Leuven, Belgium; Sirris, Charleroi, Belgium; Amitek Prototyping, De Meern, The Netherlands) and were sterilised before use in the operating room.

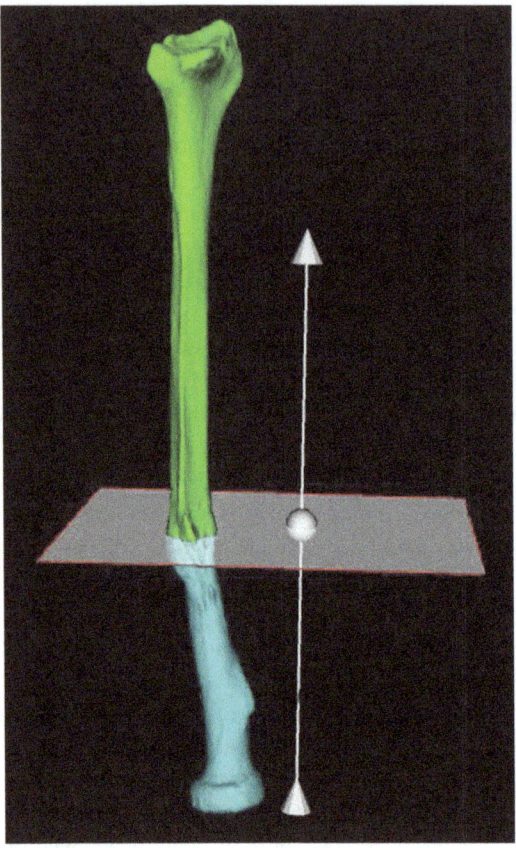

Fig. 1 Positioning of cutting plane

Surgical procedure

Depending on the complexity of the malunion, patients were treated with an open-wedge osteotomy or an oblique single-cut rotation osteotomy (OSCRO) [14]. Both osteotomy types were planned by using virtual or physical synthetic models of both radii and/or assisted by intraoperative use of patient-specific cutting guides and jigs (Fig. 2). In the latter method, the sterilised surgical guide was positioned at the specific bone surface and was fixated with Kirschner wires, using the planned fixation holes. In the case of an oblique single-cut rotation osteotomy (OSCRO), the guide was removed after the osteotomy and a stainless steel jig served to set the angle between the proximal and distal bone segment [14]. Rotational alignment was achieved by rotating the malunited distal bone segment over the planned angle. Regular plate and screw fixation was performed to maintain the position. Postoperative management varied from direct mobilisation to 2 weeks of plaster of Paris immobilisation.

Data collection and outcome

Patients were evaluated postoperatively after a minimum follow-up of 6 months. The main outcome was residual 3D

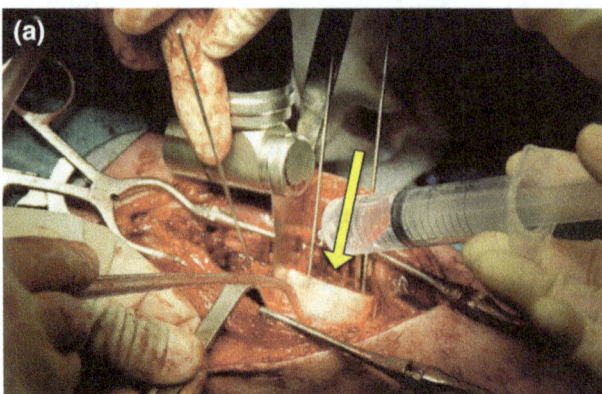

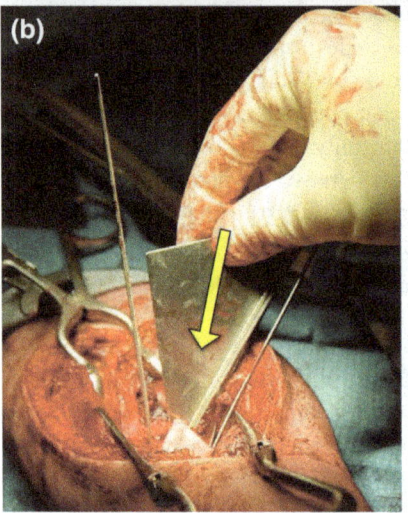

Fig. 2 a Intra-operative correction of deformation with cutting guide (*yellow arrow*). **b** Intra-operative correction of deformation with angled jig (*yellow arrow*) (colour figure online)

malpositioning based on a postoperative CT scan of both forearms. Residual malpositioning was again expressed in terms of six positioning parameters. These residual malpositioning parameters were quantified in exactly the same way as described for preoperative planning, with the one difference that the postoperative image was used for segmentation of the bone instead of the preoperative image. Secondary outcome was the postoperative range of motion of the wrist measured on both sides with a handheld goniometer.

This study was approved by the Medical Ethical Review Committee of the Academic Medical Centre of the University of Amsterdam. All subjects gave informed consent before participation in this study.

Statistical analysis

We reported medians and interquartile range (IQR) for nonparametric variables, and means and standard deviations (SD) for normally distributed variables. The absolute value of each malalignment parameter served to represent the residual error. The Kolmogorov–Smirnov test was used for the determination of the distribution form. The Wilcoxon signed rank test was used to compare the medians of each of the six malpositioning parameters before and after correction.

Results

A total of 16 patients were treated for a symptomatic malunion with a computer-assisted 3D planned corrective osteotomy of the radius.

Five patients were treated recently, and their follow-up was shorter than 6 months. Two patients did not want to participate in postoperative position evaluation, and one patient had moved abroad. This resulted in a total of eight patients who were included in this series.

Of the included patients, three had originally developed a malunion after sustaining an extra-articular distal radius fracture. Five patients had sustained a forearm fracture

(three antebrachial fractures and two isolated radius fractures), all of whom developed a diaphyseal malunion of the radius. The demographics of the study group are depicted in Table 1. We performed an opening-wedge osteotomy on four patients, and the other four patients received an oblique single-cut rotation osteotomy (OSCRO). All patients achieved primary osseous union. The median duration of follow-up was 26 months (IQR 12–34). No complications occurred.

The median pre- and postoperative malalignment per dimension is depicted in Table 2. Improvement in dorsopalmar tilt showed statistical significance ($p = 0.05$, Wilcoxon signed rank test). The median residual malalignment was smallest for radial length (-0.6 mm) and axial rotation ($-2.6°$).

The individual changes in preoperative and postoperative deformations are depicted in Fig. 3. In two adolescent patients (Cases 7 and 8), the radial length (translation in proximodistal direction) was not reliable due to the patients' growing skeleton between pre- and postoperative

Table 1 Demographics of study population

Case	Sex	Age[a]	Location malunion	Dominant hand affected	Indication	Technique[b]	Osteotomy type	Follow-up (months)
1	F	64	Distal, extra-articular	Yes	Pain	Cutting guide	Opening	32
2	F	53	Distal, extra-articular	Yes	Pain	Simulation	Opening	56
3	F	18	Distal, extra-articular	No	Pain, DRUJ instability	Simulation	Opening	8
4	M	32	Diaphyseal	Yes	Restricted supination	Cutting guide	OSCRO	34
5	F	18	Diaphyseal	Yes	Restricted pronation	Simulation	OSCRO	12
6	F	41	Diaphyseal + ulna	No	Restricted ROM (all directions)	Simulation	OSCRO	29
7	M	18	Diaphyseal + ulna	No	Restricted pronation/supination	Cutting guide	OSCRO	13
8	M	13	Diaphyseal + ulna	Yes	Restricted supination	Cutting guide	Opening	23

F female, *M* male, *ROM* range of motion, *DRUJ* distal radioulnar joint, *Opening* opening-wedge osteotomy, *OSCRO* oblique single-cut rotation osteotomy

[a] Age in years at time of surgery

[b] Technique consisted of either pre- and intra-operative simulation of the osteotomy using virtual or physical 3D models of both radii sometimes with intra-operative use of a custom-made cutting guide and angled jig

Table 2 Residual malalignment

Malalignment parameter	Median (IQR)			Significance[a]
	Pre-op	Post-op	Difference	
Ulnoradial shift in mm, ulnar (−), radial (+)	3.8 (1.4 to 9.9)	7.0 (1.1 to 11.0)	2.1 (−2.7 to 5.0)	0.327
Volodorsal shift in mm, volar (−), dorsal (+)	7.2 (−5.6 to 30.3)	4.0 (2.8 to 10.3)	−3.2 (−11.6 to 11.2)	0.069
Proximodistal shift in mm, shortened (−), lengthened (+)	−5.3 (−17.0 to 13.9)	−0.6 (−3.8 to 0.2)	2.9 (−0.0 to 5.4)	0.123
Dorsopalmar tilt in deg, dorsal (−), volar (−)	−9.0 (−16.8 to 13.9)	−6.4 (−7.9 to 0.4)	5.5 (−6.9 to 10.3)	**0.050**
Radial inclination in deg, ulnar (−), radial (+)	5.6 (0.4 to 8.8)	3.2 (−1.4 to 8.8)	−1.4 (−9.3 to 5.3)	0.208
Axial rotation in deg, pronation (−), supination (+)	−7.6 (−36.4 to 2.0)	−2.6 (−13.2 to 12.3)	15.0 (1.2 to −30.6)	0.484

IQR interquartile range, *deg* degrees, *mm* millimetre

[a] Related samples Wilcoxon signed rank test

Bold value indicates statistical significance ($p < 0.05$)

Fig. 3 Pre- and postoperative positioning

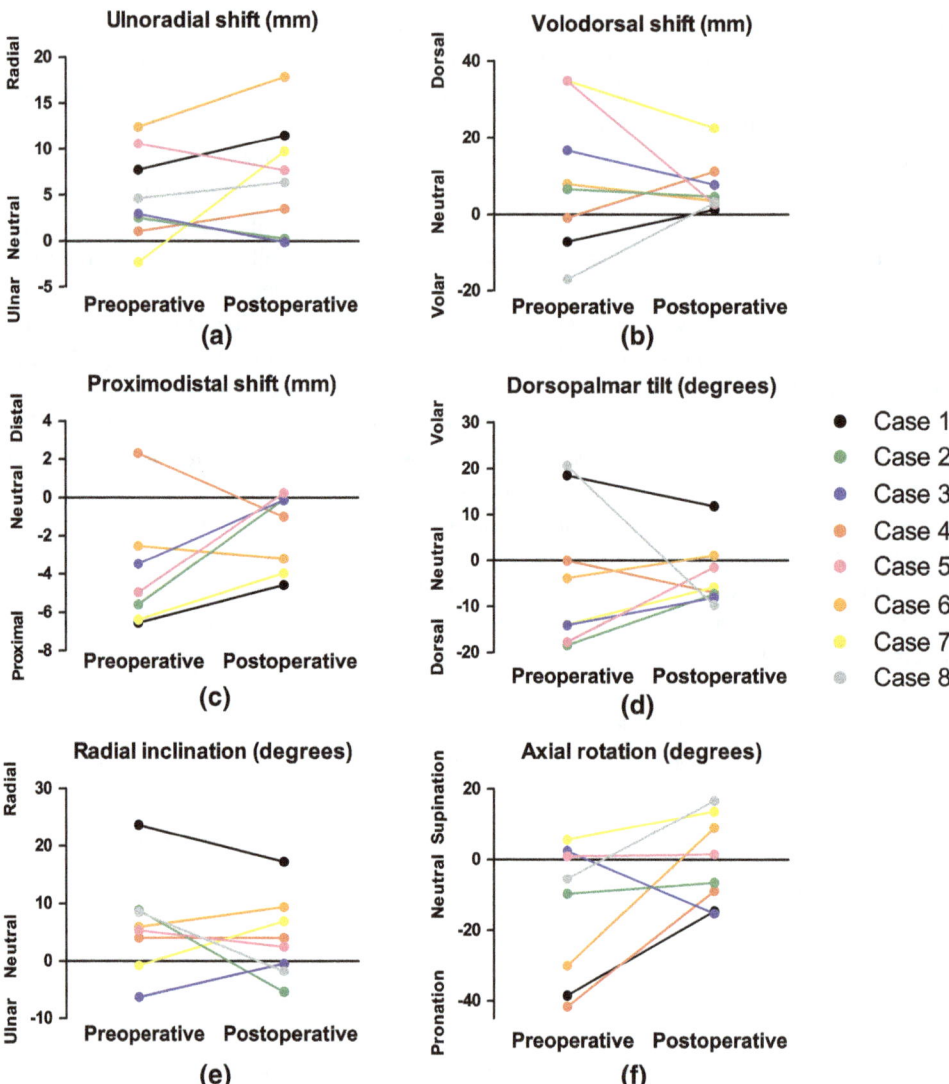

CT scans. Volodorsal translation showed improvement (correction towards neutral) in all but one patient (88 %). In six patients (75 %), ulnoradial shift increased by the correction osteotomy. In two patients, this shift was corrected to nearly neutral.

Dorsopalmar tilt was improved in seven out of eight patients (88 %): in one patient (Case 8), tilt was overcorrected from volar to dorsal. In one patient (Case 4), the preoperative neutral position was corrected to dorsal angulation (Fig. 4). Five patients originally had a malunion in pronation. In those five cases, rotations were corrected, although an overcorrection to supination was present in two patients (Cases 6 and 8). Radial inclination was improved in six out of eight patients (88 %).

Six patients (88 %) experienced a postoperative increased range of motion (Table 3). One patient (Case 3) slightly deteriorated. In addition to a distal radius fracture, this patient had sustained a triangular fibrocartilage complex (TFCC) tear that resulted in instability of the distal

radioulnar joint (DRUJ). The performed correction osteotomy itself did not provide enough stability, and reinsertion of the TFCC was attempted 2 months after the corrective osteotomy, but was not successful. In one patient (Case 2), the indication for treatment was based on pain, instead of restricted ROM. The preoperative range of motion (ROM) was therefore not measured. There was no statistically significant difference in terms of malalignment parameters between the cases that were corrected with use of a cutting guide versus the corrections that were visualised (Table 4).

Discussion

Postoperative 3D evaluation revealed improved positioning parameters for most patients in dorsopalmar tilt, axial rotation (pronation and supination), radial inclination, proximodistal shift and volodorsal shift. Dorsopalmar tilt

Computer-assisted 3D planning techniques are expected to optimise preoperative treatment plans and therefore minimise residual malalignment [7]. In our study, alignment improved in five of the six positioning parameters, of which improvement in dorsopalmar tilt reached significance despite the small number of patients.

There are several explanations for the residual malalignment. Firstly, the transfer from the virtual plan to the actual realignment and fixation might leave room for error. Although in half of the patients, we used patient-specific cutting jigs to transfer the planned correction onto the patients' radius and used a jig to indicate the angle of the osteotomy, reduction and fixation were done in a freehand manner with K-wires. Although cutting guides generally show beneficial in reconstructive surgery [18], based on our results we cannot yet draw conclusions on its added value. For accurate bone repositioning in future corrective osteotomy treatment, we recommend using reduction guides [15] or patient-specific fixation plates [19].

The advantage of using an oblique single-cut rotation osteotomy is the correction of angular deformities in three dimensions while maintaining optimal bone contact. However, the method does not aim to correct translational displacements. Small rotational errors after corrective osteotomy of a diaphyseal malunion may scale to relatively large translational displacements at the distal articular level. This could partly explain the residual displacements in ulnoradial and volodorsal shifts.

Secondly, the preoperative plan does not take into account the soft tissue issues many of these deformed forearms have. Earlier (surgical) trauma often causes scar formation to structures like the interosseous membrane and makes the planned repositioning difficult to realise. Additionally, full geometric restoration of bony structures may hamper full mobility if there is too much stress on the soft tissue. Therefore, in some cases, complete correction was not obtained. Despite this issue, previously published data suggest a statistically significant correlation between residual malalignment and clinical outcome [7]. When soft tissue allows, we expect that increased precision in radiological outcome will further optimise postoperative functional results.

The strength of this study is that we examined the postoperative positioning using 3D techniques. Only a few previous studies assessed postoperative results in 3D [7, 20, 21]. However, they focussed on intra-articular distal radius malunions and expressed their findings in terms of postoperative articular displacement. Another study by Vroemen et al. [7] evaluated the postoperative malalignment in 25 patients after a 2D planned corrective osteotomy using 3D imaging techniques. The median residual malalignments we presented in this study are comparable, but not

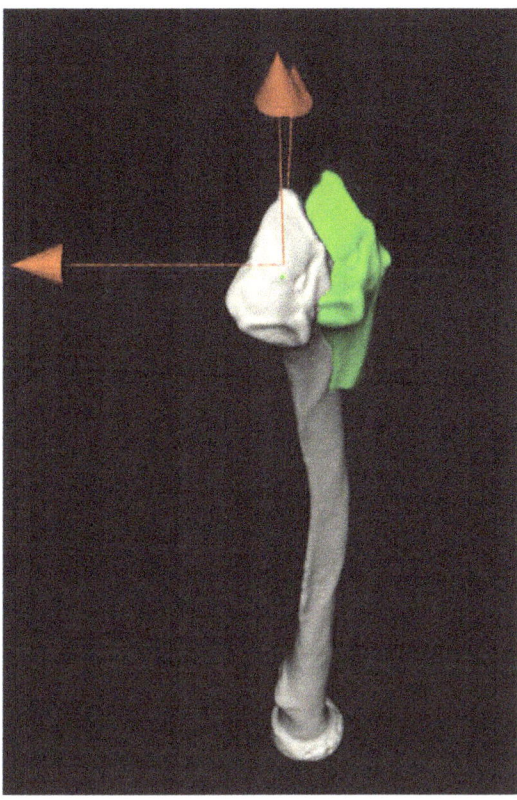

Fig. 4 Postoperative alignment in virtual model. Postoperative malalignment of the distal radius segment (*green*) of Case 4 compared to the mirrored contralateral radius (colour figure online)

Table 3 Functional results

| Case | Preoperative | | Postoperative | |
| | Range of wrist[a] | | Range of wrist[a] | |
	Pronation/supination	Flexion/extension	Pronation/supination	Flexion/extension
1	150	150	165	135
2	NA	NA	180	175
3	180	155	180	150
4	115	100	145	180
5	90	NA	155	180
6	40	55	175	175
7	80	NA	135	180
8	125	180	180	180
Average	111	128	164	169

NA not available

[a] Expressed in degrees and measured with a handheld goniometer

significantly improved. However, ulnoradial translation was worsened by the correction osteotomy. Both over- and undercorrection occurred in individual patients. All but one patient experienced improved range of motion.

Table 4 Differences in malalignment parameters compared to pre-op for patients treated with cutting guide versus visualisation

Malalignment parameter	Difference compared to pre-op Median (IQR)		Significance[a]
	Cutting guide ($n = 4$)	Visualisation ($n = 4$)	
Coronal shift in mm, ulnar (−), radial (+)	3.1 (1.9 to 10.0)	−2.6 (−3.0 to 3.5)	0.200
Sagittal shift in mm, volar (−), dorsal (+)	10.2 (−7.3 to 18.1)	−6.7 (−26.4 to −2.6)	0.200
Radial length in mm	2.2 (−2.0 to 15.7)	4.3 (0.3 to 5.4)	0.686
Palmar tilt in deg, dorsal (−), volar (−)	−6.8 (−24.5 to 4.4)	8.5 (5.2 to 14.9)	0.114
Radial inclination in deg, ulnar (−), radial (+)	−3.2 (−9.3 to 5.7)	0.3 (−11.4 to 5.3)	1.000
Axial rotation in deg, pronation (−), supination (+)	23.0 (11.5 to 30.6)	1.8 (−13.1 to 30.0)	0.343

IQR interquartile range, *deg* degrees, *mm* millimetre

[a] Independent samples Mann–Whitney *U* test

per se superior to their results after a 2D planned corrective osteotomy. However, due to the lack of preoperative 3D malpositioning of their series and a potential selection of relatively complex cases in ours, full comparison is not possible.

The postoperative range of motion we found is better than previous studies with computer-assisted 3D planned corrective osteotomy in radial malunions [22, 23]. Athwal et al. [22] included six patients with a distal radius malunion. They found an average postoperative range of motion of 89° of flexion–extension, 78 % of pronation and 74 % of supination after a mean follow-up of 25 months. Miyake et al. included 20 patients and reported a range of motion of 152° pronation and supination after a mean follow-up of 24 months.

Our functional results are also superior to published results of conventional 2D planned corrective osteotomies. A previous study that investigated the long-term results after 2D planned corrective osteotomy of distal malunions demonstrated a range of motion of 109 degrees of flexion–extension and 142° of pronation and supination after a mean follow-up of 13 years [24].

This study has several limitations. Due to the retrospective nature of this study, there was no predefined protocol for selecting patients. The decision to perform a computer-assisted 3D planned corrective osteotomy was made by the surgeon. Only patients with complex malunions were selected for this type of treatment. This approach has resulted in a selection bias and potentially limits the generalisability of our results. Due to the retrospective nature of this study, we were not able to acquire preoperative grip strength or functional questionnaires (e.g. DASH, PRWE), thus limiting the evaluation of functional outcome of the procedure. Another limitation is the heterogeneity of the population. We included subjects with both diaphyseal and extra-articular distal radius malunions.

Distal malunions commonly show axial malalignment in pronation [25], whereas diaphyseal malunions typically involve angular deformation [23]. Individual cases require different goals of correction. As mentioned, an oblique single-cut rotation osteotomy (OSCRO) aims to correct rotational deformities and is limited in providing ulnoradial or volodorsal shifts. This phenomenon—in combination with the low number of cases—may explain the lack of statistically significant improvement in individual directional parameters.

Some patients may benefit more from this 3D planned osteotomy than others. Future studies should focus on determining the appropriate indication for the use of 3D planning techniques in corrective osteotomy. This study suggests that virtual 3D planning of corrective osteotomies of radial malunions ameliorates alignment. Further enhancement of this technique is required to improve transfer of the preoperatively planned position to the intraoperative bone.

Research involving human participants and/or animals This study was approved by the Medical Ethical Review Committee of the Academic Medical Centre of the University of Amsterdam. All procedures performed in studies involving human participants were in accordance with the ethical standards of the institutional and/or national research committee and with the 1964 Helsinki Declaration and its later amendments or comparable ethical standards.

Informed consent Informed consent was obtained from all individual participants included in the study.

Author contributions All authors have made substantial contributions to the design of this paper, revising the manuscript, approved the final version and are accountable for all aspects of the work.

References

1. Cooney W, Dobyns J, Linscheid R (1980) Complications of Colles' fractures. J Bone Joint Surg 62:613–619

2. McKay SD, MacDermid JC, Roth JH, Richards RS (2001) Assessment of complications of distal radius fractures and development of a complication checklist. J Hand Surg Am 26:916–922. doi:10.1053/jhsu.2001.26662

3. Crisco JJ, Moore DC, Marai GE, Laidlaw DH, Akelman E, Weiss AC et al (2007) Effects of distal radius malunion on distal radioulnar joint mechanics—an in vivo study. J Orthop Res. doi:10.1002/jor

4. Buijze G, Prommersberger K-J, González Del Pino J, Fernandez DL, Jupiter JB (2012) Corrective osteotomy for combined intra- and extra-articular distal radius malunion. J Hand Surg Am 37:2041–2049. doi:10.1016/j.jhsa.2012.07.013

5. Fernandez DL (1982) Correction of post-traumatic wrist deformity in adults by osteotomy, bone-grafting, and internal fixation. J Bone Joint Surg 64:1164–1178

6. Prommersberger K-J, van Schoonhoven J, Lanz UB (2002) Outcome after corrective osteotomy for malunited fractures of the distal end of the radius. J Hand Surg Am 27B:55–60

7. Vroemen JC, Dobbe JGG, Strackee SD, Streekstra GJ (2013) Positioning evaluation of corrective osteotomy for the malunited radius: 3-D CT versus 2-D radiographs. Orthopedics 36:e193–e199. doi:10.3928/01477447-20130122-22

8. Miyake J, Murase T, Yamanaka Y, Moritomo H, Sugamoto K, Yoshikawa H (2013) Comparison of three dimensional and radiographic measurements in the analysis of distal radius malunion. J Hand Surg Eur 38:133–143. doi:10.1177/1753193412451383

9. Bilic R, Zdravkovic V, Boljevic Z (1994) Osteotomy for deformity of the radius: computer-assisted three-dimensional modelling. J Bone Joint Surg 76-B:150–154

10. Cirpar M, Gudemez E, Cetik O, Turker M, Eksioglu F (2010) Rotational deformity affects radiographic measurements in distal radius malunion. Eur J Orthop Surg Traumatol 21:13–20. doi:10.1007/s00590-010-0653-1

11. Capo JT, Accousti K, Jacob G, Tan V (2009) The effect of rotational malalignment on X-rays of the wrist. J Hand Surg Eur 34:166–172. doi:10.1177/1753193408090393

12. Pennock A, Phillips C, Matzon J, Daley E (2005) The effects of forearm rotation on three wrist measurements: radial inclination, radial height and palmar tilt. Hand Surg 10:17–22. doi:10.3928/01477447-20130122-22

13. Leong NL, Buijze G, Fu EC, Stockmans F, Jupiter JB (2010) Computer-assisted versus non-computer-assisted preoperative planning of corrective osteotomy for extra-articular distal radius malunions: a randomized controlled trial. BMC Musculoskelet Disord 11:282. doi:10.1186/1471-2474-11-282

14. Dobbe J, du Pré K, Kloen P, Blankevoort L, Streekstra G (2011) Computer-assisted and patient-specific 3-D planning and evaluation of a single-cut rotational osteotomy for complex long-bone deformities. Med Biol Eng Comput 49:1363–1370. doi:10.1007/s11517-011-0830-3

15. Murase T, Oka K, Moritomo H, Goto A, Yoshikawa H, Sugamoto K (2008) Three-dimensional corrective osteotomy of malunited fractures of the upper extremity with use of a computer simulation system. J Bone Joint Surg Am 90:2375–2389. doi:10.2106/JBJS.G.01299

16. Stockmans F, Dezillie M, Vanhaecke J (2013) Accuracy of 3D virtual planning of corrective osteotomies of the distal radius. J Wrist Surg 2:306–314

17. Dobbe JGG, Strackee SD, Schreurs AW, Jonges R, Carelsen B, Vroemen JC et al (2011) Computer-assisted planning and navigation for corrective distal radius osteotomy, based on pre- and intraoperative imaging. IEEE Trans Biomed Eng 58:182–190. doi:10.1109/TBME.2010.2084576

18. Krishnan S, Dawood A, Richards R, Henckel J, Hart A (2012) A review of rapid prototyped surgical guides for patient-specific total knee replacement. J Bone Joint Surg Br 94:1457–1461

19. Dobbe J, Vroemen J, Strackee S, Streekstra G (2014) Patient-specific distal radius locking plate for fixation and accurate 3D positioning in corrective osteotomy. Strateg Trauma Limb Reconstr 9:179–183

20. Schweizer A, Fürnstahl P, Nagy L (2013) Three-dimensional correction of distal radius intra-articular malunions using patient-specific drill guides. J Hand Surg Am 38:2339–2347. doi:10.1016/j.jhsa.2013.09.023

21. Vroemen JC, Dobbe JGG, Sierevelt IN, Strackee SD, Streekstra GJ (2013) Accuracy of distal radius positioning using an anatomical plate. Orthopedics 36:457–462. doi:10.3928/01477447-20130327-22

22. Athwal GS, Ellis RE, Small CF, Pichora DR (2003) Computer-assisted distal radius osteotomy. J Hand Surg Am 28:951–958. doi:10.1016/S0363-5023(03)00375-7

23. Miyake J, Murase T, Oka K, Moritomo H, Sugamoto K, Yoshikawa H (2012) Computer-assisted corrective osteotomy for malunited diaphyseal forearm fractures. J Bone Joint Surg 94:1–11

24. Lozano-Calderón SA, Brouwer KM, Doornberg JN, Goslings JC, Kloen P, Jupiter JB (2010) Long-term outcomes of corrective osteotomy for the treatment of distal radius malunion. J Hand Surg Eur 35:370–380. doi:10.1177/1753193409357373

25. Miyake J, Murase T, Yamanaka Y, Moritomo H, Sugamoto K, Yoshikawa H (2012) Three-dimensional deformity analysis of malunited distal radius fractures and their influence on wrist and forearm motion. J Hand Surg Eur 37:506–512. doi:10.1177/1753193412443644

31

Valgus osteotomy by external fixation for treatment for developmental coxa vara

Hany Hefny · Elhussein Mohamed Elmoatasem · Wael Nassar

Abstract Valgus subtrochanteric osteotomy is the standard surgical treatment for coxa vara. Nevertheless, there is no consensus on the method of fixation and osteotomy technique. There are some reports on employing rigid internal fixation methods that preclude the need of postoperative immobilization. This is a technical description of a valgus osteotomy performed using external fixation with preoperative and postoperative data on a cohort of 9 patients. In this study, 9 hips in 9 patients with the diagnosis of developmental coxa vara underwent a subtrochanteric osteotomy with stabilization by an external fixator. The planned correction angle was obtained for all 9 patients with the osteotomies healing primarily. Radiographic analysis showed an improvement in Hilgenreiner's epiphyseal angle and the neck-shaft angle. There were no major complications associated with use of this method of stabilization. Minimal access surgery using external fixation for a valgus osteotomy of the proximal femur is safe and effective for the treatment for coxa vara and limb length discrepancy. It has potential advantages over commonly used open techniques and provides available alternative to currently applied methods used for fixation of proximal femoral osteotomies.

Keywords Coxa vara · Osteotomy · External fixator · Ilizarov

H. Hefny · E. M. Elmoatasem (✉) · W. Nassar
Ain Shams University, Cairo, Egypt
e-mail: hmoatasem@yahoo.com

H. Hefny
e-mail: hhefny@yahoo.com

W. Nassar
e-mail: wgnassar@hotmail.com

Introduction

Classically defined as a femoral neck-shaft angle of <110°, coxa vara is relatively uncommon and is present in approximately 1/25,000 children [1]. This deformity results from a heterogeneous group of conditions that can be classified as congenital, developmental, dysplastic and traumatic [1]. The natural history of coxa vara may be debilitating as the child develops progressive limb length discrepancy, limp, pain, abductor weakness, and restricted motion. Secondary acetabular dysplasia and genu valgum may compound the problem. With the exception of some forms of developmental coxa vara which can resolve, a variety of surgical methods have evolved to deal with progressive coxa vara [1–5]. Despite well-executed osteotomies, recurrence is cited in the literature as ranging from 30 to 70 % [1, 3, 4, 6]. The high recurrence rate can be explained by the biomechanics of the underlying disorder. Coxa vara lends itself to progression as the physis assumes a more vertical position. Resultant forces across the hip then become shearing rather than compressive [7]. This bending moment is damaging not only to the mechanical properties of stability of the epiphysis but also to normal continued physeal growth. Thus, unlike the normal hip where these resultant forces are compressive, in coxa vara, the shearing forces cause the deformity to recur unless the osteotomy addresses the physeal position satisfactorily [8]. Adequate surgical correction of coxa vara can be difficult, requiring careful clinical and radiographic assessment, preoperative planning, proper implant selection and meticulous surgical technique. Restoration of the femoral capital physis to a relatively horizontal position will aid to normalize the biomechanical forces. This correction of Hilgenreiner's epiphyseal angle (HEA) to <38° is the goal of intraoperative correction. This has been shown to reduce the risk of recurrent coxa vara, regardless of the etiology of the deformity and the age of the patient [4, 8]. Achieving corrections of limb deformities and length discrepancies through less invasive means is increasingly popular [9]. Recently, good results have been reported using external fixator systems for the correction of proximal femoral deformities secondary to slipped capital femoral epiphysis (SCFE), Perthes' disease in children and percutaneous proximal femoral osteotomy for coxa vara [10–12]. We describe the surgical technique of a minimally invasive percutaneous approach for correction of severe coxa vara using external fixation.

Patients and methods

Between 2002 and 2010, nine subtrochanteric femoral osteotomies were performed in nine consecutive patients for treatment for coxa vara using external fixator systems for stabilization. Two different types of external fixation were used: the monolateral limb reconstruction system (LRS) fixator in 2 cases and the multiplanar Ilizarov fixator in 7 cases. The age at initial surgery was averaged 10.1 years (range 6–16 years). All the patients included in the study had developmental coxa vara. Any patient with coxa vara due to other etiologies, viz, acquired, dysplastic or congenital (e.g., fracture neck femur, fibrous dysplasia or proximal femoral focal deficiency, respectively) was excluded from the study. Patients included in this study presented with the chief complaint of a limp, with minimal or no pain. Physical examination revealed a short leg gait with an abductor lurch, a positive Trendelenburg test, limitation of abduction and internal rotation of the involved hip in all patients. Standard radiographs, including an anteroposterior (AP) view of the pelvis and frog lateral of the affected hip, were done before and 1, 3, 6 and 12 months after surgery. Limb scanograms were available preoperatively in all patients. HEA and the neck-shaft angle were measured before surgery, immediately after surgery and at latest follow-up on the AP pelvis radiograph. All patients had a HEA of more than 60°, a femoral neck-shaft angle (FNSA) of <95° and an obliterated or reversed articulo-trochanteric distance (ATD, Fig. 1). Six patients had preoperative shortening averaging 3.4 cm (range 2–5). In 3 patients, an additional diaphyseal femoral osteotomy was done to correct limb length discrepancy and mechanical axis deviation (Fig. 1). The mean duration of follow-up was 4.2 years (range 2–8 years).

Operative technique

All patients were operated under general anesthesia. Patients were positioned in lateral decubitus. The involved lower extremity was prepared and draped. With the affected limb held in hip neutral position, a true AP view of

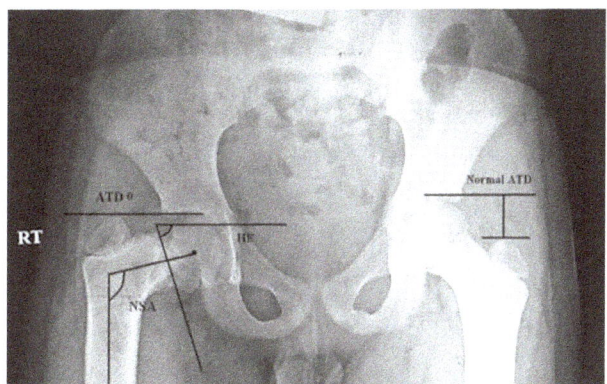

Fig. 1 Radiographic evaluations on the standing anteroposterior radiographs with the hips in neutral position were performed. *a* Measurements of the Hilgenreiner's epiphyseal angle (HE), neck-shaft angle (NSA), articulo-trochanteric distance (ATD)

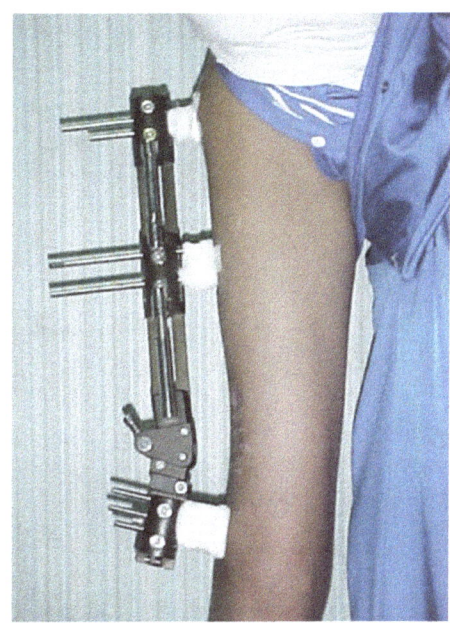

Fig. 2 Clinical photograph showing application of Orthofix fixator after distal femoral osteotomy for limb lengthening and correction of mechanical axis

the involved hip was reproduced on the C-arm monitor. Placing the half-pins in the proximal segment with the limb in the hip neutral position avoids the need for extensive skin release around the half-pins after the corrective osteotomy. The proximal half-pin was placed in a direction from superolateral to inferomedial. We used a modified technique by inserting a Kirschner wire, followed by cannulated drill and finally the half-pin inserted under C-arm control (Fig. 2). In the case of using the Ilizarov fixator, the half-pins were mounted on femoral arch and care was taken to allow at least 2 finger breadths between the arch and the underlying skin (Fig. 3). Next, with the limb in neutral alignment in the frontal, sagittal and

Fig. 3 Application of proximal half-pin in direction from superolateral to inferomedial

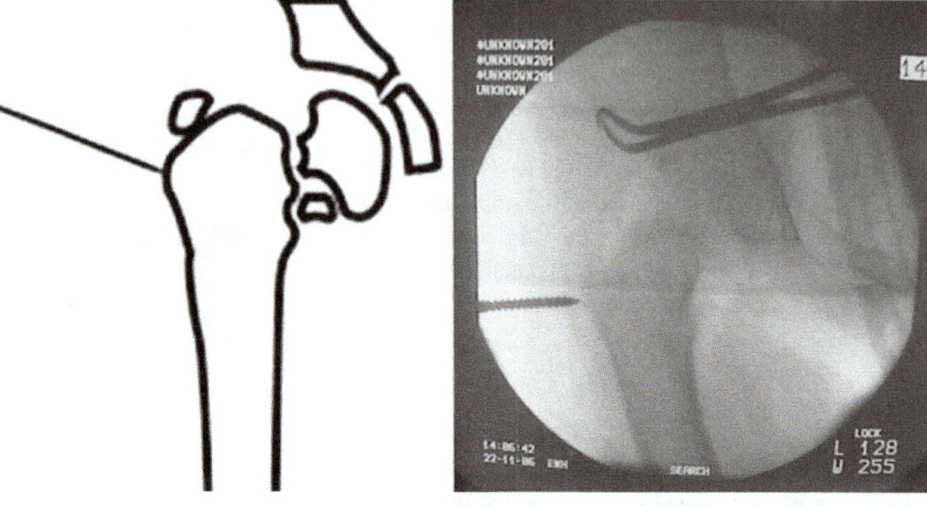

Fig. 4 Distal half-pin inserted in a perpendicular angle with the anatomical axis of the proximal femur

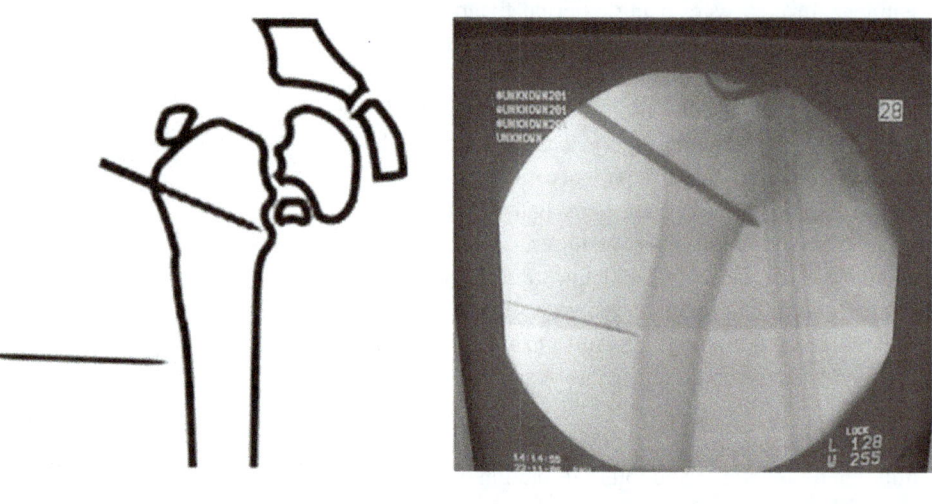

Fig. 5 Osteotomy site at the subtrochanteric area

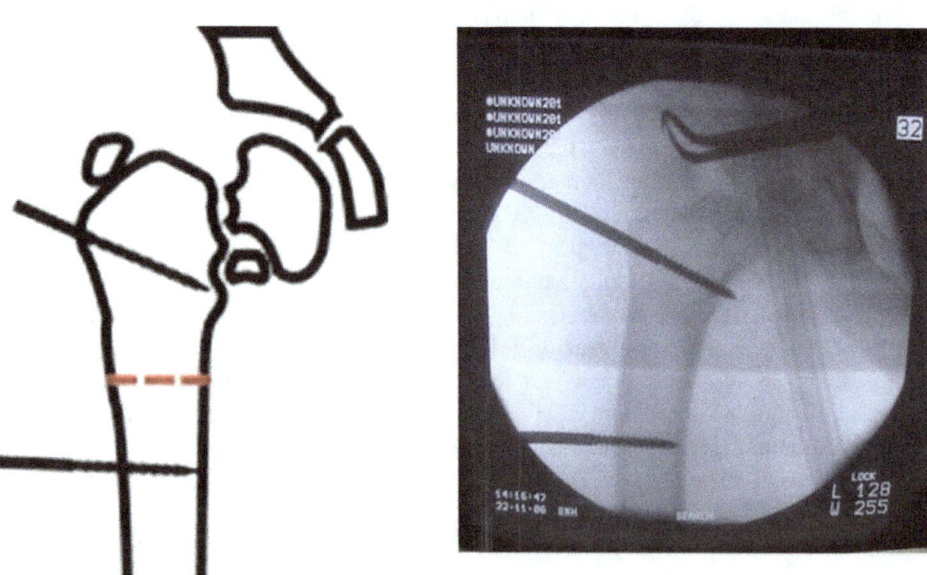

transverse planes (i.e., knee neutral position), distal half-pins to the osteotomy site were placed at right angles to the femoral shaft, mounted on one or more arches according to the size of the limb (Fig. 4). For better control of the proximal fragment of the femur and to avoid uncontrolled displacement, the frame was mounted and the connecting

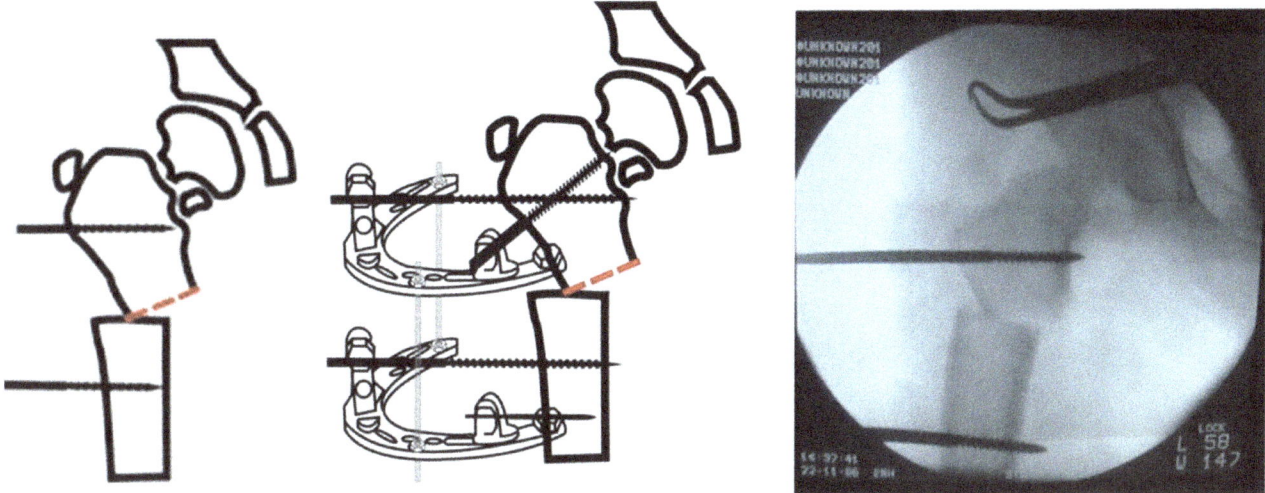

Fig. 6 Acute correction through a subtrochanteric osteotomy

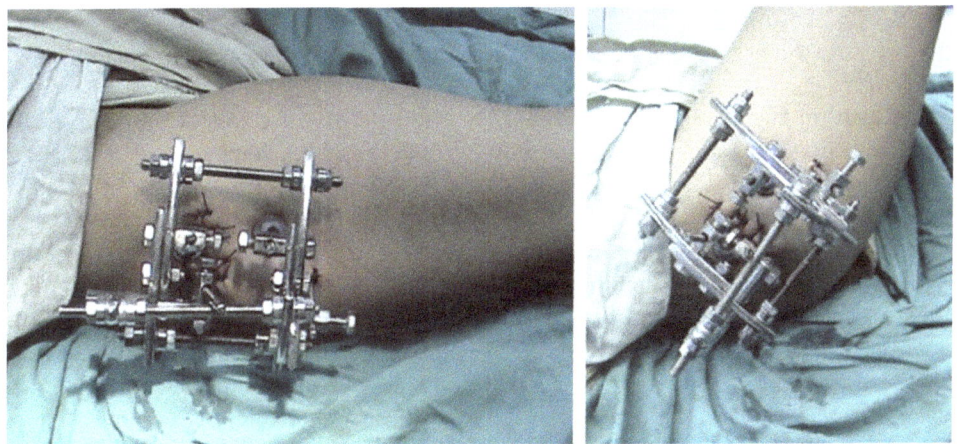

Fig. 7 Clinical photograph showing the application of 2 arches and 3 connecting rods

rods between the 2 arches were not tightened until the osteotomy was made.

A 2-cm transverse incision was made at the level of the proposed osteotomy site in the subtrochanteric area. Multiple drill holes were made, which were then connected by an osteotome or using a Gigli saw (Fig. 5). Once the osteotomy was complete, the correction was achieved by approximating the 2 arches using the 3 connecting rods so that the arches became parallel or by using the swiveling clamp on the LRS fixator (Figs. 6, 7).

Results

A total of 9 subtrochanteric osteotomies were performed with coxa vara of the same etiology. One patient had revision surgery for a failed subtrochanteric osteotomy with plate and screws. All osteotomies achieved the planned correction angle (Fig. 8). Radiographic analysis revealed an average correction of Hilgenreiner's epiphyseal angle by 41.3° (range 30°–64°) from 75.2° (range 60°–102°) before surgery to 33.8° (range 30°–38° degrees) after surgery. The FNSA improved by an average of 48.2° (range 45°–55°); this was from an average of 82° (range 70°–95°) before surgery to an average of 132.3° (range 125°–140°) after surgery. The ATD improved from −8 mm (range −12 to 1 mm) before surgery to +10 mm (range +8 to +18 mm) after surgery. The minimum follow-up was 2 years. At latest follow-up, no loss of correction was measured.

There were no intraoperative fractures or neurovascular injuries. Evaluation of follow-up radiographs showed that all osteotomies had healed by 4 months after surgery with no nonunions, malunions, device failures or avascular

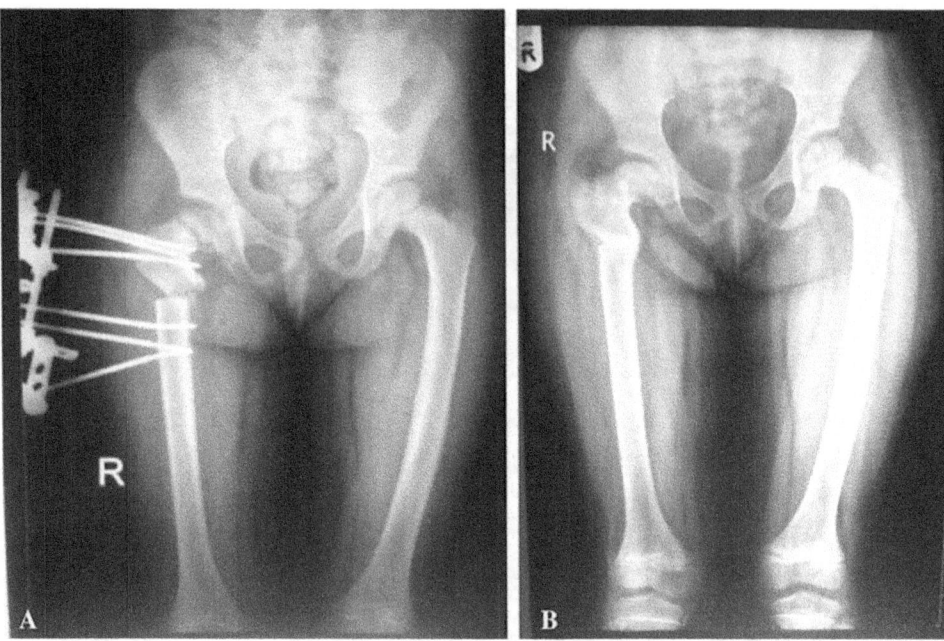

Fig. 8 a X-ray for postoperative follow-up of osteotomy after acute correction, **b** healed osteotomy with correction of neck-shaft angle

necrosis. Position changes in bony fragments were not noted in any patients after surgery. Complications occurred in 4 (44.4 %) of 9 hips. Three (33.3 %) hips had postoperative pin tract infections; 2 (22.2 %) were superficial; and 1 (11.1 %) was deep. All five superficial infections were treated by intravenous administration of antibiotics and frequent dressing changes and healed uneventfully. In the deep infection case, removal of the half-pin and debridement were performed 2 months after the primary operation, which did not jeopardize the fixation of the frame.

Discussion

Multiple surgical techniques have been described for correction of coxa vara. These include the Langenskiold intertrochanteric osteotomy, the interlocking intertrochanteric osteotomy, the valgus subtrochanteric osteotomy with blade plate fixation and the Pauwel's Y-shaped intertrochanteric osteotomy [3, 4, 6, 8, 13–15]. Excellent long-term follow-up has been reported with both the Pauwel's osteotomy and valgus subtrochanteric osteotomy fixed with a blade plate [4, 6, 8]. Desai and Johnson reported excellent long-term results of treatment for congenital coxa vara utilizing a valgus subtrochanteric osteotomy in 20 hips of 12 patients [8]. Their mean postoperative correction of the FNSA to 136° and the HEA to 30° is comparable with our series (132.3° and 33.8°, respectively). Outstanding long-term results of the Pauwel's osteotomy were reported by Cordes et al. in a series of 14 children and 18 hips with coxa vara of multiple etiologies [6]. Their mean

postoperative correction of the FNSA to 141° and the HEA to 29° was comparable to the results of this series. Recurrence of deformity occurred in a single case in that series due to loss of fixation postoperatively; this did not occur in our group of patients.

There are several pitfalls with current techniques for proximal femoral osteotomies. These include the need for an open procedure with removal of a trapezoidal fragment of bone from the subtrochanteric area, producing blood loss and further shortening of an already short extremity [15]. There are limited choices of implants to allow secure fixation of the underlying bone, which can be quite small in young children. Furthermore, any fixation device needs to avoid the proximal femoral growth plate, leaving a limited length of bone available for secure fixation. Typically, the implant is rigidly applied to the underlying bone, making appropriate lateral translation of the distal fragment and minor adjustments after fixation very difficult. Depending on the stability achieved at surgery, some of these children may need a hip spica cast for several weeks after surgery to protect against displacement at the osteotomy site. All will need a second operation to remove the internal fixation device [3].

The ideal fixation device for a multiplanar femoral trochanteric osteotomy is one that allows the surgeon to perform an accurate correction, is easily applied, maintains rigid fixation, permits early joint motion and mobilization of the patient and avoids another operation for removal [10]. The external fixator technique fits this description. There are several potential benefits of this technique, which include avoidance of a large open exposure, decreased potential for significant blood loss and the ability to achieve an accurate and sustained correction of the multiplanar deformity. Using a low-energy osteotomy in this technique, limb length discrepancy can be improved without compromising the quality and time for bony union. Early mobilization with a short hospital stay is possible by avoiding the need for any supplemental cast immobilization. Problems associated with internal fixation such as prominent hardware, implant failure, the possibility of violating the proximal femoral growth plate, the need for a second major surgical procedure for removing an internal implant and the potential for deep infection are significantly decreased. However, there are potential obstacles to this technique. These include a need to be familiar with the use of external fixators capable of using deformity correction, e.g., the Ilizarov fixator or Orthofix LRS fixator, although other external fixator systems can be used as long as the principles outlined above are followed. The inconvenience of pin sites with the possibility of drainage or infection around the pins is another drawback and must be discussed with the patient and relatives beforehand. By using hydroxyapatite-coated half-pins, our modified technique of pin insertion [16], avoiding thermal necrosis while drilling, oral antibiotics early for pin site drainage and doing appropriate pin site releases and care, we have recorded few deep pin-related complaints. With preoperative education and counseling, the patients adapt well to the external fixator.

Despite well-performed osteotomies, the literature cites recurrence rates of 30–70 % [9, 16]. This is in contrast to this report where none of the 9 hips had to be revised. In a study of valgus osteotomies for coxa vara, Carroll et al. reported a recurrence rate of nearly 50 % [6]. If the Hilgenreiner's epiphyseal angle is corrected to 38° or less, 95 % of the children had no recurrence of their varus deformity [6]. The most important factor in reducing the likelihood of recurrent varus is restoration of the femoral neck physis to an anatomic position (a HE angle of 38° or less), thereby normalizing the forces across the physis [4, 8]. It may be to achieve an overcorrection of the HE angle to the normal (anatomic) value of 22° to ensure no recurrences. Although we report no recurrences until the latest follow-up, a weakness in this study is a longer minimum follow-up period for all patients in order to fully assess the long-term impact of our technique on the incidence of recurrence.

In the event a repeat osteotomy is required, this technique avoids the increased morbidity from the absence of large incisions or retained hardware. This technique may also have a role in the treatment for other proximal femoral deformities in children such as those associated with SCFE, Perthes' disease and developmental dysplasia of the hip.

The valgus osteotomy produced a reduction in leg length discrepancy, but 3 patients required a distal femoral osteotomy to address additional length discrepancies and angular deformities near the knee. Shim et al. [17] noted that patients with progressive coxa vara often develop ipsilateral compensatory genu valgum. This highlights the need to avoid medial displacement of the osteotomy, which will exacerbate loading of the lateral compartment and distal femoral physis. This problem has not been addressed in more recent articles on the subject, such as those by Sabharwal et al. [12], Skaggs et al. [18] and Kim et al. [19]. When the coxa vara is corrected, the genu valgum may be unmasked and therefore recommend a full-length standing radiograph or CT scanogram to document alignment and leg length problems preoperatively. In this study, we addressed mechanical axis correction by subtrochanteric and distal femoral osteotomies enabling correction of the coxa vara, mechanical axis deviation and limb length inequality.

Conclusion

A percutaneous external fixator-based technique is described for the treatment for developmental coxa vara and limb length discrepancy in a pediatric cohort. It has potential advantages over commonly used open techniques in being minimally invasive, easily reproducible and provides a versatile alternative to currently available methods for fixation of proximal femoral osteotomies.

References

1. Amstutz HC (1970) Developmental (infantile) coxa vara: a distinct entity. Report of two patients with previously normal roentgenograms. Clin Orthop 72:242–247
2. Beals RK (1998) Coxa vara in childhood: evaluation and management. J Am Acad Orthop Surg 2:93–99
3. Borden J, Spencer G Jr, Herndon C (1966) Treatment of coxa vara in children by means of a modified osteotomy. J Bone Joint Surg Am 48:1106–1110
4. Cordes S, Dickens DR, Cole WG (1991) Correction of coxa vara in childhood. J Bone Joint Surg Br 1:3–6
5. Weighill F (1976) The treatment of developmental coxa vara by abduction subtrochanteric and intertrochanteric femoral osteotomy with special reference to the role of adductor tenotomy. Clin Orthop 116:116–124
6. Desai S, Johnson L (1993) Long-term results of valgus osteotomy for congenital coxa vara. Clin Orthop 294:204–210
7. Pauwels F (1976) Biomechanics of the normal and diseased hip. Springer, New York, pp 24–29
8. Carroll K, Coleman S, Stevens PM (1997) Coxa vara: surgical outcomes of valgus osteotomies. J Pediatr Orthop 17:220–224
9. Behrens F, Sabharwal S (2000) Deformity correction and reconstructive procedures using percutaneous techniques. Clin Orthop 375:133–139
10. Colyer RA (1980) Compression external fixation after biplane femoral trochanteric osteotomy for severe slipped capital femoral epiphysis. J Bone Joint Surg [Am] 62:557–560

11. Ito H, Minami A, Suzuki K, Matsuno T (2001) Three-dimensionally corrective external fixator system for proximal femoral osteotomy. J Pediatr Orthop 21:652–656

12. Sabharwal S, Mittal R, Cox G (2005) Percutaneous triplanar femoral osteotomy correction for developmental coxa vara: a new technique. J Pediatr Orthop 25:28–33

13. Amstutz HD, Wilson PD (1962) Dysgenesis of the proximal femur (coxa vara) and its surgical management. J Bone Joint Surg Am 44:1–24

14. Lahdenranta U, Pylkkanen P (1977) Early and late results of Brackett's operation for pseudarthrosis of the neck of the femur in infantile coxa vara. A review of 30 pseudarthrosis of the neck of the femur in infantile coxa vara. A review of 30 operations. Acta Orthop Scand 48:74–79

15. El Ghazaly SA (2008) Femoral subtrochanteric dome osteotomy in the treatment of coxa vara. Egypt Orthop J 43(2):316–326. ISSN: 1110-1148

16. Kishan S, Sabharwal S, Behrens F, Reilly M, Sirkin M (2002) External fixation of the femur: basic concepts. Tech Orthop 17(2):239–244

17. Shim JS, Kim HT, Mubarak SJ, Wenger DR (1997) Genu valgum in children with coxa vara resulting from hip disease. J Pediatr Orthop 2:225–229

18. Skaggs DL, DuBois B, Kay RM, Hale JM, Tolo VT (2000) A simplified valgus osteotomy of the proximal femur in children. J Pediatr Orthop (Part B) 9:115–118

19. Kim HT, Chambers HG, Mubarak SJ, Wenger DR (2000) Congenital coxa vara: computed tomographic analysis of femoral retroversion and the triangular metaphyseal fragment. J Pediatr Orthop 20:551–556

32

Operative treatment and outcome of unstable distal radial fractures using a palmar T-miniplate at a non-specialized institution

E. Skouras · Y. Hosseini · V. Berger ·
K. Wegmann · T. C. Koslowsky

Abstract Treatment options for displaced distal radial fractures are still a controversial topic of discussion. Although good results for the palmar plating of high-volume centers have been published, evidence of its successful use in smaller institutions is still lacking. We report the clinical and radiological results of the treatment for 84 distal radial fractures with a single 2.4-mm T-miniplate in an institution performing <30 procedures per year. According to the AO classification system, there were 30 A, 5 B, and 49 C fractures with a patients mean age of 64 years. After a minimum of 12-month follow-up, we found very good and good results according to the Gardland and Sarmiento scores and a DASH of 5.6. Only five patients were classified as having a moderate outcome. A remaining intra-articular step-off of more than 1 mm was seen in 15 patients. In a comparison of grip strength between the injured and uninjured hands, we saw a difference of 6.8 % less on the injured side. We saw two instances of tendon rupture and one of tendon irritation due to prominent dorsal screws and necessitating revision surgery. Flexor tendon irritation was noted in one patient, requiring a second operation. Modern treatment for distal radial fractures can be performed successfully and with good clinical outcome in smaller institutions. Based on the high and increasing incidence of distal radial fractures, there is no need to transfer these patients into high-volume centers.

Level of evidence Case study, Level IV.

Keywords Distal radial fractures · T-miniplate osteosynthesis

Introduction

Distal radial fractures seem to be the most common fracture entity currently seen in accident and emergency units, with an annual estimated incidence of 36.6 women/10,000 and 8.9 men/10,000 per year [1]. A significantly growing elderly population with a markedly increasing life expectancy may increase the fracture incidence by a further 50 % by the year 2030 [2]. Non-operative treatment using a plaster cast is usually chosen for non-displaced fractures. A stable reduction in displaced fractures may also be treated non-operatively [3]. Unstable and displaced radial fractures are treated operatively. Besides stability and displacement, intra-articular or extra-articular fracture type may also be important for the decision. The ideal method for surgical management of these fractures has been a controversial topic of discussion, and numerous procedures are available. Percutaneous Kirschner wire fixation, joint-bridging and non-joint-bridging external fixation, or a combination of both can be used successfully [4–6]. The palmar locking plate has recently become popular [5, 7, 8] for treatment for distal radial fractures, and good to excellent clinical results have been published [8–11]. In fact, there are a number of studies demonstrating good results in the treatment for distal radial fractures with palmar locked angle plates at a large, specialized institution. The limited number of specialized institutions coupled with the increasing number of

E. Skouras · K. Wegmann
Klinik und Poliklinik für Orthopädie und Unfallchirurgie,
Universtsklinikum Köln, Kerpener Straße 62,
50937 Cologne, Germany

Y. Hosseini · V. Berger · T. C. Koslowsky (✉)
Department of Surgery, St. Elisabeth-Hospital,
Werthmannstraße 1, 50935 Cologne, Germany
e-mail: tkoslowsky@web.de

distal radial fractures may be leading to a lack of treatment capacity of this injury. The purpose of this prospective study was to evaluate the subjective and objective outcome after operative treatment for distal radial fractures using a palmar locked angle miniplate (Koenigsee, 2.4 mm T-miniplate) by a smaller, non-specialized institution to evaluate the necessity for referral to high-volume services.

Patients and methods

This study was performed at a hospital with a non-specialized trauma service with the healthcare level of basic trauma and reconstructive surgery. Over a period of 3 years (2005–2007), a total of 82 patients with 84 distal radial fractures (mean age 64 years (18–94 years); 15 males and 67 females) were followed prospectively. Preoperative work-up included a clinical examination and standard two-plane X-rays. After initial sandwich casting, the operation was performed as an elective procedure with a mean of 4 days (injury day to day seven) after trauma, except for those patients with open fractures (four patients) and/or neurological affection (one patient). Besides these emergency criteria, indications for surgical intervention were the following: radial shortening of more than 3 mm; dorsal comminution; dislocation of more than 20° in extra-articular fractures; or an intra-articular step-off of more than 2 mm. According to the AO classification system, there were 30 A (eight A2, 22 A3), 5 B (one B1, one B2, and three B3) and 49 C (18 C1, 24 C2, and seven C3) fractures. A total of 77 patients were right-handed and five were left-handed. Thirty-six patients had injured the dominant hand; 46 patients had injured the non-dominant hand. Two patients had injured both hands.

There were two distal ulna fractures, which were treated additionally with a descending intramedullar elastic nail.

Two patients had suffered proximal femur fractures that were treated simultaneously by prosthetic replacement or a Y-nail, respectively.

All patients were treated by two surgeons with a 3 year of special training in trauma and orthopedic surgery with the same type of implant: the 2.4-mm T-miniplate (Koenigsee Implantate, Aschau, Germany) with either three or four holes in the shaft bar for conventional 3.5-mm cortical screws and six 2.2-mm fine-threaded locked angle miniscrews for the diagonal distal bar. Figure 1 shows the dimensions of the plate and screw placed on a sawbone model via an intraoperative X-ray. Operative procedures were performed using a tourniquet, and a standard distal Henry approach was used for fracture exposure. In extra-articular fractures, distal screws were placed parallel to the joint surface, and reduction was performed using the "lift technique" [12]. Intra-articular fractures were reduced beginning with the distal radioulnar fragment, where a guiding K-wire was placed precisely into the radio-ulna corner with the use of an image intensifier, again parallel to the radiocarpal and radioulnar joint surface. Then, a miniplate with the locked angle guiding drill holder was placed over the K-wire. A stepwise reduction and fixation of the joint block was performed with the locked angle 2.2-mm miniscrews until the initial K-wire was exchanged for another miniscrew. As the next step, the whole joint block was reduced and reaffixed to the shaft using the "lift technique." Here, special care was taken with the reduction in the distal radioulnar joint. Finally, the pronator quadratus muscle was reaffixed as far radial as possible, at least enough to protect the plate from the flexor pollicis longus tendon. Postoperative casting was performed for 6 days to initiate regular wound healing. Hospitalization was 6 days in mean (1–25 days). Then, functional treatment without casting or splinting with additional physiotherapy was performed twice weekly. X-rays were taken on days two,

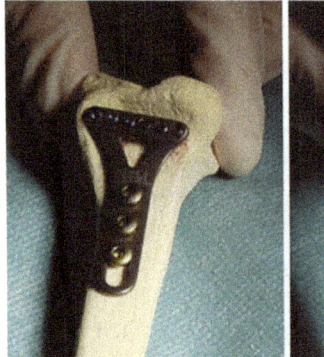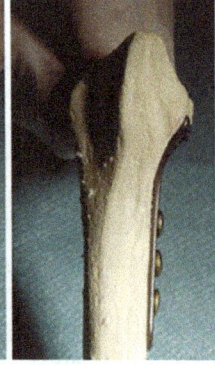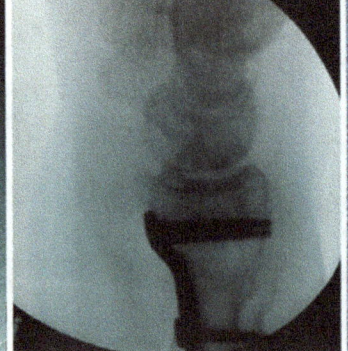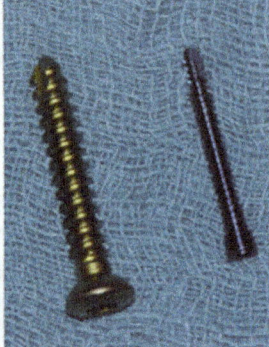

Fig. 1 A fluoroscopy of the dimensions of the palmar miniplate on a sawbone model. The right side of the picture shows the self-cutting 3.5-mm screws for the long bar of the plate. Six smaller 2.2-mm locked angle miniscrews have been placed at the distal part of the plate, each addressing as many fracture fragments as possible

seven, and 42 after the operation and at the time of follow-up. Degenerative changes were detected according to Knirk and Jupiter [13].

Follow-up was performed by the first and second authors, MS and YH, including a radiological and clinical work-up. The radiological work-up was performed on a PACS system and included the congruency of the joint surface, dorsal angulation, and loss of dorsal angulation. Radial shortening was measured as a vertical distance between the ulna border of the distal radius and the most distal point of the ulna head [14]. Malunion was defined as a dorsal angle less than zero degrees, a palmar angle <15°, a carpal malalignment [15], a distal radial shortening of more than 3 mm, or a combination of these parameters [8].

The clinical follow-up included a standardized examination of the injured and contralateral side. Range of motion of the wrist was determined on the frontal and sagittal planes, and pronation and supination were measured according to the neutral 0 method with a standard goniometer. To determine the functional results, we used the Sarmiento [16], Gardland [17], and DASH [18] scores.

Grip strength in Newtons was measured on both sides using a computer-assisted hydraulic hand goniometer (Vernier Software & Technology®, Beaverton, Oregon).

Results were analyzed with a Student's t test, and significance was granted for $p < 0.05$. For patient with double-side fractures, only one clinical score was performed.

Results

The clinical and radiological data are summarized in Tables 1, 2, 3, and 4. At the time of follow-up, clinical results were very good or good according to the Gardland and Sarmiento scores with a DASH score of 5.6. Only five patients were classified as having a moderate outcome. Function was almost unlimited. We saw an anatomical reduction in the distal radius including the joint surfaces and, in Typ A Fractures, in the metaphyseal area in 58 fractures. A remaining intra-articular step-off of more than one mm was seen in 15 fractures at the first postoperative X-ray, whereas four patients had an intra-articular step-off in the radiocarpal joint and 11 in the distal radioulnar joint;

arthritic changes were seen in 42 fractures at the time of follow-up. Compared to the first postoperative X-ray, we saw a loss of radial length of 2 mm [from −2.41 mm (−7–5 mm) to −0.23 (−4–6 mm)] at the time of follow-up. There was no significant loss of palmar tilt and radial inclination (see Table 1). In comparing grip strength between the injured (78.5 N; 8.9–216 N) and uninjured hands (84.2 N; 24.9–236.2 N), we saw a difference of 6.8 % less strength on the injured side. At the time of follow-up, we could identify a total number of two tendon ruptures and one case of tendon irritation due to prominent dorsal screws, leading to revision surgery. Flexor tendon irritation was noted in one patient, necessitating a second operation. The two tendon ruptures were treated with an indicis proprius transfer. No complex regional pain syndrome (CRPS) and no infection were seen in this study. Figure 2 shows a typical prä and postoperative X-ray of a AO C2 distal radial fracture treated with a miniplate.

Discussion

A significantly growing population of elderly patients and their increasing life expectancy will lead to an increase in osteoporotic fractures. Besides fractures of the proximal femur, proximal humerus, and vertebral column, distal radial fractures play an important role in the medical treatment of this age group. The patients treated by our hospital with an incidence of 49 (out of 84) AO type C

Table 2 Arthritic changes detected at the time of follow-up in the postoperative X-ray

Arthritic changes	Grade 0	Grade 1	Grade 2	Grade 3
Initial post OP X-ray	49	26	9	0
At follow-up	42	33	9	0

Table 3 The clinical scores obtained at the time of follow-up

Clinical data	Excellent	Good	Moderate	Bad
Sarmiento score	67	15	0	0
Gardland score	52	25	5	0

Table 1 Radiological results at the time of follow-up

	At first X-ray post OP	At follow-up
Palmar tilt	11.75° (5°–15°)	11.60° (5°–14°)
Radial inclination	20.09° (15°–29°)	20.98° (15°–29°)
Radial shortening	−2.41 mm (−7–5 mm)	−0.23 mm (−4–6 mm)
Joint surface incongruency (radiocarpal > 1 mm)	4 × >1 mm	
Joint surface incongruency (radioulnar > 1 mm)	11 > 1 mm	

Table 4 The functional results obtained at the time of follow-up

	Injured side mean (min–max)	Uninjured side mean (min–max)
Supination (°)	86.19° (20°–90°)	88.1° (40°–90°)
Pronation (°)	87.67° (45°–90°)	88.5° (40°–90°)
Extension (°)	56.72°(30°–70°)	60.3° (40°–80°)
Flexion (°)	· 62.5° (30°–90°)	68.1° (55°–90°)
Radial abduction (°)	25.29° (10°–35°)	29.6° (20°–40°)
Ulna abduction (°)	34.16° (15°–50°)	38.9° (20°–55°)

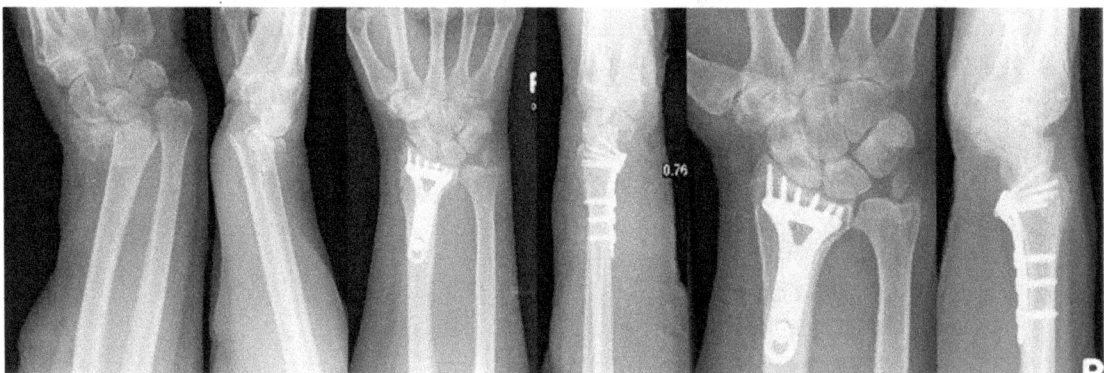

Fig. 2 A complex AO C2 distal radial fracture and its reconstruction with a locked angle miniplate. The clinical result shows a free and unlimited function of the wrist. The patient only complains a prominent ulnar head without pain due to the nonunion of the ulnar styloid and minimal ulnar plus. The increased radial inclination was asymptomatic

fractures and a mean age of 64 years are comparable to those reported by other institutions [8, 10]. The high incidence of osteoporosis in this age group and the sex distribution of 67 women to 15 men may be the reason for the high incidence of complex fracture patterns: Figl et al. [10] report a number of 34 (out of 85) AO type C fractures, and their incidence has increased from 31 (out of 46) C type fractures as reported by Wei et al. [5] to 71 % as reported by Jupiter et al. in 2010 [9]. The treatment for distal radial fractures is a controversial topic of discussion. Despite evidence that an unsatisfactory radiological outcome does not necessarily predict deficient clinical results after non-operative treatment for distal radial fractures in senior citizen patients [19], the current literature on this fracture pattern shows a trend toward operative treatment [20]. Operative treatment options range from isolated pin fixation to external fixation to locked angle plate fixation [6, 9, 21]. Isolated pinning was reported by Goften and Liew [6]. The authors report this method to be effective for fractures that are too unstable for non-operative treatment. In the recent literature, several authors compare external fixation to palmar locking plate fixation.

Wei et al. [5] published a DASH of 18 12 months after external fixation compared to five in the volar locking plate group. A standard deviation of 14 and four, respectively, led to an insignificant difference between these two groups. Grip strength after 12 months was 18 kg (external fixation)

versus 16.9 kg (volar plating), again without any significant differences, including the same ranges of motion in the two fixation groups. In contrast to these almost identical results at the end point of the study after 1 year, the authors saw favorable results in the volar plating groups just 3 months after fixation: in other words, the volar plating group reached their final good results earlier.

These results were supported by Rizzo et al. [22]: they found similar grip strength and range of motion after a follow-up of 29 months in a total of 41 patients, whereas DASH and radiographic outcomes were better in the volar plating group compared to the external fixation and pinning group. They concluded that volar plating seemed to be favorable to external fixation.

On the other hand, Abramo et al. [4] did not find any subjective difference between volar plating and isolated external fixation, but grip strength and ROM were better in the volar plating group 1 year after surgery.

Although the results of objective and subjective outcomes might be confusing regarding these two methods of treatment, at least there is evidence that in the best cases, external fixation is comparable to if not worse than volar plating [4, 22]. The good results achieved in these studies with volar plating compared to other implants are also supported by isolated clinical and radiological outcome studies: Knight et al. [8] report good clinical results after following 40 patients for 59 weeks with a mean DASH of

23, and Figl et al. [10] report a grip strength of 65 % on the contralateral ineffective side with a DASH of 25. They saw a volar loss of reduction of 2° from the initial postoperative X-ray to the study end point and a loss of radial length of one mm a mean of 59 weeks after surgery. Interestingly, they saw carpal malalignment in six of their 40 patients. The authors explained this fact with a high grade of comminution in the metaphyseal area. Jupiter et al. [9] reviewed 117 patients 2 years after surgery with a mean DASH of seven and a Gardland–Werley score of four together with the AO LCP study group. They saw a remaining intra-articular step-off of more than two mm in five out of 71 intra-articular fractures at the 2-year follow-up, but saw no changes in the radial length or radial angle of palmar tilt from the immediate postoperative X-ray to the final follow-up.

In our clinical follow-up, we could confirm the good to very good clinical results reported above: a loss of grip strength between the uninjured and injured side of <10 % might be the objective reason for the DASH of 5.6 place our results at the upper level of the results reported in the current literature. This is also true for weaker scores like the Gardland–Werley and Sarmiento scores only obtaining four different items including movement, pain, arthritis, and deformity. Radiologically, we had an immediate postoperative intra-articular step-off of less or more than 1 mm in 15 patients. We did not see any correlation with the clinical outcome of these patients. This was also true for arthritic changes observed 1 year after surgery. Furthermore, we saw secondary dislocation with a loss of radial length a mean of 2 mm, again without any effect on the clinical outcome. As suspected by others, the small amount of secondary dislocation might be due to the relative distal, almost subchondral screw position of the distal 2.2-mm fine-threaded miniscrews [23]. In reviewing our clinical results together with the radiological outcome, the reason for the minor influence of radiological deficiencies might be impossible to measure clinically, a fact that was also seen by others.

Despite the euphoria of the good and very good clinical results in addition to the lower complication rates of the volar plate system compared to an external fixation technique [24–26], surgeons must keep in mind that the use of this implant may cause serious complications: tendon irritation to rupture is a major problem with a rate of 0 to 38 % [8] reported in the current literature. Flexor tendon irritation to rupture is due to very distal plate positioning, whereas extensor problems are the consequence of a screw too long in length [8]. As we had a high incidence of very distal osteoporotic fractures and did not use other implants throughout the duration of this study, we found adequate soft tissue coverage of even the very low profile plate to be important. Although the pronator quadratus muscle might

often be insufficient to cover the implant completely, we found it large enough in most cases to cover at least the ulnar parts of the plate to prevent damage to the most radial positioned flexor pollicis longus tendon. The orthopedic and trauma surgeon's technique of intraoperative observation of the flexor pollicis longus tendon during thumb movement might be the reason for the relatively low incidence of one patient with flexor irritation, even in distal plate application.

Dorsally prominent screw tips have been identified as a cause of extensor tendon injuries: Beson et al. [27] reported screw penetration into the third dorsal compartment and fracture-related bony spurs or gapping at the fracture side as potential causes of the extensor pollicis longus tendon (EPL). We saw a total of four EPL problems: one patient had an initial traumatic rupture of the EPL tendon that was repaired during the first operation; two of our patients reported an insufficient thumb elevation in a period of 2–16 weeks after surgery. Here, prominent screw tips have been indentified as the reason for this problem. In a fourth patient with the same symptoms of thumb weakness, an early revision of the EPL tendon could exclude an alteration due a postoperative problem. Although the EPL tendon is especially known to be a typical problem, paying high operative attention may lead to fewer problems. In contrast to our high incidence of this complication, others do report less to zero tendon problems [4, 9]. A continuous intraoperative fluoroscopy with respect to the complicated dorsal shape of the distal radius, especially in the region of Lister's tubercle, in addition to an aggressive treatment or revision in the situation of tendon irritation might prevent the major complication of a delayed or missed EPL rupture necessitating tendon transfer. Besides these highly relevant tendon problems, we saw one screw break leading to a secondary revision. Other common problems as described by others [4, 8, 10] such as CRPS, nerve irritation, carpal tunnel syndrome, and wound infections were not seen in our series.

Outcome scores, typically performed in follow-up studies of distal radius fractures, are highly prone to subjective influence [18], and objective radiological outcome measurements often do not correlate with the clinical outcome [28]. Today, grip strength measurements are often performed in order to objectively document functional outcomes [4, 8].

Due to its high incidence, operative treatment for distal radius fractures is performed in almost every trauma center. Good and very good results using palmar locking T-plates have been published by many, but mainly by large institutions [9, 11]. A smaller institution, with an incidence of <30 distal radial fractures necessitating operative treatment per year, obtained the good clinical, functional, and radiological results presented in this study. That fact that our results were obtained using a single implant for different fracture patterns supports the idea that a palmar locked angle implant can be used independently of the fracture type—for extra-articular as well as for comminuted intra-articular fractures. This may lead to a simplified treatment algorithm with a single implant for almost every distal radial fracture needing operative intervention. According to our results, it would generally not be necessary to refer displaced, distal radial fractures to a high-volume center.

References

1. O'Neil TW, Cooper C, Fin JD et al (2001) Incidence of distal forearm fractures in British men and women. Osteoporos Int 12:555–558

2. Rueger M, Linhardt W, Sommerfeld DW (1998) Differenzialindikation zur Behandlung der distalen Radiusfraktur Trauma und Berufskrankheit 1:6–14

3. Handoll HH, Madhock R (2003) Conservative interventions for treating distal radial fractures in adults. Cochrane Database Syst Rev, CD003209

4. Abramo A, Kopylov P, Geijer M, Tugil M (2009) Open reduction and internal fixation compared to closed reduction and external fixation in distal radial fractures: a randomized study of 50 patients. Acta Orthop 80(4):478–485

5. Wei DH, Raizman NM, Bottino CJ, Jobin CM, Strauch RJ, Rosenwasser MP (2009) Unstable distal radial fractures treated with external fixation, a radial column plate, or a volar plate. A prospective randomized trial. J Bone Joint Surg Am 91(7):1568–1577

6. Gofton W, Liew A (2010) Distal radius fractures: nonoperative and percutaneous pinning treatment options. Hand Clin 26(1):43–53

7. Rosental TD, Beredjikian PK, Bozentka GJ (2003) Function outcome and complications following two types of plating fort he distal part of the radius. J Bone Joint Surg Am 85:1956–1965

8. Knight D, Hajducka C, Will E, McQueen M (2010) Locked volar plating for unstable distal radial fractures: clinical and radiological outcomes. Injury 41(2):184–189

9. Jupiter JB, Marent-Huber M, LCP Study Group (2009) Operative management of distal radial fractures with 2.4-millimeter locking plates. A multicenter prospective case series. J Bone Joint Surg Am 91(1):55–65

10. Figl M, Weninger P, Jurkowitsch J, Hofbauer M, Schauer J, Leixnering M (2010) Unstable distal radius fractures in the elderly patient–volar fixed-angle plate osteosynthesis prevents secondary loss of reduction. J Trauma 68(4):992–998

11. Jupiter JB, Marent-Huber M, LCP Study Group (2010) Operative management of distal radial fractures with 2.4-millimeter locking plates: a multicenter prospective case series. Surgical technique. J Bone Joint Surg Am 92(Suppl):1

12. Smith DW, Henry MH (2005) Volar fixed angle plating of distal radial fractures. JAAOS 13:28–36

13. Knirk JL (1986) Jupiter JB Intra-articular fractures of the distal end of the radius in young adults. J Bone Joint Surg Am 68(5):647–659

14. Melone CP (1984) Articular fractures of the distal radius. Orthop Clin North Am 15:215–236

15. McQueen MM, Hajducka C, Court-Brown CM (1988) Redisplaced unstable fractures of the distal radius, randomized comparison of four treatment methods. J Bone Joint Surg Br 70:649–651

16. Sarmiento A, Pratt GW, Berry NC et al (1975) Colles fractures. Functional bracing in supination. JBJS (Am) 57(3):311–317

17. Gardland JJ Jr, Werley CW (1951) Evaluation of healde 'Colles' fractures. J Bone Joint Surg 33:895–907

18. Hudak Pl, Amadino PC, Bombardier C (1996) Development of an upper extremity outcome measure: the DASH (disability of the arm, shoulder and hand). The Upper Extremity Collaborative Group (UECG). Am J Ind Med 29:602–608

19. Egol KA, Walsh M, Romo-Cardoso S, Dorsky S, Paksima N (2010) Distal radial fractures in the elderly: operative compared with nonoperative treatment. J Bone Joint Surg Am 92(9):1851–1857

20. Koenig KM, Davis GC, Grove MR, Tosteson AN, Koval KJ (2009) Is early internal fixation preferred to cast treatment for well-reduced unstable distal radial fractures? J Bone Joint Surg Am 91(9):2086–2093

21. Tyllianakis M, Mylonas S, Saridis A, Kallivokas A, Kouzelis A, Megas P (2010) Treatment of unstable distal radius fractures with Ilizarov circular, nonbridging external fixator. Injury 41(3):306–311

22. Rizzo M, Katt BA, Carothers JT (2008) Comparison of locked volar plating versus pinning and external fixation in the treatment of unstable intraarticular distal radius fractures. Hand (N Y) 3(2):111–117

23. Drobetz H, Bryant AL, Pokorny T, Spitaler R, Leixnering M, Jupiter JB (2006) Volar fixed-angle plating of distal radius extension fractures: influence of plate position on secondary loss of reduction–a biomechanic study in a cadaveric model. J Hand Surg Am 31(4):615–622

24. Anderson TJ, Lucas GL, Buhr BR (2004) Complications of treating distal radius fractures with external fixation: a community experience. Iowa Orthop J 24:53–59

25. Capo JT, Swan GK Jr, Tan V (2006) External fixation techniques for distal radius fractures. Clin Orthop 445:30–41

26. Margilot Z, Haase SC, Kotis SV, Kim HM, Chung KC (2005) A metaanalysis of outcomes of external fixation versus plate osteosynthesis for unstable distal radius fractures. J Hand Surg (Am) 30(6):1185–1199

27. Beson EC, De Carvalho A, Mikola EA et al (2006) Two potential causes of EPL rupture after distal radius volar plating. Clin Orthop 451:218–222

28. Arora R, Gabl M, Gschwentner M, Deml C, Krappinger D, Lutz M (2009) A comparative study of clinical and radiologic outcomes of unstable colles type distal radius fractures in patients older than 70 years: nonoperative treatment versus volar locking plating. J Orthop Trauma 23(4):237–242

33

Outcome after modified Putti-Platt procedure for recurrent traumatic anterior shoulder dislocations

Gijs I. T. Iordens · Esther M. M. Van Lieshout ·
Bernd C. Van Es · Niels W. L. Schep · Roelf S. Breederveld ·
Peter Patka · Dennis Den Hartog

Abstract Most recent studies on procedures for stabiliz-ing the glenohumeral joint focus on arthroscopic tech-niques. A relatively simple open procedure is the modified Putti-Platt procedure. The aim of these retrospective case series was to evaluate the functional outcome, patient sat-isfaction, and quality of life of patients who underwent this procedure. After a median follow-up time of 4.7 (P_{25}–P_{75} 1.7–6.8) years, fifty-one patients could be enrolled with a mean age of 25 (21–39) years. Five patients (10 %) reported re-dislocations. The median Constant score for the affected side was 84 (P_{25}–P_{75} 75–91). Median loss of motion in abduction, elevation, external rotation, and external rotation in 90° of abduction did not exceed 10° when compared to the healthy shoulder. A median Rowe score of 92 (P_{25}–P_{75} 75–95) was measured. The WOSI score and SF-36 showed excellent quality of life. The VAS proved high patient satisfaction with the outcome; 7.9 (6.8–9.5). We concluded that the modified Putti-Platt pro-cedure leads to excellent outcome scores and only marginal restriction in range of motion combined with a high patient satisfaction. Our data prove that excellent results can be obtained with a relatively simple open procedure.

G. I. T. Iordens · E. M. M. Van Lieshout ·
B. C. Van Es · P. Patka · D. Den Hartog (✉)
Department of Surgery-Traumatology, Erasmus MC,
University Medical Center Rotterdam, PO Box 2040,
3000 CA Rotterdam, The Netherlands
e-mail: d.denhartog@erasmusmc.nl

N. W. L. Schep
Trauma Unit Department of Surgery, AMC,
Amsterdam, The Netherlands

R. S. Breederveld
Department of Surgery, Red Cross Hospital,
Beverwijk, The Netherlands

Keywords Shoulder · Instability · Bankert ·
Putti-Platt · Procedure

Introduction

The incidence of recurrent instability after a first-time shoulder dislocation ranges from 10 % in patients older than 40 years to almost 90 % in patients younger than 20 years [1–3]. To durably treat an unstable shoulder, it requires surgical intervention. Despite the growing expe-rience with arthroscopic techniques, open procedures still render similar results [4–6]. One of the oldest open "non-anatomic" techniques for this purpose is the Putti-Platt procedure. This procedure was designed to shorten the subscapularis muscle and the anterior capsule in order to stabilize the glenohumeral joint. However, underlying pathologic lesions like a labral tear is not addressed [7–9]. This method frequently resulted in significant loss of external rotation and concomitant osteoarthritis [8, 10, 11]. During the past two decades, several modifications of the original Putti-Platt procedure have been developed [12–15]. Since 2000, a specific modification of the Putti-Platt procedure is the preferred treatment for recurrent anterior glenohumeral instability in one academic and one nonac-ademic teaching hospital in The Netherlands. This modi-fication implies imbrication of the subscapularis muscle and capsule along with anatomic repair of underlying pathology.

Most studies on modified Putti-Platt procedures focused on recurrent instability and functional outcome. Data on patient satisfaction with the outcome and quality of life after a modified Putti-Platt procedure are not available. The aim of this retrospective study was to evaluate these spe-cific aspects of recovery as well as the functional outcome after a modified Putti-Platt procedure for recurrent shoulder instability.

Materials and methods

Patients

This is a retrospective case series including all adult patients (aged 18 years or older) that were treated with a modified Putti-Platt procedure after recurrent (i.e., two or more) anterior shoulder dislocation between 2000 and 2010. All consecutive patients were selected from two hospital databases, one academic center, and one teaching hospital. This procedure was standard care in the treatment of recurrent anterior glenohumeral instability in both clinics. Patients with insufficient comprehension of the Dutch language to complete the questionnaires were excluded. All patients gave written informed consent to participate in this study, which was approved by the medical research ethics committees of both participating hospitals.

Surgical procedure

An approximately 7 cm incision from slightly lateral to the coracoid process was made running along the deltopectoral groove. The posterolateral surface of the humeral head was carefully inspected by palpation for the presence of an impression fracture (Hill-Sachs lesion). After exposing the tendon of the subscapularis muscle, it was vertically transected, 1–2 cm proximal from its insertion on the minor tubercle. After incising the capsule, a Fukuda retractor was used facilitating inspection of the glenoid surface. When a labral detachment (i.e., Bankart lesion) was identified, it was repaired in the following way. The labrum was reattached to the anterior glenoidal rim together with the capsule using suture anchors. In case of a capsular tear, a capsular repair was performed. Subsequently, the subscapularis muscle was shortened by transferring the medial part under the lateral part; consequently, imbrication of the capsule was achieved in all patients. Over-tightening of the subscapularis muscle may lead to an undue post-operative restriction in range of motion. In order to asses whether the subscapularis muscle and capsule were not too tight or too loose, the arm was placed alongside the body with the elbow in 90° flexion with the thumb pointing up during subscapularis reefing. In this position, the shoulder was required to reach neutral position (0° of external rotation). However, when unsupported, gravity was not expected to externally rotate the arm any further. It should be noted that the lateral stump of the subscapularis muscle was not attached to the anterior glenoid rim as customary in the original Putti-Platt procedure. This modified Putti-Platt procedure, which was used for all patients in this study, has also been described elsewhere [12–14]. Post-operatively, all patients received an immobilizing sling (e.g., Polysling or Gilchrist). Between weeks two and six, only circumduction exercises were allowed. From 6 weeks onward, patients were permitted external rotation and strength-enhancing exercises if tolerated.

Outcomes assessment and data collection

The shoulder function was assessed primarily using the Constant score. This scoring system consists of four variables, reflecting function, range of motion, pain, and strength of the shoulder joint [16]. A secondary functional outcome measures were the disability of arm, shoulder, and hand (DASH) score. Scores ranged from zero points (representing no disability) to 100 points (representing severe disability) [17–19]. In addition, the Rowe score was used. This is a tool for the assessment of shoulder instability after shoulder-stabilizing procedures [20]. The range of motion (ROM) at the time of follow-up was measured using a goniometer. Furthermore, the injury-related quality of life was assessed using the Western Ontario Shoulder Index (WOSI). It was calculated as a percentage of the maximum possible score, with a higher score indicating less quality of life [21]. The health-related quality of life was measured using the Short Form-36; the scores for the physical and mental components were converted to a norm-based score and compared with the norms for the general population of the United States [22]. Patient satisfaction with the outcome of treatment was measured using a visual analog scale (VAS), in which zero indicated full dissatisfaction and 10 indicated full satisfaction.

Data were collected from medical charts and a questionnaire completed by the patients. Baseline data included age at the time of surgery, dominant side, gender, tobacco and alcohol consumption, and medical history at the time of surgery. Injury-related variables included initial trauma mechanism, affected side, duration of instability, number of dislocations before surgery, previous stabilizing procedures, and presence of a labral lesion or Hill-Sachs lesion. Intervention-related variables included number of anchors used, institution, post-operative treatment, and duration and type of immobilization and physical therapy. All intra- and post-operative complications and secondary interventions were recorded.

Statistical analysis

Data were analyzed using the statistical package for the social sciences (SPSS) version 16.0 or higher (SPSS, Chicago, Ill., USA). Normality of continuous data was tested with the Shapiro–Wilk test, and homogeneity of variances was tested using the Levene's test. Descriptive analysis was performed in order to describe baseline characteristics (intrinsic, injury, and intervention-related variables) and outcome measures. Continuous data are reported as medians and percentiles (nonparametric data) or as means and standard deviation (parametric data), and categorical data as numbers with percentages. A Mann–Whitney U test (numeric variables) or chi-squared analysis was performed in order to assess whether there were differences in characteristics and outcome if surgery was performed on the dominant side versus the nondominant side. We also assessed whether outcome differed between the two hospitals. A multivariable linear regression analysis was performed in order to model the relation between different covariates and the Constant score. Intrinsic, injury, and intervention-related variables were added as covariate. Similar models were made for the other numeric outcome measures.

Results

Patient and intervention characteristics

Sixty patients underwent a modified Putti-Platt procedure between 2000 and 2010, and nine patients could not be retrieved ($N = 7$) or did not consent to participate ($N = 2$). The remaining 51 patients, of which 37 (73 %) were male, could be enrolled after a median follow-up time of 4.7 (P_{25}–P_{75} 1.7–6.8) years (Table 1). All of these patients completed every questionnaire. Most patients sustained their initial dislocation during sporting activities ($N = 30$, 59 %). Intervention characteristics are also outlined in Table 2. Of all patients' standard shoulder X-rays were made prior to surgery. In a subset of patients, additional MRI scans ($N = 33$, 65 %) or CT scans ($N = 8$, 16 %) were made. Thirty-one (61 %) patients had radiological signs of a Hill-Sach's lesion, none of which required surgical repair. Forty-five patients (88 %) had a Bankart lesion (Table 2), and three patients (6 %) had SLAP lesions. All labral lesions were repaired upon recognition with a median of two (P_{25}–P_{75} 2–3) suture anchors. Unfortunately, intra-operative range of motion was only rarely recorded. No intra-operative complications were encountered. Eight patients (16 %) developed recurrent instability; five of these patients (10 %) reported a recurrent dislocation after 6, 5, 3, and 1 year, respectively. For the fifth patient, the dislocation date was not recorded. Multivariable binary logistic regression analysis showed a positive relation between the occurrence of a recurrent dislocation after surgery (dependent variable) and the duration of the post-

Table 1 Baseline characteristics of the study population

Total number of patients	51
Male[a]	37 (72.5)
Age at first dislocation (year)[b]	21 (13–24)
Age at surgery (year)[b]	25 (21–39)
Time between first dislocation and surgery (months)[b]	24 (12–96)
Length of follow-up (months)[b]	56 (20–81)
Right side affected*	28 (54.9)
Dominant side affected*	25 (55.6)
Total number of dislocations[a]	
<5	23 (45.1)
5–10	14 (27.5)
10–15	5 (9.8)
>15	9 (17.6)
Trauma mechanism[a]	
Low-energy trauma; fall from standing height	3 (5.8)
High-energy trauma	8 (15.6)
Sports	30 (58.8)
Assault	3 (5.8)
Pulling or lifting	4 (7.8)
Other	3 (5.8)
Smoking at time of surgery[a]	21 (41.2)
Alcohol consumption at time of surgery[a]	37 (72.5)

* In six patients the dominance was unknown, therefore this percentage was calculated for 45 patients instead of 51

Data are shown as [a] numbers with percentages or as [b] median with P_{25}–P_{75} between brackets

Table 2 Pathologic lesions and intervention characteristics

Bankart lesion[a]	45 (88.2)
Labral tear	33 (73.3)
Bony	12 (26.7)
SLAP lesion[a]	3 (5.9)
Capsule tear	3 (5.9)
Hill-Sachs lesion[a]	31 (60.8)
Suture anchors[a]	48 (94.1)
Number[b]	2 (2–3)

Data are shown as [a] numbers with percentages or as [b] median with P_{25}–P_{75} between brackets

operative period in years. The adjusted Exp(b) value, after correction for age, duration of symptoms prior to surgery, surgery of the dominant side, and gender, was 1.806 (95 % CI 1.077–3.029; $p = 0.025$;) per year. Two patients with recurrent dislocations required a secondary intervention; one patient underwent a second-modified Putti-Platt procedure, and the other patient was treated with a Bristow-Latarjet procedure. Both patients currently have a stable shoulder. The three patients who did not experience actual re-dislocations reported subluxation or complained of subjective instability. Patient and intervention characteristics did not differ between the two hospitals.

Table 3 Functional outcome, quality of life, and patient satisfaction with the result of the modified Putti-Platt procedure

Data are shown for all patients, for patients whose dominant side was affected and for patients whose nondominant side was affected

Data are shown as median with P_{25}–P_{75} between brackets. Differences between both groups were assessed using the Mann–Whitney U test. In all tests, the p value was >0.050

DASH disabilities of the arm, shoulder and hand, *ROM* range of motion *VAS* visual analog score, *WOSI* Western Ontario shoulder index

* In six patients the dominance was unknown, therefore this percentage was calculated for 45 patients instead of 51

[a] Data were expressed as differences in ROM of the operated minus the nonoperated side

	Overall ($N = 51$)	Dominant side affected ($N = 25$)*	Nondominant side affected ($N = 20$)*
Loss of ROM (degrees)[a]			
Abduction	7 (0–15)	5 (0–8)	10 (0–22)
Elevation	6 (0–10)	6 (0–10)	9 (0–10)
External rotation	10 (0–20)	10 (0–20)	13 (0–29)
External rotation in abduction	8 (0–15)	7 (0–10)	12 (0–24)
Constant score			
Affected side	84 (75–91)	83 (75–93)	89 (83–93)
Contralateral side	92 (84–95)	92 (86–97)	95 (87–98)
Percentage of unaffected arm	94 (88–99)	91 (91–97)	95 (91–97)
DASH score			
Total	5.0 (0.8–10.8)	5.0 (0.8–10.4)	1.6 (0.2–11.0)
Work	0.0 (0.0–15.6)	0.0 (0.0–9.4)	0.0 (0.0–0.0)
Sports/Music	0.0 (0.0–25.0)	0.0 (0.0–7.8)	6.3 (0.0–75.0)
Rowe score			
Total	92 (75–95)	95 (75–95)	92 (75–95)
Stability	50 (50–50)	50 (50–50)	50 (50–50)
ROM	15 (15–15)	15 (15–15)	15 (5–15)
Function	30 (25–30)	30 (25–30)	30 (25–30)
WOSI			
Total score	8.9 (6.8–9.4)	8.8 (6.8–9.4)	9.1 (7.9–9.5)
Physical	8.8 (7.5–9.5)	8.7 (7.5–9.5)	9.1 (7.8–9.5)
Sports/recreation/work	8.4 (6.3–9.5)	8.5 (6.4–9.5)	8.4 (6.5–9.5)
Lifestyle	8.5 (7.5–9.5)	8.4 (7.3–9.6)	9.1 (7.8–9.6)
Emotion	8.8 (6.8–9.4)	8.0 (7.2–9.4)	9.1 (7.3–9.6)
VAS for patient satisfaction	7.9 (6.8–9.5)	8.0 (6.8–9.6)	7.9 (7.3–9.8)

Range of motion and strength

A median loss of seven (P_{25}–P_{75} 0–15) degrees of abduction and six (P_{25}–P_{75} 0–10) degrees of elevation was measured when comparing the affected side with the contralateral side (Table 3). A median loss of 10 (P_{25}–P_{75} 0–20) degrees of external rotation and eight (P_{25}–P_{75} 0–15) degrees of external rotation in 90° of abduction was observed. The motion restriction was consistently lower when the dominant side was affected than when the nondominant side was affected ($p > 0.05$). The median strength of abduction as measured at an arm's length in 90° of abduction was 7.5 (P_{25}–P_{75} 6.0–10.0) kg for the operated arm versus 9.5 (P_{25}–P_{75} 7.0–11.0) kg for the contralateral arm. Range of motion and strength was not significantly different when comparing the two hospitals.

Functional outcome and quality of life

Overall, the median DASH score was 5.0 (P_{25}–P_{75} 0.8–10.8) indicating very little disability. Patients whose dominant side was affected scored 3.4 points more than patients whose nondominant side was affected (Table 3).

Both subgroups reported a median score of 0.0 in the high performance section for work. Patients whose dominant side was affected also reported a median of 0.0 points in the high performance section for sports/music, whereas patients whose nondominant side was affected scored 6.3 (P_{25}–P_{75} 0.0–75) points.

The median Constant score for the whole group was 84 (P_{25}–P_{75} 75–91) points. Furthermore, the relative Constant score was calculated as the score of the affected arm as a percentage of the patient's healthy arm; this was 94 % (P_{25}–P_{75} 88–99).

A median ROWE score of 92 (P_{25}–P_{75} 75–95) was measured for the whole group, which is considered as an excellent result. Forty patients (78 %) scored more than 74 points, which is the threshold for a good or excellent result.

The median WOSI score was 8.9 (P_{25}–P_{75} 6.8–9.4) with none of the sub-domains (physical, sports/recreation/work, lifestyle, and emotions) scoring a loss of injury-related quality of live greater than 10 % (median). Scores were similar in patients whose dominant or nondominant shoulder had been treated. The overall SF-36 score was 107.7 (P_{25}–P_{75} 93.0–113.1). Both the physical and mental components of the SF-36 were within the population norm of 50 ± 10 (SD) points and were independent of the affected side. Patients reported a high satisfaction with the outcome on the VAS score; 76 % of all patients scored seven or more points out of 10. Functional scores and quality of life were not significantly different when comparing the two hospitals.

Discussion

Our results show that the modified Putti-Platt procedure, as performed in our case series, is an effective treatment for recurrent anterior shoulder instability, leading to acceptable recurrence rates and satisfactory functional outcome, quality of life, and patient satisfaction.

In the literature, an anterior labral detachment (i.e., Bankart lesions) is present in approximately from 65 to 90 % of the shoulders that are surgically treated for anterior instability [4, 10, 20, 23]. In 88 % of the patients in this study, a Bankart lesion was present and subsequently treated. Bankart lesions contribute to recurrent shoulder instability [24–26]. Nevertheless, most modifications of the original Putti-Platt procedure do not address any contributing anatomic pathology (i.e., labrum and glenoid pathology) apart from capsular laxity and subscapularis muscle redundancy. On the other hand, despite their important roles in shoulder instability, capsular laxity and subscapularis muscle redundancy are neglected subjects in most reports on Bankart repairs [20, 27]. For these reasons, both aspects of glenohumeral instability were addressed in the current study. Several authors have described Bankart repairs in combination with a capsular shift procedure [9, 20, 28]. However, shortening of the subscapularis muscle is often not performed. Only one retrospective report of 30 patients was found in which all three aspects of shoulder instability were addressed [29].

Although most surgically stabilized shoulders remain stable over time, recurrent dislocations are important complications to take into account. Recurrent dislocations occurred in 10 % of our patients, which is in line with the 10 % found by Pelet et al. [29] who used a similar technique. Hayes et al. [1] reported a mean re-dislocation rate of 11 % after a mean follow-up of 4.3 years in seven studies following open Bankart repair. Re-dislocation rates of up to 36 %, most of which were higher than 20 %, have been reported in several studies after a Putti-Platt procedure [9, 30–33]. Recurrences tend to occur even after a longer post-operative time [6, 34]. However, most recurrent dislocations occur within the first 5 years following surgery [29].

Arthroscopic treatment has evolved greatly over the past decades, gaining in interest over open procedures. Potential benefits of minimally invasive procedures include less surgical dissection and post-operative pain and an improved range of motion. However, in a meta-analysis on open versus

arthroscopic stabilization by Lenters et al. [35], 97 of the 527 (18 %) arthroscopically treated patients experienced recurrent stability. A meta-analysis from 2004 studying the same subject also demonstrated a higher recurrence rate in patients treated arthroscopically (3 vs. 13 %) [36]. Another meta-analysis from 2010 on this topic found a recurrence rate of only 2.9 % in the arthroscopic group when only including trials from later than 2002 [37]. This suggests that arthroscopic techniques have evidently improved over time. Unfortunately, functional outcome and range of motion could not be adequately addressed.

Particularly, loss of range of motion has been labeled as the greatest disadvantage of the original procedure. Even after the modification as described by Symeonides et al., restrictions in external rotation of up to 29° have been reported [10, 38, 39]. Pelet et al. [29] who used a different modification even found a mean loss of 33° of external rotation and a mean loss of 24° loss of external rotation in 90° of abduction ($N = 39$) as opposed to 10° and 8°, respectively, in the current study. The limited restriction of external rotation as encountered in the current study could be explained by the fact that extra care was taken not to over-shorten the subscapularis muscle. Another explanation could lie in the duration of follow-up since surgery. The restriction in ROM has proven to diminish during the course of the post-operative period [38, 40].

The median DASH score in our population was 5.0 points, which is comparable to the 4.3 points that Hovelius et al. [41] found in 17 patients, 25 years after a (simplified) Putti-Platt procedure. The slightly inferior result for the Constant score was largely attributed to a median difference in strength of 2.0 kg between the affected and healthy shoulder. To the best of our knowledge, no previous studies have reported on the health-related quality of life after stabilizing procedures of the glenohumeral joint.

All procedures in these series were performed by three surgeons. This could be considered as a drawback that might have introduced a bias, but also as strength because all procedures were performed in a consistent way. The fact that satisfactory results were obtained in most patients, irrespective of the hospital where the surgery was performed, emphasizes the generalizability of this modification of the Putti-Platt procedure. A limitation of this study is that we performed multiple statistical comparisons on a relatively small population, which has a risk of accepting a spurious relation. However, applying the Bonferroni correction would be too stringent and might falsely reject true effects.

Ahmad et al. [24] stated that "the ideal surgical goals in treating shoulder instability are to anatomically correct all of the contributing pathology encountered, preserve range of motion, and preserve or restore normal joint mechanics". Our data show that the modified Putti-Platt procedure as performed in our series closely meets these criteria;

motion restriction is marginal, outcome scores are satisfactory, and the patients are highly satisfied with the end result. The modified Putti-Platt procedure can therefore be considered as an effective treatment option for recurrent anterior traumatic shoulder instability.

References

1. Hayes K et al (2002) Shoulder instability: management and rehabilitation. J Orthop Sports Phys Ther 32:497–509
2. Pensak M et al (2010) Management of acute anterior shoulder instability in adolescents. Orthop Nurs 29:237–43; quiz 244–5
3. Robinson CM et al (2006) Functional outcome and risk of recurrent instability after primary traumatic anterior shoulder dislocation in young patients. J Bone Joint Surg Am 88:2326–2336
4. Bottoni CR et al (2006) Arthroscopic versus open shoulder stabilization for recurrent anterior instability: a prospective randomized clinical trial. Am J Sports Med 34:1730–1737
5. Fabbriciani C et al (2004) Arthroscopic versus open treatment of Bankart lesion of the shoulder: a prospective randomized study. Arthroscopy 20:456–462
6. Sperber A et al (2001) Comparison of an arthroscopic and an open procedure for posttraumatic instability of the shoulder: a prospective, randomized multicenter study. J Shoulder Elbow Surg 10:105–108
7. Kiss J et al (1998) The results of the Putti-Platt operation with particular reference to arthritis, pain, and limitation of external rotation. J Shoulder Elbow Surg 7:495–500
8. Osmond-Clarke H (1948) Habitual dislocation of the shoulder; the Putti-Platt operation. J Bone Joint Surg Br 30B:19–25
9. Salomonsson B et al (2009) The Bankart repair versus the Putti-Platt procedure: a randomized study with WOSI score at 10-year follow-up in 62 patients. Acta Orthop 80:351–356
10. Gill TJ, Zarins B (2003) Open repairs for the treatment of anterior shoulder instability. Am J Sports Med 31:142–153
11. van der Zwaag HM et al (1999) Glenohumeral osteoarthrosis after Putti-Platt repair. J Shoulder Elbow Surg 8:252–258
12. Brav EA, Jeffress VH (1952) Simplified Putti-Platt reconstruction for recurrent shoulder dislocation; a preliminary report. West J Surg Obstet Gynecol 60:93–97
13. Leach RE, et al (1982) Results of a modified Putti-Platt operation for recurrent shoulder dislocations and subluxations. Clin Orthop Relat Res 164:20–25
14. Symeonides PP (1972) The significance of the subscapularis muscle in the pathogenesis of recurrent anterior dislocation of the shoulder. J Bone Joint Surg Br 54:476–483
15. Symeonides PP (1989) Reconsideration of the Putti-Platt procedure and its mode of action in recurrent traumatic anterior dislocation of the shoulder. Clin Orthop Relat Res 246:8–15
16. Constant CR, Murley AH (1987) A clinical method of functional assessment of the shoulder. Clin Orthop Relat Res 214:160–164
17. Beaton DE et al (2001) Measuring the whole or the parts? Validity, reliability, and responsiveness of the disabilities of the arm, shoulder and hand outcome measure in different regions of the upper extremity. J Hand Ther 14:128–146
18. Hudak PL, Amadio PC, Bombardier C (1996) Development of an upper extremity outcome measure: the DASH (disabilities of the arm, shoulder and hand) [corrected]. The Upper Extremity Collaborative Group (UECG). Am J Ind Med 29:602–608
19. Kocher MS et al (2005) Reliability, validity, and responsiveness of the American shoulder and elbow surgeons subjective shoulder scale in patients with shoulder instability, rotator cuff disease,

and glenohumeral arthritis. J Bone Joint Surg Am 87:2006–2011
20. Rowe CR, Patel D, Southmayd WW (1978) The Bankart procedure: a long-term end-result study. J Bone Joint Surg Am 60:1–16
21. Kirkley A et al (1998) The development and evaluation of a disease-specific quality of life measurement tool for shoulder instability. The Western Ontario Shoulder Instability Index (WOSI). Am J Sports Med 26:764–772
22. Ware JE Jr, Sherbourne CD (1992) The MOS 36-item short-form health survey (SF-36). I. Conceptual framework and item selection. Med Care 30:473–483
23. Rowe CR, Zarins B (1981) Recurrent transient subluxation of the shoulder. J Bone Joint Surg Am 63:863–872
24. Ahmad CS et al (2005) Biomechanics of shoulder capsulorrhaphy procedures. J Shoulder Elbow Surg 14:12S–18S
25. Hawkins RH, Hawkins RJ (1985) Failed anterior reconstruction for shoulder instability. J Bone Joint Surg Br 67:709–714
26. Shah AS, Karadsheh MS, Sekiya JK (2011) Failure of operative treatment for glenohumeral instability: etiology and management. Arthroscopy 27:681–694
27. Chen S et al (2005) The effects of thermal capsular shrinkage on the outcomes of arthroscopic stabilization for primary anterior shoulder instability. Am J Sports Med 33:705–711
28. Protzman RR (1980) Anterior instability of the shoulder. J Bone Joint Surg Am 62:909–918
29. Pelet S, Jolles BM, Farron A (2006) Bankart repair for recurrent anterior glenohumeral instability: results at twenty-nine years' follow-up. J Shoulder Elbow Surg 15:203–207
30. Fredriksson AS, Tegner Y (1991) Results of the Putti-Platt operation for recurrent anterior dislocation of the shoulder. Int Orthop 15:185–188
31. Hovelius L, Thorling J, Fredin H (1979) Recurrent anterior dislocation of the shoulder. Results after the Bankart and Putti-Platt operations. J Bone Joint Surg Am 61:566–569
32. Konig DP et al (1997) Osteoarthritis and recurrences after Putti-Platt and Eden-Hybbinette operations for recurrent dislocation of the shoulder. Int Orthop 21:72–76
33. Varmarken JE, Jensen CH (1989) Recurrent anterior dislocation of the shoulder. A comparison of the results after the Bankart and the Putti-Platt procedures. Orthopedics 12:453–455
34. Magnusson L et al (2002) Revisiting the open Bankart experience: a four- to nine-year follow-up. Am J Sports Med 30:778–782
35. Lenters TR et al (2007) Arthroscopic compared with open repairs for recurrent anterior shoulder instability. A systematic review and meta-analysis of the literature. J Bone Joint Surg Am 89:244–254
36. Freedman KB et al (2004) Open Bankart repair versus arthroscopic repair with transglenoid sutures or bioabsorbable tacks for recurrent anterior instability of the shoulder: a meta-analysis. Am J Sports Med 32:1520–1527
37. Petrera M et al (2010) A meta-analysis of open versus arthroscopic Bankart repair using suture anchors. Knee Surg Sports Traumatol Arthrosc 18:1742–1747
38. MacDonald PB et al (1992) Release of the subscapularis for internal rotation contracture and pain after anterior repair for recurrent anterior dislocation of the shoulder. J Bone Joint Surg Am 74:734–737
39. Regan WD Jr et al (1989) Comparative functional analysis of the Bristow, Magnuson-Stack, and Putti-Platt procedures for recurrent dislocation of the shoulder. Am J Sports Med 17:42–48
40. Hashiuchi T et al (2000) The changes occurring after the Putti-Platt procedure using magnetic resonance imaging. Arch Orthop Trauma Surg 120:286–289

Permissions

The contributors of this book come from diverse backgrounds, making this book a truly international effort. This book will bring forth new frontiers with its revolutionizing research information and detailed analysis of the nascent developments around the world.

We would like to thank all the contributing authors for lending their expertise to make the book truly unique. They have played a crucial role in the development of this book. Without their invaluable contributions this book wouldn't have been possible. They have made vital efforts to compile up to date information on the varied aspects of this subject to make this book a valuable addition to the collection of many professionals and students.

This book was conceptualized with the vision of imparting up-to-date information and advanced data in this field. To ensure the same, a matchless editorial board was set up. Every individual on the board went through rigorous rounds of assessment to prove their worth. After which they invested a large part of their time researching and compiling the most relevant data for our readers.

The editorial board has been involved in producing this book since its inception. They have spent rigorous hours researching and exploring the diverse topics which have resulted in the successful publishing of this book. They have passed on their knowledge of decades through this book. To expedite this challenging task, the publisher supported the team at every step. A small team of assistant editors was also appointed to further simplify the editing procedure and attain best results for the readers.

Apart from the editorial board, the designing team has also invested a significant amount of their time in understanding the subject and creating the most relevant covers. They scrutinized every image to scout for the most suitable representation of the subject and create an appropriate cover for the book.

The publishing team has been an ardent support to the editorial, designing and production team. Their endless efforts to recruit the best for this project, has resulted in the accomplishment of this book. They are a veteran in the field of academics and their pool of knowledge is as vast as their experience in printing. Their expertise and guidance has proved useful at every step. Their uncompromising quality standards have made this book an exceptional effort. Their encouragement from time to time has been an inspiration for everyone.

The publisher and the editorial board hope that this book will prove to be a valuable piece of knowledge for researchers, students, practitioners and scholars across the globe.

List of Contributors

Ram Chander Siwach, Rajesh Rohilla, Roop Singh, Rohit Singla, Sukhbir Singh Sangwan and Paritosh Gogna
Department of Orthopaedic Surgery, Paraplegia and Rehabilitation, Pt. B.D. Sharma PGIMS, 9-J/28, Medical Enclave, Rohtak 124001, Haryana, India

Andreas Leonidou, Konstantinos Antonis and Omiros Leonidou
First Department of Trauma and Orthopaedics, Athens Paediatric Hospital "Agia Sophia", Thivon and Papadiamantopoulou, Goudi, 11527 Athens, Greece

Andreas Leonidou, Krissen Chettiar, Simon Graham, Pouya Akhbari and Eleftherios Tsiridis
Division of Surgery, Academic Department of Orthopaedics and Trauma, Aristotle University Medical School, Thessaloníki, Greece

C. Biz and C. Iacobellis
Orthopaedic Clinic, Department of Surgery, Oncology and Gastroenterology DiSCOG, University of Padua, Via Giustiniani 2, 35128 Padua, Italy

Ahmet Aslan, Mehmet Nuri Konya, Aykut Özdemir, Hüseyin Yorgancigil, Gökhan Maralcan and Emin Uysal
Department of Orthopedics and Traumatology, Afyonkarahisar
State Hospital, Orhangazi Mh. Nedim Helvacıoğlu Cd. Uydukent, 03100 Afyonkarahisar, Turkey

Ashraf A. Khanfour and Mohamed M. El-Sayed
Department of Orthopaedic Surgery, Damanhur National Medical Institute, Damanhur, Egypt

Gemma Humm, Saqib Noor, Philippa Bridgeman and Michael David
Queen Elizabeth Hospital, University Hospitals Birmingham NHS Foundation Trust, Mindelsohn Way, Birmingham B15 2GW, UK

Deepa Bose
East and North Hertfordshire NHS Trust, Lister Hospital, Coreys Mill Lane, Stevenage SG1 4AB, UK

Andreas Leonidou, Zoltan Kiraly, Hristifor Gality, Shane Apperley, Sean Vanstone and David A. Woods
Department of Trauma and Orthopaedic Surgery, Great Western
Hospitals NHS Foundation Trust, Marlborough Road, Swindon SN3 6BB, UK

David J. S. Roberts
London North West Healthcare NHS Trust, Harrow, UK

Anna Panagiotidou
UCL Institute of Biomedical Engineering, London, UK

Ramsagar Pandit, Yatinder Kharbanda, Vikas Birla and Yashwant Singh Tanwar
Department of Orthopedics, Apollo Hospital, HNo299, Pocket B, DDA Flats, Sarita Vihar, New Delhi, Delhi 110076, India

Vishal Srivastava and Ashok Rajput
Department of Orthopedics, Dr. RML Hospital and PGIMER, New Delhi, Delhi 110001, India

Birgitta Svernlöv
Department of Plastic Surgery, Hand Surgery and Burns, Linköping University Hospital, 581 85 Linköping, Sweden
Faculty of Experimental and Clinical Medicine, Linköping University, Linköping, Sweden

Jens Nestorson and Lars Adolfsson
Department of Orthopedic Surgery, Linköping University Hospital, 581 85 Linköping, Sweden
Faculty of Health Science, Linköping University, Linköping, Sweden

B. M. Naveen, G. R. Joshi and B. Harikrishnan
Department of Orthopaedics, Armed Forces Medical College (AFMC), Pune 411040, India

Peter M. Stevens, Lucas Anderson, Bruce A. MacWilliams, Christian J. Gaffney and Heather Fillerup
Department of Orthopaedics, University of Utah, Salt Lake City, UT 84113, USA

J. K. Wiggers and R. M. Snijders
Trauma Unit, Department of Surgery, Academic Medical Center, Meibergdreef 9, 1105 AZ Amsterdam, The Netherlands

J. G. G. Dobbe and G. J. Streekstra
Department of Biomedical Engineering and Physics, Academic Medical Center, Amsterdam, The Netherlands
Department of Radiology, Academic Medical Centre, University of Amsterdam, Amsterdam, The Netherlands

D. den Hartog
Trauma Research Unit, Department of Surgery, Erasmus Medical Center, Rotterdam, The Netherlands

N. W. L. Schep
Trauma Unit, Department of Surgery, Academic Medical Center, Meibergdreef 9, 1105 AZ Amsterdam, The Netherlands
Department of Surgery, Maasstad Hospital, Rotterdam, The Netherlands

Leonard C. Marais and Nando Ferreira
Tumour, Sepsis and Reconstruction Unit, Department of Orthopaedic Surgery, School of Clinical Medicine, Grey's Hospital, University of KwaZulu-Natal, Private Bag X9001, Pietermaritzburg 3201, South Africa

Colleen Aldous
School of Clinical Medicine, College of Health Sciences, University of KwaZulu-Natal, Durban, South Africa

Theo L. B. Le Roux
Department of Orthopaedics, I Military Hospital, University of Pretoria, Pretoria, South Africa

Kamilcan Oflazoglu
Massachusetts General Hospital, 55 Fruit Street, 02114 Boston, United States

Nienke Koenrades and Matthijs P. Somford
Department of Orthopaedic Surgery, Medisch Spectrum Twente, Haaksbergerstraat 55, 7513 ER Enschede, The Netherlands

Michel P. J. van den Bekerom
Department of Orthopaedic Surgery, Onze Lieve Vrouwe Gasthuis Amsterdam, Oosterpark 9, 1091 AC Amsterdam, The Netherlands

Nikolai Briffa, Raju Karthickeyan, Joshua Jacob and Arshad Khaleel
Trauma and Orthopaedic Department, Ashford and St. Peter's Hospital NHS Trust, London, UK

Alexios Dimitrios Iliadis, David Goodier, Peter Calder, Matthew Sewell and Parag Kumar Jaiswal
Limb Reconstruction Unit, Royal National Orthopaedic Hospital NHS, Brockley Hill, Stanmore, Middlesex HA7 4LP, UK

Jay Meswania and Gordon Blunn
University College London - Institute of Orthopaedics and Musculoskeletal Science, Royal National Orthopaedic Hospital (RNOH), Brockley Hill, Stanmore HA7 4LP, UK

S. Salih, C. Blakey, D. Chan, J. C. McGregor-Riley, S. L. Royston and M. G. Dennison
Department of Trauma and Orthopaedics, Northern General Hospital, Herres Rd, Sheffield S5 7AU, UK

S. Gowlett and D. Moore
Department of Radiology, Northern General Hospital, Sheffield, UK

Jesse M. van Buijtenen, Mischa L. C. van Tunen and Wietse P. Zuidema
Department of Surgery, VU University Medical Centre, 1007 MB Amsterdam, The Netherlands

Emile A. Heilbron
Department of Radiology, VU University Medical Centre, Amsterdam, The Netherlands

Jeroen de Haan
Department of Surgery, Westfriesgasthuis, Hoorn, The Netherlands

Henrica C. W. de Vet
Department of Epidemiology and Biostatistics and the EMGO Institute for Health and Care Research, VU University Medical Centre, Amsterdam, The Netherlands

Robert J. Derksen
Department of Surgery, Zaandam Medical Centre, Zaandam, The Netherlands

Madhavan C. Papanna, K. A. Saldanha, Binu Kurian, James A. Fernandes and Stan Jones
Department of Trauma and Orthopaedics, Sheffield Children Hospital, Sheffield S10 2TH, UK

Sherif Galal
Department of Orthopaedic Surgery and Traumatology, Faculty of Medicine, Kasr AL-Ainy School of Medicine, Cairo University, Cairo 11559, Egypt

N. Ferreira
Department of Orthopaedic Surgery, Tygerberg Hospital, University of Stellenbosch, Cape Town 7505, South Africa

L. C. Marais
Tumour, Sepsis and Reconstruction Unit, Department of Orthopaedic Surgery, Greys Hospital, Nelson R. Mandela School of Medicine, University of KwaZulu Natal, Pietermaritzburg, South Africa

D. Tiren and D. I. Vos
Department of General and Trauma Surgery, Amphia Hospital, 4800 RK Breda, The Netherlands

James Youngman
Department of Trauma and Orthopaedic Surgery, University College London Hospital, 235 Euston Road, London NW1 2BU, UK

Dimitri Raptis
University Hospital Zurich, Zurich, Switzerland

Khalid Al-Dadah
Department of Trauma and Orthopaedic Surgery, University College London Hospital, 235 Euston Road, London NW1 2BU, UK
Imperial College London, London, UK

Fergal Monsell
Bristol Royal Hospital for Children, Bristol, UK

Alfred O. Ogbemudia and Anirejuoritse Bafor
Department of Orthopaedics and Trauma, University of Benin Teaching Hospital, PMB 1111, Benin City, Edo State, Nigeria

Ehimwenma J. Ogbemudia
Department of Medicine, University of Benin, Benin City, Edo State, Nigeria

Edwin Edomwonyi
Department of Orthopaedics and Trauma, Irrua Specialist Teaching Hospital, Irrua, Edo State, Nigeria

Andras Heijink
Department of Orthopaedic Surgery, Academic Medical Center (AMC), Meibergdreef 9, 1105 AZ Amsterdam, The Netherlands
Department of Orthopaedic Surgery, Amphia Hospital, Breda, The Netherlands

Marc L. Wagener
Department of Orthopaedic Surgery, St. Radboud University Hospital, Nijmegen, The Netherlands

Maarten J. de Vos
Department of Orthopaedic Surgery, Tergooi Hospitals, Hilversum, The Netherlands

Denise Eygendaal
Department of Orthopaedic Surgery, Amphia Hospital, Breda, The Netherlands

M. M. J. Walenkamp, R. J. O. de Muinck Keizer and J. C. Goslings
Trauma Unit, Department of Surgery, Academic Medical Centre, University of Amsterdam, room G4-137, 1100 DD Amsterdam, The Netherlands

P. Kloen
Department of Orthopaedic Surgery, Academic Medical Centre, University of Amsterdam, Amsterdam, The Netherlands

S. D. Strackee
Department of Plastic, Reconstructive and Hand Surgery, Academic Medical Centre, University of Amsterdam, Amsterdam, The Netherlands

Hany Hefny, Elhussein Mohamed Elmoatasem and Wael Nassar
Ain Shams University, Cairo, Egypt

E. Skouras and K. Wegmann
Klinik und Poliklinik für Orthopädie und Unfallchirurgie, Universitsklinikum Köln, Kerpener Straße 62, 50937 Cologne, Germany

Y. Hosseini, V. Berger and T. C. Koslowsky
Department of Surgery, St. Elisabeth-Hospital, Werthmannstraße 1, 50935 Cologne, Germany

Gijs I. T. Iordens, Esther M. M. Van Lieshout, Bernd C. Van Es, Peter Patka and Dennis Den Hartog
Department of Surgery-Traumatology, Erasmus MC, University Medical Center Rotterdam, 3000 CA Rotterdam, The Netherlands

Niels W. L. Schep
Trauma Unit Department of Surgery, AMC, Amsterdam, The Netherlands

Roelf S. Breederveld
Department of Surgery, Red Cross Hospital, Beverwijk, The Netherlands

Index